OUR ENEMY, THE GOVERNMENT:

HOW COVID ENABLED THE EXPANSION AND ABUSE OF STATE POWER

2nd EDITION

RAMESH THAKUR

Our Enemy The Government:
How Covid Enabled the Expansion and Abuse of State Power

2nd Edition

Print ISBN: 978-1-7638845-7-1
Ebook ISBN: 978-1-7638845-6-4

Published by A Sense of Place Publishing in conjunction with the Brownstone Institute, 2026.

Original Cover Design: Vanessa Mondozzi

NATIONAL LIBRARY OF AUSTRALIA

A catalogue record for this book is available from the National Library of Australia

TABLE OF CONTENTS

TABLES AND FIGURES

PROLOGUE

It is one of the greatest medical scandals of the century according to a leading health expert in Brussels. The Council of Europe Health Chief has accused major pharmaceutical firms of organising a campaign of panic and unduly influencing World Health Organisation decisions.

John Snow, Channel 4 News (UK), 2010 (*sic*), as quoted by Tom Jefferson and Carl Heneghan, 14 June 2023.

European Parliament, *REPORT on evaluation of the management of H1N1 influenza in 2009–2010 in the EU*, Report A7-0035/2011, 9 February 2011

European Parliament Resolution, Committee on the Environment, Public Health and Food Safety, adopted on 25 January 2011 by a 58-2 vote.

Excerpts

The European Parliament,

D. whereas the criteria for defining a 'pandemic', as revised by the WHO in 2009, are based solely on the spread of the virus while disregarding the severity of the illness caused by it,

E. whereas Member States, the European Commission and … the WHO should take into account the virulence of a future influenza outbreak as well as the propagation of the virus when making public health decisions which may affect public health and social policies,

J. whereas the pharmaceutical industry had to respond to a sudden, pressing and exponential demand for the supply of vaccines by the Member States; whereas the industry had to develop with very great urgency a new vaccine likely to be effective against the virus,

L. whereas the expenditure committed by certain Member States to the response plans drawn up relates mainly to the purchase of vast quantities of vaccines and antiviral treatments, and whereas purchasing procedures led to concerns regarding compliance with rules on public procurement and transparency in some Member States,

N. whereas lawsuits were taken in various Member States, alleging corruption and conspiracy on the part of civil servants in relation to contracts signed in summer 2009 between ministries of public health and manufacturers of H1N1 influenza vaccines,

O. whereas according to the Commission the reluctance of vaccine suppliers to bear full product liability may have contributed to reducing citizens' trust in vaccine safety; whereas confidence in vaccines against H1N1 influenza was also undermined by incomplete and contradictory communication on the benefits and risks of vaccination and the potential risks of H1N1 influenza to the public,

Q. whereas pandemic influenza preparedness planning relies to a great extent on vaccination strategies; whereas vaccination strategies should rely on three conditions to be successful: efficacy of the vaccine, a positive benefit-risk balance for the vaccine, and targeting of risk groups,

R. whereas there needs to be transparency about the fulfilment of these conditions,

T. whereas there is a need for studies on vaccines and antiviral medications that are independent from pharmaceutical companies so as to have a balance between private and publicly funded studies,

X. whereas despite the repeated requests made by the European Ombudsman to the European Medicines Agency (EMA), the documents held by the EMA relating to research protocols, clinical trials and the undesirable effects of medicinal products submitted to it for assessment are not always accessible to the public,

Y. whereas the information and communication concerning H1N1 influenza in 2009-2010 in the EU have demonstrated the crucial role played by the media in relaying public health precautions and recommendations, but also in emphasising selected aspects of the outbreak and its consequences, thus potentially altering public opinion perceptions and the public authorities' responses,

8. Urges the WHO to revise the definition of a pandemic, taking into consideration not only its geographical spread but also its severity;

13. Recalls that according to current Union legislation on medicinal products, liability for the quality, safety and efficacy concerning the authorised indications of a medicinal product rests with the manufacturer, and calls for full application of this rule by Member States in all contracts for the procurement of vaccines, as an important factor in maintaining/regaining citizens' trust in vaccine safety;;

14. Requests, ... that consideration be given to the possibility of easing access for developing countries to vaccine products in the event of a pandemic;

15. Takes the view that the European Centre for Disease Prevention and Control (ECDC) has to exercise its powers as an independent agency to assess and communicate the severity of infection risk and be given adequate means for all its tasks;

17. Demands that increased vigilance and complete transparency be assured with regard to the evaluation of, and reporting on, medicinal products recommended in the event of health emergencies, and more particularly in genuine pandemic situations;

18. Underscores the need for studies independent of the pharmaceutical companies on vaccines and antiviral medications;

19. Wishes to ensure that scientific experts have no financial or other interests in the pharmaceutical industry that could affect their impartiality; requests the development of a European code of conduct relating to the exercise of the function of a scientific expert in any European authority in charge of safety and of the management and anticipation of risks; requires that each expert subscribe to the ethical principles of this code of conduct before taking up his or her duties;

21. Calls in particular on the European Commission, with the support of the EMA, to improve the accelerated authorisation procedures for the placing on the market of medicinal products designed to respond to a health crisis … in such a way that proper clinical trials are carried out before a pandemic occurs, in order to ensure a full assessment of the risk-benefit balance associated with the use of those medicinal products for the relevant target groups and to come up with corresponding legislative proposals where necessary;

25. Reminds the EMA of the regulatory requirement to make access available to all the documents relating to clinical trials, research protocols and undesirable effects of the medicinal products evaluated by its experts, including the vaccines and anti-viral drugs;

26. Recognises that conflicts of interest among experts who advise European public health authorities lead to suspicions of undue influence and harm the overall credibility of these public health authorities and their recommendations;

30. Is aware of the need to communicate risks and benefits more clearly and transparently to the public;

EXPLANATORY STATEMENT

A[I]nfluenza A(H1N1) 2009 caused 2 900 deaths in Europe. These figures are low in comparison to the official mortality estimates for seasonal influenza, which the Commission put at 40 000 deaths in a moderate year and 220 000 in a particularly severe season. They are also significantly less than the most optimistic forecasts suggested by the health services of the EU Member States ....

[A] raft of measures that were very costly ... and disproportionate to the actual—and known—severity of H1N1 influenza.

The rapporteur pointed to the case of Poland, where the government did not proceed to vaccination against H1N1, and where nevertheless the death rate was comparable to those countries which decided to go for national vaccination campaigns....

According to the rapporteur, the analysis of the management of H1N1 influenza in Europe highlights an underlying problem: a lack of independent evaluation by our national and/or European health authorities, and a resulting failure to adapt the public health measures, as best as possible and in real time, to the actual clinical and epidemiological statistics available ....

[V]accination strategies should rely on three conditions to be successful: that the vaccine is efficacious, that it has a positive risk-benefit balance and that it is targeted to the risk groups. ....

1: A WORLD IN PANIC

Let us begin with the deep history following the initial lockdowns. What follows are my initial postings and intuitions, trying to work out the extent to which the panic response was justified.

Coronavirus pandemic: sceptical question marks make for better policy than excitable exclamation marks [1]

When did the world's media and politicians become collective versions of Lance Corporal Jones in the British comedy series *Dad's Army*, screaming "Don't panic! Don't panic!'? Colour me contrarian, but since the 2003 Iraq war, my working motto has been: when you come across excitable exclamation marks, substitute sceptical question marks and you'll be right.

According to World Life Expectancy, Australia's annual death toll is around 170,000. Heart diseases kill more than 23,000 people. The number of deaths from flu and pneumonia is over 4,000 and from road fatalities around 1,300. Averaging the total, about 40,000 Australians will have died as at 26 March. As of that date, 12 Australians had died with the coronavirus affliction.

---

[1] *Pearls and Irritations*, 30 March 2020 https://johnmenadue.com/ramesh-thakur-coronavirus-pandemic-sceptical-question-marks-make-for-better-policy-than-excitable-exclamation-marks/

Led by the media, panic set in to drive public policy before data was collected to show that, for most people, the Covid-19 virus will be worse than seasonal flu. The crisis escalated with an Imperial College study of 16 March which described Covid-19 as "a virus with comparable lethality to H1N1 influenza in 1918" (the Spanish flu that killed upwards of 50mn people, one-sixth to one-third of them Indians). Without an aggressive suppression strategy of prolonged lockdown, it could cause 0.5mn deaths in the UK and 2.2mn in the US. This caused Prime Minister (PM) Boris Johnson to switch dramatically from the initial herd immunity strategy—let the virus spread through the community because the mortality rate is well within the parameters of a seasonal flu—to a drastic nationwide lockdown. Other governments were soon infected by the panic virus and the favoured strategy became to prioritise citizen's health over the nation's economy. As a total lockdown leads to economic shutdown, the pain is alleviated through industry bailout and social benefit packages.

To kill the virus, must we kill the economy?

In earlier flu epidemics (Asian Flu 1956–58, Hong Kong Flu 1968, SARS 2003, avian flu 2008, swine flu 2009), the numbers infected and killed were sufficient to produce a severe impact on society. But governments didn't shut down their country, destroy the economy nor jeopardise their way of life. People suffered but endured. This too shall pass.

In responding to an epidemic, there is a trade-off between public health and economic stability. It is the duty of health professionals to focus solely on the former. It is the responsibility of governments to balance the two and intuit the social fulcrum: the sweet spot at the intersection of dangerous complacency, alarmist panic and reasonable precautions. The injunction to first do no harm implies that governments should be wary of prolonged economic lockdowns: the cure might indeed be worse than the disease.

Public policy must be based on a balance of risks and benefits, often amidst uncertainty, incomplete information and unintended and perverse human, health and economic consequences. The health of citizens and the health of the national economy are closely connected and interdependent. A healthy economy requires a healthy workforce. Conversely, most wealthy industrial countries have greatly superior public health systems and outcomes because a strong economy makes it possible to invest in the entire infrastructure of health delivery. Supply chain disruptions can elevate the risks of death from other potentially life-threatening ailments, including heart problems, diabetes, chronic lung disease and overlap between these (comorbidities).

In the US, people at risk from these illnesses total 70-80mn. At 1% excess fatality in this group caused by shortages resulting from the economic shutdowns, another 750,000 Americans will die. On the other side of this necessarily grim ledger, for those who are not elderly, *after infection*, the mortality rate is about equal to the risk of dying from all other causes. In addition, layoffs and income losses will cause a spike in long-term mental health problems and suicides. Australia has already begun developing a major mental health package to address heightened anxiety caused by job losses, wage cutbacks, isolation and loneliness. Prolonged house-bound isolation could also see a surge in domestic violence cases.

Meanwhile the rushed returns home from overseas in confined planes to crowded immigration lines, the panic buying in supermarkets to hoard up and the long queues at CentreLink offices have contributed their share to the cross-infection.

Modelling is assumption-driven and data-limited

Was the panic caused by flawed, inflated mortality statistics? The original Imperial College paper used sketchy data and heroic assumptions. More sceptical voices have emerged since then. One team finally got around to testing an entire village of 3,000 people near Florence for the SARS-CoV-2 virus which causes Covid-19. The results show that 50%-75% of those infected were asymptomatic and thus would not be tested in most jurisdictions. This is fully consistent with an Oxford modelling that maps a range of different outcomes using different assumptions.

The limited early observational data suggest that the true infection rate may be thirty (Wuhan) or hundred (Italy) times higher than the number of confirmed cases, which would drop the fatality rate, of the total infected population, to one-thirtieth or one-hundredth. On the basis of the existing albeit inadequate data, Eran Bendavid and Jay Bhattacharya, professors of medicine at Stanford University, conclude that the Covid-19 mortality rate could be as low as 0.01% of all those infected, one-tenth the average flu mortality of 0.1%: "Such a low death rate would be cause for optimism." Hence their conclusion: "A universal quarantine may not be worth the costs it imposes on the economy, community and individual mental and physical health. We should undertake immediate steps to evaluate the empirical basis of the current lockdowns."

According to the RealClearPolitics running tally, as of 29 March, the total deaths were 30,627 from a total confirmed cases of 659,435. Italy had the highest number of fatalities at 10,023. Among countries with a recorded number of deaths over 100, the confirmed cases per million people varied from 4.3 in Indonesia, 18.6 in Brazil and 58.4 in China, to a high of over 1,500 each in Italy and Spain. The fatality rate compared to confirmed cases similarly varied widely, from 0.75% in Germany, 1.67% in the US and 4.05% in China, to 8.83% in Indonesia and 10.84% in Italy. The extreme variability of all these merely confirm the widely disparate standards of health-related surveillance and data collection around the world. Reliable data are simply not available of the total numbers of those actually infected and those dying from Covid-19.

According to the Centers for Disease Control and Prevention (CDC), as of 28 March, the total US Covid-19 cases were 103,321, of whom 1,668 people had died. By that date, according to the World Health Organisation (WHO), the total global deaths from Covid-19, the first case of which was reported to WHO on 31 Dec 2019, was 26,654. Meanwhile the CDC data show that in the first ten weeks of 2020, 40,149 Americans had died from influenza and pneumonia. On 25 March Neil Ferguson, lead author of the fateful Imperial College report, gave evidence to a parliamentary select committee inquiring into Britain's response to Covid-19: "UK deaths from the disease are now unlikely to exceed 20,000… and could be much lower." Moreover, between 50%-67% of them would likely have died within one year anyway owing to old age and comorbidities.

Between them, these examples show firstly the perils and pitfalls of modelling, and secondly the problems and risks of basing public policy on models before sufficient data is available to test their assumptions and conclusions.

In the meantime we have imposed devastating social and economic costs. The sensible strategy would have been to isolate the elderly and vulnerable and let everyone else get on with their lives. Dr David L. Katz of Yale University, an expert in public health and preventive medicine, calls this a "vertical interdiction" strategy to distinguish it from the "horizontal interdiction" strategy of mass social distancing. The end result of such a strategy, to which we can still pivot, would be to achieve herd immunity for the population at large, but without the social and economic costs that will be with us for some time, with significant long term physical and mental health damage as well.

Influenza and pneumonia cause 3.2mn deaths worldwide annually. If each individual case around the world was tallied daily on the front page of all newspapers, a similar panic would arise. Road accidents kill another 1.3mn annually that could be saved by banning all automobiles. Sensibly, we hold the resulting disruption to everyday life to be too high a price to pay.

Similarly, life and death is part of an eternal cycle. Take sensible precautions, carry on calmly and put in place emergency measures only after the facts are in. But retain built-in flexibility to adjust policy interventions continually in line with the threat's evolution, spread and gravity; the collection and analysis of facts and evidence; and the availability of diagnostic tools and preventive and therapeutic interventions.

To be clear, we may yet get to the stage where truly draconian measures are necessary to control a Spanish flu-like epidemic. But as of now, the limited data we do have don't seem to support such extreme measures. Where most Western governments proved negligent was in failing to use the time after the outbreak in China to build up their response capacity across the board in order to be able to scale up emergency measures as required, if and when an epidemic hits.

Balancing risks, costs, and benefits

The first balance a government must assess is the risk of creating mass hysteria and panic with premature reporting and the risk of losing control by delaying public announcements of the true scale, gravity and urgency of a nascent epidemiological emergency. They can then settle on the optimal balance between sufficiently slowing the disease, preventing an economic meltdown, and maintaining a functioning society while the threat and responses evolve and the virus spreads.

I write as someone in the high risk category of over 70 with cardiovascular comorbidity. I have no wish to live for an extra year or two at the cost of crushing my children's careers, plans and dreams.

Coronavirus postscript[2]

Two brief comments as a follow up to my article on coronavirus on 30 March.

First, I noted the puzzling variance in the fatality rates, from 0.75% in Germany to 10.84% in Italy. Here is a plausible explanation. In Italy, every person who dies with a coronavirus infection is recorded as dying from it, but only 12% of these deaths have actually been caused by coronavirus. The latter would imply a mortality rate of a more credible 1.3%. A similar point is made about the UK by John Lee, a recently-retired Professor of Pathology who spent most of his adult life in healthcare and science, regarding the relative mortality rates of flu and coronavirus with only the latter listed as a notifiable disease.

Incidentally, having scaled down its estimate of the maximum death toll from 500,000 to 20,000, Imperial College now puts the figure of 5,700 as the likely number of coronavirus deaths, of whom up to two-thirds would have died from other causes within one year anyway. So *5,700 will die with coronavirus* in the UK but *under 2,000 will die due to coronavirus.*

In Germany, by contrast, the underlying health conditions are recorded as the cause of death, not coronavirus. And Germany has tested a broader spectrum of the population, including children and those with very mild symptoms, rather than the Italian practice of testing the very sick who have been hospitalised.

Second, more and more medical-scientific-epidemiological experts are speaking out questioning the mass hysteria and the panicky responses. The diversion of resources to fight coronavirus on a

---

[2] *Pearls and Irritations*, 1 April 2020, https://johnmenadue.com/ramesh-thakur-coronavirus-postscript/

war footing, the damage inflicted on the economy as a result, the rise in serious mental health problems, and the degrading of health services with sharp economic losses, mean that the true moral debate is not "lives vs money," but "lives vs lives."

Flattening the economy costs lives, livelihoods and freedoms, too[3]

Confronted by the coronavirus pandemic as a "black swan" event, most countries have chosen the hard suppression strategy with variably stringent lockdown measures. This is based on modelling that shows a dramatic shortage of intensive care beds and ventilators and other crucial medical equipment to treat the numbers afflicted under worst-case scenarios. Panicked by the prospect of health systems being overwhelmed and millions dropping like flies as in the 1918 "Spanish flu" pandemic, they have shuttered entire economies and populations.

While this is understandable in conditions of extreme uncertainty with a novel virus, there should have been more caution because of a history of failed catastrophist warnings, the massive economic costs which also have deadly impacts, the draconian infringement on individual freedoms, and the availability of other strategies rather than the mythical "do nothing" alternative.

Health professionals are duty-bound to map the best- and worst-case scenarios. Governments bear the responsibility to balance health, economic, and social policies. Once these are included in the decision calculus, the political and ethical justification for the hard suppression strategy is less obvious.

First, there are many "known unknowns" about the coronavirus: the true infection- and case-fatality rates; the variable reliability of

---

[3] *The Lowy Interpreter*, 17 April 2020, https://www.lowyinstitute.org/the-interpreter/flattening-economy-costs-lives-livelihoods-and-freedoms-too

statistics from different countries that are not always measuring the same things with a standardised methodology; the risks of (re)infection rates as social-distancing restrictions are lifted, and more.

In a series of articles in *The Spectator*, John Lee discusses the non-comparable ways in which coronavirus infections and deaths are recorded in different countries, and the relative mortality rates of flu and coronavirus. He is highly critical of the modelling to date used as the basis of current UK policy. Teams from Oxford and Stanford mapped a range of different outcomes using different assumptions.

Because of the acceleration with which the initial surge in infections comes, governments have been worried that without control measures, they will not have time to react and hence have implemented preventive lockdowns. Better safe than sorry is a good prudential policy. Yet we also lack reliable data about the retransmission rate. High levels of testing means more policy options for social mobility and economic reopening. If the average number of new cases generated by a single infected individual is above one, an outbreak spreads, but contracts below one. The challenge becomes to keep the combined new infections and retransmission rates constant or falling, rather than exponential and explosive. By mid-April Asian countries were fearing a second wave of infections and on Thursday Japan declared a nationwide state of emergency to suppress the virus. A gentle exit strategy will be accompanied by an intensive "test, trace and isolate" regime to detect and kill new outbreaks.

Second, catastrophism on previous epidemics proved false. In 1999, European Union scientists suggested up to 500,000 people could die from the UK mad cow disease. By October 2013, 177 deaths were recorded from the disease. In 2005, the UN's coordinator David Nabarro warned between 5 to 150mn people could die from avian flu. The WHO's official estimates were 2–7.4mn. Only 455 people died of bird flu from 2003–2019.

With the 2009 swine flu, instead of the feared 1.3% fatality rate, the actual rate was 0.02%, comparable to the US 2007–09 seasonal flus.

In the UK, against the "reasonable worst-case scenario" of 65,000 deaths, there were only 457. And the government spent £1.2bn on flu remedies that were not needed. The WHO came under severe criticism for having served the interests of "Big Pharma" in selling unnecessary vaccines.

UK fatality estimates for Covid-19 were scaled down dramatically by Imperial College London within two weeks, from 510,000 to 20,000 and then 5,700. On 12 April the UK was reported as having crossed the 10,000 mark in numbers killed. But this is misleading for, like Italy, the UK records someone dying with virus as dying of it: patients who "had tested positive for Covid-19 at time of death." By contrast, Germany attributes the deaths to the comorbidity. The *Financial Times* helpfully explores this issue in an article "The mystery of the true coronavirus death rate."

The *Financial Times* had another interesting analysis of whether the UK government has been captured by epidemiologists over other experts, treating them like demigods. At least 22 experts have questioned the high casualty projections of the dominant models. The high-end estimates have so far proven to be exaggerated.

According to the National Center for Health Statistics, the annual fatality toll from flu and pneumonia in 2017 was 55,672 and from diabetes another 83,564. Australia recorded 158,493 deaths in total in 2018 from all causes. In the 45 days from Australia's first Covid-19 death on 1 March to 63 deaths on 16 April, around 19,500 Australians would have died from all causes, but there was no daily chart on the front page of the newspapers recording the mounting toll every day. Against Australia's maximum capacity of 6,636 ICU beds, on 15 April there were just 214 coronavirus patients in hospital, with 76 in an intensive care unit.

Third, at some point the cure becomes worse than the disease. The harshness has been justified as prioritising lives over jobs. But "flattening the epidemic curve" comes at the cost of flattening economies. A spate of reports from Goldman Sachs, the International Labour

Organization, International Monetary Fund, Oxfam, World Bank , and World Trade Organization warn of dramatic decelerations and contractions in GDP and trade from the pre-pandemic forecasts, with a resulting ballooning of poverty with job losses and income falls..

Grave and prolonged economic damage takes its own tragic toll on lost livelihoods and lives. This is seen at its most acute and more immediately in developing countries whose people "fear hunger may kill us before coronavirus".

However, advanced economies are not immune. The UK has recorded a sharp rise in the number of people dying at home, including from cardiac arrests, because people are reluctant to call for an ambulance. They fear that beds may not be available, or that they might contract the virus in hospital. Because an efficient and universal-access health system operates inside a robust and resilient economy, decreased wealth will inevitably lead to degraded public health infrastructure and a resulting loss of life.

Most elective surgery is postponed while hospital beds lie idle awaiting coronavirus patients. An article in *Lancet Psychiatry* says Covid-19 could have "profound and pervasive impact on mental health " caused by loneliness and anxiety. On 16 April the US Department of Labor reported that unemployment claims had risen by more than 20mn over the previous four weeks, around the number of jobs added over the past decade. The lockdown also puts women at much greater risk of domestic violence.

Many heroic assumptions are also being made: about the capacity of national governments to contain short-term damage and revive the economy from induced coma in the medium term; about the Trump administration's skill in managing the economic and trade fallout; and about the limited global damage from economic downturns in China, Europe, and US.

Fourth, asserting state control over swathes of economic activities is not the only curtailment of freedoms. The extreme measures of quarantining entire populations also constitute de facto mass house arrests.

The physical, mental, and emotional health benefits of open-air exercise are universally acknowledged. A court in Germany has reversed a regional government's ban on people going to the beach as a disproportionate curb on freedoms. In a BBC interview on 30 March, former UK Supreme Court Justice Lord Sumption warned : "when human societies lose their freedom, it's not usually because tyrants have taken it away. It's usually because people willingly surrender their freedom in return for protection against some external threat."

We have both the right and a duty as citizens to be vigilant against government over-reach. Democratic accountability generally improves public policy outcomes.

Fifth, Europe and the US have been less successful in their interventions than the East Asian states, which have mostly avoided generalised hard lockdowns.

Lockdowns slow the peaking and help to ensure an even distribution of cases, but may not reduce the final numbers significantly. Anthony Costello of University College London claims alternative public health measures such as identification of cases and contact tracing could have softened the lockdown. Rigorous social distancing has shut down large parts of the economy and also left the UK vulnerable to a recurrence of the disease when restrictions are lifted because few people will have acquired immunity.

Indiscriminate shutdowns require the least and most vulnerable—the young and fit versus the elderly and infirm—to shoulder equally the risk of the virus spreading. The fatality rates in the big congested regions such as London, New York City, and New Jersey are the worst affected. And overwhelmingly the elderly and people with existing comorbidities are the most at risk. In Canada half the deaths have been in aged care homes. New York, with many traits the opposite of Australia's, was initially too casual about the virus and in the second week of April it resorted to mass burials . A strategy that makes sense for the biggest and most densely packed cities may be less appropriate elsewhere.

Australia's low toll is better explained by physical isolation, vast open spaces, low density living, few multigenerational households, high use of private cars instead of mass transit, and sociocultural practices.

Australia's collateral costs could have been reduced and the health outcomes might not have been dissimilar with a policy of early checks at air and sea ports of entry by mid-February; isolating the elderly, infirm and vulnerable; quarantining the infected with serious symptoms; putting in place testing facilities at office complexes, shopping malls and other crowded public spaces; and leaving individuals responsible for personal hygiene and social-distancing precautions.

Responding to Covid-19 1: Can we save lives and preserve our quality of life at the same time?[4]

In an open letter to Prime Minister Scott Morrison on 19 April, more than 200 economists rejected commentators' calls for a rapid return to work and labelled the notion of a "trade-off" between public health and the economy a "false distinction." They said that while the measures adopted to contain the spread of Covid-19 had caused economic damage, those negative effects were far outweighed by the lives saved.

Their charge that this is a false distinction is correct, but it needs further examination. To someone from a poor country, people on moral high horses can appear to be so far from the ground that they can no longer see reality. There are different policy pathways to saving lives while allowing them to be lived in dignity.

As of 4 May, India's Covid-19 death toll was 1,566 and confirmed cases were at 46,437 (though those figures may be understated.)

4 *The Strategist*, 5 May 2020, https://www.aspistrategist.org.au/responding-to-covid-19-can-we-save-lives-and-preserve-our-quality-of-life-at-the-same-time/

UN estimates show that more than 800,000 Indian infants died in 2019, a mortality rate of 3%. Nearly 1mn children under the age of 5 years died, an even higher mortality rate of 3.7%. Those figures are 10 times higher than the infant and child mortality rates in Australasia. Most of these Indian children died from preventable causes—nutritional deficiencies, lack of sanitation and lack of access to healthcare.

Oxfam has warned that the Covid-19 pandemic could push an extra half billion people into poverty, and the UN estimated in mid-April that the global economic downturn could cause hundreds of thousands of additional child deaths in 2020.

Jayant Menon, a visiting fellow at the ISEAS–Yusof Ishak Institute in Singapore, has raised the need to flatten the "misery curve" in poor countries. The inflection point for the virus curve is when the health system is overwhelmed. Menon says that the analogous point on the misery curve is when the harm caused by the curtailment measures starts impinging on health or survival.

Both curves must be kept below their tipping points—but in poor countries, misery has outpaced data. Because both curves are highly sensitive to rapid changes in a highly dynamic environment, policy measures must be adjusted as circumstances evolve.

The signatories on the letter to Australia's prime minister are concerned experts engaging in a vital public debate about saving lives even at some cost to the economy. Some political heavyweights in the UK are also talking the language of trade-offs. Scotland's First Minister Nicola Sturgeon has called for a "better balance" between tackling the disease and protecting the economy. Former Chancellor George Osborne agrees, urging an open discussion about the hard trade-offs that may be needed in a nation that will be living with the virus for the foreseeable future.

Multiple reports have documented the immediate and likely long-term economic harm caused by lockdowns. The World Trade Organization warns of dramatic decelerations and contractions in GDP and trade, with a resulting ballooning of job losses and fall in incomes. The IMF estimates that the global economy will shed around $9 trillion in 2020. World output will contract by 3%, hitting both advanced and emerging economies and sparking steep rises in unemployment, debt and bankruptcies.

For this pain to be justified, lockdowns must be effective in saving lives in big numbers. Conversely, if health gains are negligible but economic, social, and even healthcare costs are high, the economists are right, but for the opposite reason to what they meant.

The onus is on the proponents of lockdowns to prove the case for the extensive cessation of economic activities, suspension of individual freedoms and mass house arrest of entire populations. As Sweden's chief epidemiologist Anders Tegnell has observed, shutting down and locking down have no "historical scientific basis"; the sole basis for such tough love is epidemiological modelling.

Tegnell told the BBC on 24 April that Sweden was better placed than most European countries to face a second wave of the outbreak. The strategic goal was to slow the progression of the disease so the country's healthcare system didn't become overwhelmed. Between 15% and 20% of the population is estimated to have become immune, which is enough to slow and control the spread of the disease further. Regarding Sweden's high death toll relative to its Nordic neighbours, he noted that "as many as 50% of deaths had come in care homes for the elderly, which have banned visitors," so it's "hard to know how a lockdown would have stopped that."

John Lee is sceptical about the effectiveness of lockdowns in limiting the spread of the virus and says "there isn't any direct evidence that what we are doing is actually affecting the peak." John Ioannidis, a professor at Stanford University's School of Medicine, holds multiple appointments in statistics, biomedical data, health research and policy and is ranked among the world's 100 most-cited scientists on Google Scholar. He calls the existing data on coronavirus infections "utterly unreliable" and dismisses much of the early Covid-19 epidemiological modelling, which forecast a death toll of 500,000 in the UK, over 2mn in the US and 40mn globally, as "speculation and science fiction" feeding a "mob mentality."

Viruses may be highly infectious or highly lethal, but rarely are they both. In large-scale community tests, a Stanford study of 3,200 people in California showed the number of infections to be 50 to 85 times higher than the number of confirmed cases, and a study by Gangelt in Germany showed an infection fatality rate of 0.37% rather than the modelled 0.9%. These studies indicate that Covid-19 spread earlier and much further than was initially imagined, which suggests that it is correspondingly less deadly.

There's a growing body of evidence that lockdowns are ineffective. Carl Heneghan, professor of evidence-based medicine at Oxford, argues that UK infections peaked a week *before* the lockdown was imposed on 23 March.

Examining data from all the US states, Wilfred Reilly concludes that lockdowns do not result in lower coronavirus mortality than social-distancing measures done well. Scott W. Atlas, a former chief of neuroradiology at Stanford Medical Center, looked at death rates in New York, the epicentre of US infections and deaths. He found death rates of 0% for those under 18 and 0.01% for those 18 to 45 years old without underlying conditions. Of the 6,570 killed by the virus to that date, 99.2% had underlying conditions. So even older people without pre-existing conditions may not need to self-isolate.

Localised shutdowns, targeted quarantine and sheltering in place can complement more generalised border closures and social distancing—a conclusion reinforced by a new study from the National Bureau of Economic Research in the US: "we find that optimal policies differentially targeting risk/age groups significantly outperform optimal uniform policies and most of the gains can be realized by having stricter lockdown policies on the oldest group."

Responding to Covid-19 2: Are lockdowns doing more harm than good?[5]

There appears to be no appreciable difference in fatality rates for US states that instituted lockdowns early or late, or among European countries whose social-distancing and lockdown measures varied significantly. Hong Kong, South Korea, and Taiwan seem to have managed the crisis without tough lockdowns as well as Australia and New Zealand have with lockdowns. The quality of government decision-making and the capacity of healthcare systems to respond quickly may have been more crucial than rigorously enforced sheltering in place.

On 24 April, Australia's chief medical officer, Brendan Murphy, conceded that the effective reproduction rate of the virus—the rate of new infections relative to the number of patients known to be infected—was under 1. Below that level, the infection wanes. That was the situation in every Australian state and territory in mid-March, *before* the stage 3 lockdowns took effect on 30 March. Does that mean that the economically less damaging stage 1 and 2 restrictions were working well enough that Australia didn't need to go to stage 3 lockdowns?

Murphy's answer was that, until then, about two-thirds of Australia's Covid-19 cases were imported. Once that wave had died down, there was a risk that a rapid acceleration of community transmission would take the reproduction rate above 1 again and cause an exponential explosion of fresh infections.

There are trade-offs within health as well. Total coronavirus deaths in Australia are so low that, thanks to the lockdowns, the reduction in the number of road fatalities may exceed the number of Covid-19 deaths averted.

---

[5] *The Strategist*, 6 May 2020, https://www.aspistrategist.org.au/responding-to-covid-19-are-lockdowns-doing-more-harm-than-good/

The *Wall Street Journal* reported that many hospitals and doctors in the US were grappling with an unexpected side effect: a financial squeeze that could deplete the healthcare resources needed to meet local surges in cases and threaten the operations of some financially struggling hospitals. Staff were laid off and clinics and outpatient facilities closed as elective procedures were suspended in many hospitals. Thus, a policy designed to protect the health system from being overwhelmed has instead partially crippled it.

Meanwhile, expenses soared as hospitals sought scarce supplies to cope with the anticipated surge in Covid-19 patients. Doctor visits fell by 50% on average. Hospitals were losing US$45 billion a month. According to Dr Jonathan Geach, tens of millions of patients are failing to receive the medical care they need in a timely manner. At the Mayo Clinic, 65% of hospital beds and 75% of operating rooms are empty. How many of the nearly 2mn new cancers each year in the US, as well as heart, kidney, liver and pulmonary illnesses, will go undetected for months because routine screenings and appointments have been put on hold?

In the UK, one estimate puts the number of planned and elective operations cancelled in the past three months at 2.1mn. This is in addition to the 4.5mn people who were on hospital waiting lists before the crisis. The UK has recorded a sharp rise in the number of people dying at home, including from cardiac arrests, because people are reluctant to call for an ambulance. They fear that beds may not be available, or that they might contract the virus in hospital. Fresh research shows that, owing to deferred consultations and suspended treatments of other diseases as the UK focuses on the coronavirus pandemic, almost 18,000 cancer patients could die.

A report in the *Financial Times* references an internal British government estimate that ultimately, without mitigation, up to 150,000 people in the UK could die prematurely of conditions other than Covid-19 because of the lockdown. Preliminary figures indicate that between 23 March and 10 April, 35,817 of the recorded 46,000 deaths in Britain were not directly linked to Covid-19. That's an 18% increase in the number of deaths compared with the same period in 2019.

A report in *Lancet Psychiatry* says measures taken in response to Covid-19 could have a profound and pervasive impact on mental health. US authorities and experts too are warning of an approaching "historic wave" of mental health problems caused by the months-long Covid-19-related "daily doses of death, isolation and fear." Lockdowns also put women at much greater risk of domestic violence. It will be interesting to watch the rates of divorce and births in the year following the great lockdown. In earthquake-prone countries, disaster preparedness has suffered from the nearly exclusive focus on coronavirus.

What of Australia? Ben Mol and Jonathan Karnon, professors at Monash and Flinders medical schools, confirmed that significantly fewer people have been presenting with acute heart problems and stroke and some cancer screening has also ceased.

Many life-threatening situations are discovered during routine annual check-ups and screening, which is why tests are mandated for particular age groups. Some years ago I had a stent inserted. The entire cycle from initial sense that something was wrong, to emergency consultation with the cardiologist, referral for an angiogram and emergency surgery, took about five weeks. With the same symptoms in this lockdown, it's very likely I'd have died before getting the stent.

How will citizens react to the stress of indefinite lockdown? There's a danger that some governments will take advantage of the pandemic to tighten controls to an unnecessary extent and for some police to enforce them overzealously. Jonathan Sumption, a former UK Supreme Court judge, warned, "This is what a police state is like." Amnesty International Canada demanded oversight protections for human rights during Canada's Covid-19 response. UN Secretary-General António Guterres warned that the coronavirus pandemic was becoming a human rights crisis, with authoritarian responses, surveillance, closed borders and other rights abuses.

A serious weakness in epidemiological models comes from data that are uncertain and behavioural relationships that are unstable. Human nature being what it is, increasing numbers of people will gradually begin to resocialise and governments will face a choice between tightening coercion or a collapse of their authority. It would seem better to control the timing, sequence and pace at which restrictions are eased, with built-in flexibility to bring some back should infection numbers shoot up again, than to lose control of the agenda.

Lockdowns can be cruel, heartless, and deadly[6]

Those of us who argue the coronavirus cure can indeed be worse than the disease, are sometimes accused of putting the economy ahead of lives. This is morally offensive. Unless someone is silly enough to claim saving just one life is worth a complete shutdown of the whole country, the debate is about the thresholds of mortality against the human, health, social, and economic costs of different strategies. Judged against these criteria on the evidence to date, it's a challenge to justify the hard lockdowns of Australia and New Zealand.

Jamlo the heartbreak girl

India's social, family, housing, and water-cum-sanitation realities are a nightmare for any epidemic that is both highly infectious and highly lethal. Physical distancing is impossible to implement in slums where multigenerational families sleep in one room, eat together, and share communal water and sanitation facilities. The same conditions make it impossible in a rambunctious democracy to conceal a big spike in deaths. India's surprisingly low Covid-19 mortality thus must have an explanation other than the lockdown.

---

[6] *Australian Outlook*, 15 May 2020, https://www.internationalaffairs.org.au/australianoutlook/lockdowns-can-be-cruel-heartless-and-deadly/; Part 2, 21 May 2020,

Yet India is uniquely vulnerable to lockdown shocks because of the overwhelming dominance of the informal sector. The lockdown could cripple the economy, worsening the unemployment crisis, destroying the livelihoods of daily wage workers (under 10% of Indians have salaried employment), forcing thousands of interstate migrant workers to return home under stressful conditions with mass transportation suspended, distressing the agricultural sector, and disrupting food chains. How exactly does a rickshawallah survive a seven-week lockdown?

Migrant workers from India's poorer states were caught off-guard with the four hours' notice of the total lockdown for 21 days from 25 March, and then its rolling extension thereafter. No thought was given to what they would do, how they would survive, and how they'd get home. Many decided to walk home in groups.

Jamlo Madkam was a 12-year old girl working in the fields of Karnataka state. When the lockdown was extended on 16 April, she joined a group who planned to walk the 100km to their home state of Chattisgarh. To hide from the police, they trekked through dense forest and over hills. Jamlo was carried part of the way by some adults but on 18 April, just 11km from home, her life gave out due to fatigue, hunger, and dehydration. She had worked nine and ten hour shifts every day for eight weeks at the daily wage of ₹200 (A$4.00) and saved ₹13,500 that was found in her bag. In death, she benefitted other migrant labourers trekking home as shamed authorities encouraged trucks to give migrants lifts instead of penalising them for doing so. Her story is a proxy for so much that ails India, including child labour, no social safety net, and moral apathy of the nation to the most marginalised and vulnerable communities.

Sixteen other migrants were walking home from the western state of Maharashtra to their home state of Madhya Pradesh in central India. In the early hours of 8 May, they were mowed down by a freight train while sleeping on railway tracks.

Nasty, brutish and short: life is still Hobbesian for millions of human beings. I've argued in *The Times of India* that in poor countries, the imbalance between coronavirus and other deaths, some up to nearly fifty times higher, means the singular fixation with the coronavirus is beyond perverse. If the media could show Table 1.1 as a banner headline with daily updates, people would not have lost all sense of perspective about the threat from coronavirus compared to other human insecurities.

Table 1.1: Deaths in India from selected diseases, pro-rated 25 March–12 May 2020

Flu & Pneumonia	TB	Diarrhoea	Corona
87,260	**63,356**	**58,043**	**2,415**

Of course, the equation is qualitatively different in industrialised countries. Many Westerners seem to have some strange notions about the human right to be protected from all life-threatening risks and emotional trauma. How dare we say: all life ends in death, get used to it. To my astonishment, the pandemic has brought about an expansion in state power right into our homes and across public spaces to an extent not seen previously, even in wartime.

The price paid in civil liberties and individual freedoms is eloquently expressed by Lord Sumption, former Judge of the UK Supreme Court. Saying life is priceless is a slogan, "just empty rhetoric," else the Allies would not have gone to war against Hitler. Human beings are family- and community-oriented social animals. Sharing food and drink at home or in restaurants, enjoying the cinema, watching cricket, appreciating a concert or a play are not optional add-ons but fundamental to our daily life as human beings. "Social distancing" by contrast is profoundly anti-social and rubs against every fibre of human civilisation. From everything we now know, the elderly should be free to meet, greet and hug grandchildren under 10 to bring back joy and cheer to their lives.

Debating the great lockdown[7]

Early assumptions of extraordinary SARS-CoV-2 infectiousness and lethality have proven fallacious. Some are already calling the coronavirus lockdown "the Greatest Mistake in History."

The seductive numerical precision of the Imperial College London (ICL) 16 March model, with grim forecasts of deaths in the tens of millions, provoked a herd-like panic across the world but was refuted by data collected in the following weeks that progressively reduced its policy usefulness. Early modelling of the virus was based on the initial statistics from Wuhan and Italy. Indeed, with the significant number of asymptomatic cases, the most common symptom of the virus is no symptom at all.

Has the Great Lockdown worked? Cross-jurisdiction comparisons are notoriously difficult and it's almost impossible to prove lives have been saved except by falling back tautologically on the model's own projections of mortality figures with no lockdown. It's easier to raise questions about the claimed success.

Countries with different lockdown strategies show broadly similar coronavirus curves. The model, based not on science but flawed assumptions and skewed data, has failed badly in its predictions of the evolution of the curve. Chris von Csefalvay, an epidemiologist who specialises in the virology of bat-borne illnesses, including coronaviruses, examined the code behind Neil Ferguson's model after ICL eventually and reluctantly shared a cleaned up version. He concluded its flaws fall "somewhere between negligence and unintentional but grave scientific misconduct."

---

[7] *Australian Outlook*, 21 May 2020, http://www.internationalaffairs.org.au/australianoutlook/debating-the-great-lockdown-part-two/

Across the entire population, mortality figures are within the seasonal fluctuations of flu. But unlike the flu, which tends not to discriminate between different age cohorts, coronavirus is very age-specific. The elderly, with comorbidities like heart and lung diseases, obesity, and other diseases associated with old age, are significantly more at risk. The strong association with comorbidities means that even for the elderly, coronavirus per se does not pose a significantly higher risk of death.

This is shown in a visually striking age-adjusted graph from the BBC on 6 May (Figure 1.1). For those under 20, the graph suggests the risk is negligible. Perhaps most surprisingly, children under 10 do not appear to be transmitters of the disease. Thus a boy with coronavirus did not pass it on to 170 contacts, but he did cross-infect two siblings with the common cold and flu. In New York, two-thirds of new hospital admissions were infected at home while sheltering-in-place. Prolonged exposure in enclosed environments like households is high risk; in outdoor settings the risk is under 5%. In the UK, the "vast majority" of patients had no coronavirus symptoms on admittance but picked up the disease in the hospital.

Figure 1.1: Risk of dying each year by age in Great Britain

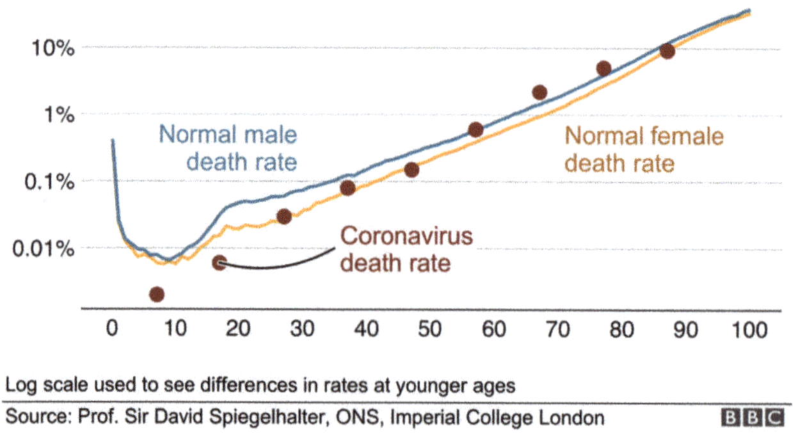

The obsession with the coronavirus has meant a neglect of other preventive screening and therapeutic interventions, producing significant numbers of excess deaths from other causes. Professor Karol Sikora, a consultant oncologist with the National Health Service, estimates up to 50,000 more UK deaths from cancer owing to the lockdown-induced pause in health screenings. The German magazine *Tichys Einblick* claims it's obtained an 86-page official report, an unofficial translation of which says the lockdown measures "apparently cost more lives, for example of cancer patients, than of those actually killed" by Covid-19. Australia's top mental health experts warn that a lockdown-induced 50% jump in suicides could kill ten times as many as the virus.

Figure 1.2: Germany's infection curve 1 March–10 May2020

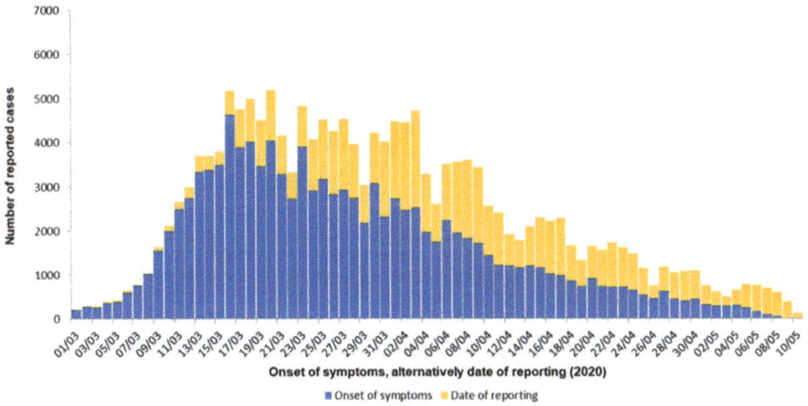

Source: Robert Koch Institute, Berlin

"R" is defined as the mean number of people cross-infected by one case. It is the magic number informing all epidemiological models of the likely progression of the virus under different scenarios and how to keep it below 1, the threshold at which infections grow in the overall population. A good example of the R number falling below 1 before a lockdown was imposed and staying so throughout comes from Germany. This chart from the Robert Koch Institute shows that by 23 March, when the most severe lockdown measures were imposed, R was already below 1 and in the following weeks did not decline any further. Thus the lockdown seems to have made no appreciable difference to R.

The geography of coronavirus

Geography seems a far more striking feature of the variance than lockdown and other policy interventions. For reasons as yet unknown, coronavirus has hit Europe and the US (especially New York) particularly hard, while Asia and the Pacific have thus far been spared its worst ravages. Europe and North America combined host only 14% of the world's population but account for 75 and 86% of the world's total coronavirus cases and deaths, respectively. By contrast Asia, with 60% of the world's population, accounts for just 16% of infections and 8% of deaths to date, while Africa's shares are 17, 1.5 and 0.8%, respectively. One line of speculation looks at the possibility that Europe and the US have been hit by a particularly virulent mutation of Covid-19. No doubt the scientific explanation will come in due course.

There are two striking European examples to date of observational data that contradict the dominant epidemiological model. Belarus has been ruled by a dictator since 1994. President Alexander Lukashenko has dismissed Covid-19 panic as a "psychosis," rejected lockdown and social distancing measures, and refused to close schools and cancel football matches. On 1 April, a WHO official warned that Belarus was entering a "concerning" new phase and urged the imposition of new measures to control the infection, but was rebuffed. By 20 May, Belarus had just 179 Covid-19 deaths.

The best-known example of a country bucking the model is Sweden. An application of the ICL model to Sweden projected that, without a lockdown instituted by 10 April, between 70,000 and 90,000 people would die by mid-May. The actual total on 20 May was

3,831—significantly higher than Sweden's Nordic neighbours but far lower than most of Europe. The two points of comparison are likely to be among the most watched over the next year.

Targeted interventions vs blunderbuss lockdowns

A study for the US National Bureau of Economic Research compared age-specific relative risks of infection, hospitalisation, and death. Its overall conclusion: "semi-targeted policies that simply apply a strict lockdown on the oldest group can achieve the majority of the gains from fully-targeted policies." This also avoids the perverse health consequences, extraordinary economic costs, and draconian curtailment of individual freedoms.

A one-size-fits all approach dissipates effort, distracts from the age-specific measures for the elderly as their special needs get lost in the noise, and, by harming the economy, diminishes the resources we have as a society to protect the most vulnerable. The cluster in Sydney's Newmarch House, with over 15 coronavirus deaths, is what happens when care is diffuse and generalised instead of focussed and targeted. Instead, governments should quarantine the elderly, direct more and better resources towards them (e.g. the quality of care in institutions and making sure they have opportunities to go outside in the sun and air while maintaining physical distancing), and be more cautious in reopening borders.

Meanwhile, they should let the 20-60 age group get back to normal activity ASAP, and perhaps the 60-69 age group with a bit more watchful caution. Governments should watch the famous effective reproduction rate (R) carefully to keep it below 1 so the cases keep falling. Serological testing will allow us to measure the gradual spread of the infection across the population. The idea of a bubble with countries with comparable and better coronavirus success indicators is a good one, starting with Australia and New Zealand, but also including some other regional neighbours.

Herd immunity, not herd mentality

A team of scientists from Edinburgh and London has suggested a segmenting-and-shielding strategy that segments the elderly and frail while shielding their carers with adequate personal protective equipment as a means to exit the lockdown with minimal risk of an overpowering second wave of infections. It is adapted from the "cocooning" of infants by immunisation of close family members that is a pillar of infection, prevention and control strategies.

This is the essence of the Swedish "model": protect the vulnerable, allowing the virus to spread slowly, within the ICU bed capacity, through the healthy population and thereby build herd immunity across the country. According to Swedish chief epidemiologist Anders Tegnell, "The more people become immune, the slower the spread of the virus in a population." The key to the herd immunity strategy is it acknowledges that the virus is serious and unstoppable, but that most people will come through fine if the vulnerable are sheltered and the seriously ill are hospitalised.

Infection curves have been falling in countries with and without hard lockdowns. PM Scott Morrison may not like the term, but unless we want a permanently drawn-up moat around Australia's shores, one way or another the only long-term viable solution is herd immunity by a combination of natural infection-cum-survival and then mixing into the general population, and vaccination. The latter may never arrive: not all past coronaviruses have a vaccine. On 14 May WHO emergencies expert Mike Ryan told an online briefing: "this virus may become just another endemic virus in our communities, and this virus may never go away."

In retrospect, Australia could have used the good fortune of the virus arriving in the latter part of its summer, instead of in the middle of the flu season as in the northern hemisphere, firstly to boost surge capacity at every bottleneck point to test, isolate, trace and treat cases; and secondly to follow the Swedish model with greater success and lower overall cost to lives, mental health, and the economy.

The tyranny of coronaphobia[8]

I've had two big worries during the pandemic, starting from the very beginning and still ongoing. Both relate to my sense that "coronaphobia" has taken over as the basis of government policy in so many countries, with a complete loss of perspective that life is a balance of risks pretty much on a daily basis.

First, the extent to which dominant majorities of peoples in countries with universal literacy can be successfully terrified into surrendering their civil liberties and individual freedoms has come as a frightening shock. There is this truly confronting video of the police in Melbourne assaulting a small young woman—for not wearing a mask!

On the one hand, the evidence base for the scale and gravity of the Covid-19 pandemic is surprisingly thin in comparison to the myriad other threats to our health that we face every year. We don't ban cars on the reasoning that every life counts and even one traffic death is one too many lives lost. Instead, we trade a level of convenience for a level of risk to life and limb.

On the other hand, the restrictions imposed on everyday life as we know it have been far more draconian than anything previously done, even during World War II or the great 1918-19 flu. In present circumstances, the argument for the crucial importance of liberties has been made most eloquently by former UK Supreme Court Justice Lord Sumption in a BBC interview on March 31st, and repeated several times since.

But it's also an argument that Benjamin Franklin, one of the founding fathers of America (and therefore suspect in the post-Black Lives Matter and statues-toppling environment), made back in the 18th century: "Those who would give up essential Liberty, to purchase a little temporary Safety, deserve neither Liberty nor Safety."

---

[8] Brownstone Institute, 5 August 2022, https://brownstone.org/articles/the-tyranny-of-coronaphobia/

Yet, the evidence for the effectiveness of draconian lockdowns is less than convincing. As one Lancet study concluded, "Rapid border closures, full lockdowns, and wide-spread testing were not associated with Covid-19 mortality per million people."

Second, the coronavirus threatens to overwhelm the health and economies of many developing countries where a billion people subsist in a Hobbesian state of nature and life is "nasty, brutish and short." In poor countries, the biggest numbers of deaths are caused by water-borne infectious diseases, nutritional deficiencies and neonatal and maternal complications.

The lockdown has produced its own version of Thucydides' dictum that the strong do what they can, the weak suffer as they must. In developing countries, saving livelihoods is no less important than saving lives. The privileged jet-setters who imported the virus can utilise the private hospitals but the poor they infect have little access to decent healthcare and will be disproportionately devastated. The rich carry the virus, the poor bear the burden since staying at home means foregoing daily income.

I remain very puzzled at how so many people I considered to be liberals have been so utterly indifferent to the plight of the poor and the casual labourers who do not have the luxury of working from home, nor savings to fall back on to tide their family over until they can earn an income again.

Celebrities posting videos and selfies of working from home in opulent mansions is positively obscene and revolting. Not surprisingly, given my Indian background, I was powerfully influenced by the visual images of the millions of migrant workers literally on the march by foot over thousands of kilometres trying desperately to make their way back to home villages as all work dried up.

Many died en route and the heartbreaking case of Jamlo Madkam in particular has never stopped haunting me.

This is not to say that high-income Western countries are immune from the deadly effects of lockdown. But the acuteness of the harsh impacts on the poor is just unconscionable and hard to comprehend intellectually as well as emotionally.

What about AFTER this pandemic? What worries you the most?

Most of my answer to this question is anticipated in the answer to the first question: the long-term impact on the health, nutritional requirements, food security, mental wellbeing of people, etcetera. I've been worried from the start by the long-term impact of lockdowns over the coming decade on the lives and livelihoods of poor people in poor countries, on schooling, on immunisation campaigns.

I wonder, too, if we have set ourselves up to repeat the folly every year with annual outbreaks of flu, especially if it is a bad flu season. If not, why not? Perhaps someone will come up with the slogan "Flu Lives Matter." Or governments could just pass laws making it illegal for anyone to fall sick and die.

How and when are we going to return to the "new normal" and what will it look like? Globalisation has underpinned unprecedented prosperity and the rise of educational and health outcomes for billions of people around the world, along with a dark underbelly of uncivil society. Will its discontents now throw away substantial benefits as the world retreats behind national moats once again?

The pandemic proves conclusively the need to demilitarise foreign policy and promote greater multilateral cooperation against grave threats that are global in nature and require global solutions. What my former boss, the late Kofi Annan, called "problems without passports" require solutions without passports. The risk is instead we will move in the opposite direction and recreate regionalised balance of power systems in various hotspots around the world.

Pandemics have long been identified as one of many global challenges for which the world should have prepared in advance. Recently *The Wall Street Journal* had a major investigative article on the failure to do so, despite ample warnings from scientists. "A Deadly Coronavirus Was Inevitable. Why Was No One Ready?" asked the authors, and quite rightly too.

Another catastrophe into which we seem to be sleepwalking is a nuclear war. And remember, the whole point of the sleepwalking analogy is that people walking in their sleep are not aware of it at the time. Other pressing global challenges include growing ecosystem imbalances and fragility, depletion of fish stocks, food and water insecurity, desertification, and of course a host of other diseases that remain the biggest killers on an annual basis.

By way of a concluding reflection, I think a common error has been to privilege the medical over all other considerations. In reality, and certainly with the benefit of hindsight but also from the very beginning in my case, this should have involved a considered assessment of what I call "A Balance of Interests" (my chapter in *The Oxford Handbook of Modern Diplomacy)*. Governments must take into account and reconcile medical, social, economic, liberal democratic, human rights, and international policies in fashioning an integrated public policy response to a pandemic.

Epilogue

The above is extracted from a long, 3,000 word full page interview featured in a Sunday edition of the Argentine daily La Nación on August 22, 2020 (in Spanish): Hugo Alconada Mon, "The Tyranny of Coronaphobia," Interview with Ramesh Thakur.

Since then Covid has mutated into multiple variants, mass vaccinations have been carried out in very many countries, and our understanding, data, and knowledge have evolved and grown. Despite that, re-reading these two worries each about the policy responses to Covid two years ago and about the possible ramifications for what the post-Covid new normal will look like, I don't think I would change a single word today.

I confess I still don't understand the global outbreak of collective panic and hysteria, the shelving of all existing pandemic management plans, the failure of medical professions to speak out, and the astonishing public compliance with authoritarian

2: COVID IN CONTEXT IN LOW INCOME COUNTRIES

It is well known by now that the timing and severity of the pandemic differed across the different regions of the world. The global media landscape is dominated by the big houses in the industrialised Western countries. Consequently few Westerners outside specialist circles realised the extent to which the impact of the pandemic was quite different in the poorer countries of the world. And so were the policy lessons and imperatives.

Africa and the pandemic panic: Facts not fear[9]

Africa is at risk of getting the worst of both worlds: failure to check the epidemic and failure to check economic collapse. Why?

First, because of a lack of state capacity, most African countries lack the administrations and health systems to implement and enforce "test, isolate, treat and trace" regimes. What exactly does social distancing mean if you live in sprawling informal settlements that characterise almost all major cities in the developing world. Second, the dominance of the informal sectors and extreme dependence on daily wages to keep families afloat mean that economic disasters will deepen the misery of millions and multiply illnesses and deaths.

[9] *ACCORD Covid-19 In-depth Analysis*, 19 May 2020, https://www.accord.org.za/analysis/africa-and-the-pandemic-panic-facts-not-fear/

SARS-CoV-2 emerged through a chain not yet fully grasped in Wuhan, China and hitched a ride on the world's flyways to insinuate itself into the very interstices of globalisation and spread rapidly to Iran, Europe and North America. As at 15 May, the total number of Covid-19 (the disease caused by the virus) cases was 4.5mn and over 300,000 people had died with it worldwide. By any criterion, that is a serious pandemic.

But in perspective, the annual global deaths from leading causes is: coronary diseases 8.7mn, stroke 6.2mn, lung cancers and diseases 4.8mn, influenza and pneumonia 3.2mn, diabetes 1.6, and diarrhoea and tuberculosis 1.4mn each. So coronavirus does not represent the end of the world. People suffer but endure. This virus too shall pass and indeed is on the way down almost everywhere.

As of 13 May, the total number killed with Covid-19 in the 55 countries that make up the African Union was 2,382, or an average of 43 and a median of just 10 deaths per country. Algeria and Egypt are the only countries to record over 500 deaths. If we exclude them, the average falls to 1.3 deaths/week per country. That should not be enough to make it even to the inside pages of most newspapers, let alone disrupt life as we know it through massive shutdowns.

In comparison, Table 2.1 shows the top three killers in South Africa are HIV/AIDS (138,000 per year), heart diseases (41,000), and influenza and pneumonia (35,000); in Kenya they are diarrhoea (33,000), HIV/AIDS (30,000) and influenza and pneumonia (27,000); and in Nigeria they are influenza and pneumonia 305,460; diarrhoea 186,218, and tuberculosis 175,124.

Table 2.1: Deaths by disease, pro-rated 1 January–13 May 2020

Country	Influenza & pneumonia	HIV/AIDS	Diarrhoea	TB	Covid-19
Kenya	9 846	10 929	12 140	3 245	36
Nigeria	111 610	61 714	68 041	63 988	152
South Africa	12 909	50 480	4 436	9 231	206

What lessons can Africa learn from the experience of others thus far?

On 14 May, Mike Ryan, emergencies expert at the World Health Organisation (WHO), told an online briefing that the novel coronavirus "may become just another endemic virus in our communities, and this virus may never go away." The statement from the WHO and the empirical reality of a very minor episode of the pandemic across Africa so far set the parameters of how Africa could address this particular "crisis": as potentially but not presently a serious human security threat.

Africa has the opportunity to lead the world in an evidence-based rather than fear-driven approach and be an oasis of sanity and calm in a world gone collectively mad.

On 16 March, Imperial College London (ICL) published a fateful paper warning of up to 510,000 Covid-19 deaths in the UK and 2.2mn in the US without government intervention, and perhaps half those numbers without hard lockdowns of national economy and society. The model has been widely criticised by software engineers for its code and by medical scientists for its flawed assumptions and distorted data. Spooked by the crisis as it unfolded in real time in Italy and elsewhere and impressed as much by China's accomplishment in suppressing it as by the grim curves of the ICL model, European, North American, Australasian and other governments imposed stringent lockdowns and social distancing requirements, often accompanied by instant heavy fines. The dominant media commentators, abandoning critical distance and objectivity, joined the herd to become pandemic panic addicts.

Figure 2.1 depicts the lack of correlation between lockdown measures and coronavirus deaths in selected countries. Restricting stringent lockdown measures to the elderly would have achieved most of the gains. Michael Levitt, a Chemistry Nobel Laureate, is on the mark with his caustic comment: "It seems that being a factor of 1,000 too high is perfectly OK in epidemiology."

The consequences of lockdown strategies for poor countries are likely to be especially tragic. A study by the Johns Hopkins School of Public Health in *Lancet* warns that in low- and middle-income countries, infant mortality could go up by 1.2mn in the next six months, and maternal mortality by 56,700, as a result of health services being disrupted by the obsession with the pandemic. This is beyond unintended and perverse consequences.

Figure 2.1: Covid deaths/mn people as at 13 May 2020, selected countries (Y/N = Yes/No to lockdown)

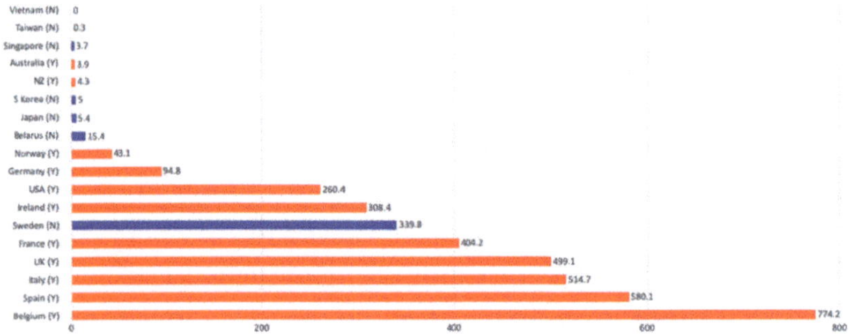

A three-pronged strategy for Africa: watch, prepare and activate

Europe and North America combined, with just 14% of the world's population, make up 75% and 86% of the world's total of the coronavirus infected and dead. Asia, with 60% of the world's population, accounts for only 16% and 8% of infections and dead. Astonishingly, Africa's shares are 17%, 1.5% and 0.8%, respectively. The science behind the pandemic is poorly understood and no one has a satisfactory explanation for Africa's great escape to date. That however is the factual reality. Accordingly, for now there is no need for African countries to take any immediate action for there is no crisis.

However, because the virus could evolve and strike suddenly and seriously, Africa should build up surveillance and testing capabilities across the continent, including at airports and seaports. Vigilance is the indispensable counterpart to caution sans panic.

It would also be prudent to undertake serological testing of population-representative samples to estimate the prevalence of antibodies and thus the spread of the infection. A second act of prudence would be to build the capacity to surge past the bottlenecks in the health and hospital systems, just in case a virulent mutation does strike suddenly.

The pandemic and the resulting socioeconomic crises also highlight the need for global circuit-breakers to identify, isolate and quarantine systemic risks early. The crisis is an opportunity to reboot the ethic of global cooperation.

WHO, which eradicated the scourge of smallpox in the 1970s, has a role in partnership with the African Union's African Center for Disease Control (African CDC) in developing state capacity in African countries to manage epidemics that is essential and non-substitutable. This is why African countries should unite in resisting US efforts to belittle and destroy WHO. Instead, they should seek WHO and African CDC assistance to establish testing facilities and protocols; stockpile essential testing and protective equipment and therapeutic medicines; and build ICU capacity to cope with sudden surges of infections so "R"—the effective rate of virus reproduction—is kept below 1 all the time to ensure the threat recedes and does not proliferate.

Taking into account the low infection rates, living conditions, and economic realities, the test, isolate, treat, and trace approach seems to be a more appropriate policy response for Africa than panic-driven lockdown strategies whose consequences could kill more people than Covid-19 itself.

"Jail Bharo!"—Channelling our inner Gandhi against the Covidcrats[10]

The evidence for the effectiveness of lockdowns is underwhelming; for the harm they cause to lives, livelihoods, mental health and civil liberties is overwhelming. Neither claim needs further substantiation for readers of this site.

Still the relentless march of lockdown folly continues, causing a growing sense of helplessness and despair. What has become clear over the course of the year is just how impervious the lockdownistas are to data, evidence, reason, and—yes—even science. Part of the explanation, I suspect, is that Western democracy has been captured by self-absorbed careerists who occupy all key positions in political parties. They have no interest in using power to advance any particular vision or achieve lofty social purposes, which is why the Australian prime minister can reject calls to defend free speech with the dismissive comment that it never created a single job. Nor do many have any experience outside of politics, putting comprehension of the real-world consequences of their decisions beyond them.

Even so, the ease with which so many well-established democracies have succumbed to pandemic fearmongering, and surrendered freedoms hard-won over centuries, is astonishing. The sickening video of a pregnant Mum handcuffed in the presence of her child for posting on Facebook about a peaceful, socially-distanced protest in a regional town in Victoria, produced victim-shaming by fellow-Victorians alongside condemnation by most other Australians.

The most eloquent defence of traditional liberties has come from Lord Jonathan Sumption—for example, in the Cambridge Freshfields Annual Law Lecture delivered on 27 October. But so far even his erudite voice and elegant reasoning are just cries in the wilderness. The

[10] *Lockdown Sceptics*, 2 December 2020, https://lockdownsceptics.org/jail-bharo-channelling-our-inner-gandhi-against-the-covidcrats/

criminalisation of the right to protest, and the advance of the totalitarian state that intrudes into the most sacred and intimate personal spaces of individuals, families, and businesses, has been backed by the ruthless deployment of the coercive apparatus of the state. I did not expect to see such scenes of confrontation between police and ordinary citizens—not militants—in Australia or Britain in my lifetime.

The failure of institutional bulwarks against the assault on freedoms has been just as dispiriting. One after another, parliaments, political parties, media, and the judiciary have abdicated their duty to hold the executive to account. The net result of the grotesquely inept, bumbling, and deeply authoritarian response of Boris Johnson to Covid-19 is the biggest attack on the lives and liberties of the freeborn English in centuries.

What then is to be done? I suggest one option is to channel our inner Gandhi against policemen indulging their inner bully and politicians indulging their inner tyrant.

Born after India's independence, I grew up with the saying the that reason the sun never set on the British Empire was that even God wouldn't trust an Englishman in the dark. In The *Government and Politics of India*, I noted that the political legacies from the Raj include civil disobedience as a legitimate and results-oriented technique of political protest.

"Civil resistance" encompasses marches, demonstrations, boycotts, strikes, and collective non-cooperation to express opposition to policies and state authorities without inflicting physical violence. This is both principled and prudent. Earlier this year, David Shor, a data analyst for the Democratic Party, was fired for tweeting a link to a scholarly paper showing that nonviolent protests have been more politically effective in redressing black minority grievances in the US than violent protests. The study, by Princeton University's Omar Wasow, looked at black-led protests from 1960-72. Wasow showed that nonviolent activism against state and vigilante repression was more effective in driving favourable media coverage and framing Congressional speech and public opinion on civil rights.

The person most associated with civil disobedience is Mahatma Gandhi. In effect, he instrumentalised, operationalised, and weaponised Henry David Thoreau's concept of civil disobedience (1849), turning it into an effective technique for peaceful mass mobilisation against a powerful opponent to end empire and win independence.

Gandhi's notion of *satyagraha*—literally, the urging of truth upon the opponent—is deeply grounded in the power of moral suasion. More recently, people have become interested in its strategic logic as a cost-effective alternative to violent resistance. In *Why Civil Resistance Works*, Erica Chenoweth and Maria Stephan showed that from 1900–2006, civil resistance campaigns outperformed armed struggles in defeating authoritarian regimes, advancing democratisation, and averting a relapse into civil war.

The British Empire's jails were the biggest training ground for the political leaders of newly independent colonies, including Jawaharlal Nehru in India. "*Jail Bharo Andolan*" is one technique of civil disobedience. It literally means "Fill the prisons movement/agitation." It's a deliberate, coordinated campaign to subvert a law or regime by courting arrest and imprisonment in numbers that physically clog the courts and overwhelm the prisons.

The fact that those imprisoned are normally law-abiding citizens adds greatly to the authorities' embarrassment. It was used frequently as part of India's independence struggle against the British. Because of that lineage, it has a legitimacy that makes it impossible for any Indian government to counter effectively. So it continues to be used in modern times, often for relatively trivial political purposes instead of in the service of a transcendental cause: to protest against corruption, price rises of essential commodities, prohibition and police brutality.

Gandhi prioritised the call of truth and conscience—"a higher court"—over the courts of justice. Delivering the annual Gandhi

Peace Foundation lecture on Gandhi's birth anniversary on 2 October in New Delhi, prominent activist-lawyer Prashant Bhushan described the serial attacks on minorities and journalists as "an assault on dissent by the use of fundamentally unjust laws". He concluded that were Gandhi alive today, he'd "surely have launched a *Jail Bharo Andolan*, daring the government to incarcerate millions of peaceful protesters from across the country".

Gandhi got habituated to being jailed by oppressive authorities in apartheid South Africa and colonial India and jail was a second home to him. British authorities would release him when he began a fast, fearing mass uprisings should he die in prison. "I always get my best bargains behind prison bars," he quipped with his trademark sense of mischief, the same that apocryphally led him to remark that European civilisation would be a very good idea.

England is "notoriously law abiding", says Nigel Jones in *The Critic*, but it also has its own heritage of successful peaceful resistance and agitation for social justice and political rights—for example, the Suffragette movement 100 years ago. As the diktats get ever more arbitrary, petty and inconsistent—you cannot hug Granny but six cops can carry her spread-eagled to a police van—citizens develop contempt for laws, lawmakers, and the principle of the rule of law.

So to those looking for what you can do: protest peacefully in large numbers, have several rungs of leaders to take the place of any who are arrested, be unfailingly polite and charmingly courteous to police officers and judges, refuse to pay fines in favour of court appearance and trial, and after the court has delivered its verdict, go to prison rather than pay fines to overwhelm the prison system until the justice system breaks down.

It requires sacrifice, courage, and steadfastness to refuse obedience to the dictates of a discredited and despised government. The dissenters must be prepared to accept the legal consequences, including imprisonment. But if you don't fight for freedom, get ready to lose it.

India's anomalous Covid-19 experience[11]

On 15 September, India had over 5.1mn Covid-19 infections, behind only the United States; and 83,000 deaths, behind the United States and Brazil. The country recorded a mortality rate of 60 deaths per million, compared to 26 for its neighbours in South Asia and 11 in Asia. The real toll might even be higher—some Indian states are undercounting Covid-19 deaths by attributing them to comorbidities, while others have weak health surveillance systems.

There are reports of discrepancies between official death tolls and counts from crematoria and burial grounds. The vast majority of Indians die at home, with last rites performed by the family. Widespread alarmism has led to stigmatisation of the virus, with some doctors and young Muslims being refused burial for fear of contagion. Families may be reluctant to take sick relatives for testing and hospitalisation, and many who succumbed to the disease have likely been cremated or buried quietly to avoid social stigma and ostracism.

On 25 March, India imposed total lockdown with just four hours of notice and no logistical preparation. Its lockdown stringency was rated 100 by Oxford University's Blavatnik School, compared to France's 88, Germany's 77, Italy's 92, and Vietnam's 58.

Covid-19 ranks only 18th among India's biggest killers, well behind heart disease, lung disease, tuberculosis, diarrhoea, diabetes, and traffic accidents. Of the 139,123 suicides in India in 2019, daily wage earners (25% of the workforce) made up 23.4%, up from 12% in 2014. The unemployed made up another 10.1%. One shudders to think what the 2020 numbers will be.

India has plummeted from the world's fastest growing major economy to the fastest shrinking. GDP contracted by 23.9% in the April–June 2020 quarter, the worst slump since India started publishing

[11] *East Asia Forum*, 18 September 2020, https://www.eastasiaforum.org/2020/09/18/indias-anomalous-covid-19-experience/

quarterly data in 1996 and the biggest drop in the G20. Unemployed migrant workers trekked home on foot during this time, leading to the tragic death of 12-year-old Jamlo Madkam. Some were sprayed with chemical disinfectants and many were harassed and extorted by corrupt police officers.

As they've returned home, migrant labourers have spread the disease deep into India's village heartland. India now has the worst of both worlds and is yet to recover on either the virus or the economy fronts. Housing, water, and sanitation realities are a nightmare for any epidemic that is both highly infectious and lethal. Physical distancing is impossible in slums where generations of families sleep in one room, eat together and share communal water and sanitation facilities.

On 30 May, despite a record daily rise of almost 8,000 cases, India announced a substantial easing of lockdown restrictions because the rise in deaths and misery caused by the lockdown was reckoned to be worse. India is now moving ahead with Unlock 4. Other poor countries have also concluded that lockdowns are not worth the economic pain.

In Europe, Asia and the United States, the effectiveness of lockdowns remains contested. One *Lancet* study concluded that "rapid border closures, full lockdowns, and wide-spread testing were not associated with Covid-19 mortality per million people." Comparing US states, another study found lockdowns did not contain the spread of the virus and opening up did not exacerbate it.

In addition to achieving herd immunity through a vaccine or the spread of the virus, scientists have been looking at the role of antibodies and pre-existing cross-immunity through T-cells in people never exposed to Covid-19.

The discrepancy between the recent spike in infections amid a fatalities plateau seen across Europe and the United States is striking. The rise in infection numbers could be an artefact of increased testing, or perhaps herd immunity has been achieved in some countries at the unexpectedly low threshold of 20% of the population being infected. One study showed the infection rate in Mumbai slums was 57%, compared to 16% in other areas—but the slums lacked commensurate fatalities, potentially indicating a low herd immunity threshold in Mumbai also.

Nobel Laureate Michael Levitt postulates a "self-flattening curve." Oxford Professor of Theoretical Epidemiology Sunetra Gupta observes that rates of infection and mortality are strikingly similar across countries with different lockdown policies, suggesting case numbers are better explained by pre-existing cross-immunity to related coronaviruses than lockdowns. Europe and the United States seem to offer more support for this thesis than for the original modelling that predicted indefinite exponential growth, with cases doubling every 3–5 days without stringent control measures.

Yet it's hard to see evidence of such self-flattening in India—or in Peru, which went into lockdown around the same time. Peru has now recorded 31,000 deaths and a mortality rate of 932 per million, despite maintaining restrictions.

India's economic slowdown began long before the pandemic hit and there was little to cushion it from the lockdown's harsh impact. The neglect of urgently needed economic and governance reforms in order to pursue a religious nationalist agenda left the country exposed to the exogenous shock. India's hospital bed capacity is only 20–25% of Western countries and it has neglected primary frontline care.

India needs to urgently upgrade its rickety public health system. There is a scandalous scarcity of epidemiologists, microbiologists, biostatisticians, and research institutes with the expertise to trace the origins of the virus, its spread and capacity gaps in the public health system. India could become "the global nerve centre of … multinational supply chains in the post-Covid-19 world" as per Prime Minister Narendra Modi's dream, but only if he acts decisively on economic and governance reforms.

India's Coronavirus emergency tells a story poorly understood[12]

The blanket and punitive travel ban for Australians returning from India is neither justified, nor does it make much sense in the efforts to curb the spreading of the virus. India's coronavirus emergency is also raising many questions of the policies imposed around the world during the pandemic.

On 1 May, Health Minister Greg Hunt invoked, for the first time ever, emergency powers under the Biosecurity Act to stop travellers from India from entering Australia. Violators face five years' jail and up to $66,600 in fines. This provoked outrage from human rights experts like former Race Discrimination Commissioner Tim Soutphommasane, media commentators normally associated with right-wing views like Chris Kenny, as well as Indo-Australians, for denying Australian citizens the inalienable right to return home and also for being racist in its selectivity.

Figure 2.2: India's seven-day rolling average of daily new Covid-19 deaths per million people in comparative perspective, 1 March 2020–30 April 2021

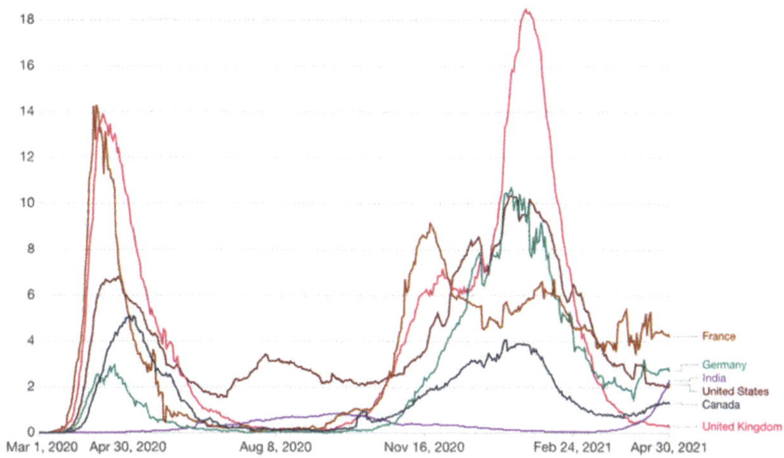

Source: Our World in Data

12 *Pearls and Irritations*, 5 May 2021, https://johnmenadue.com/indias-coronavirus-emergency-tells-a-story-poorly-understood/

When even Andrew Bolt says it's difficult to explain the policy other than as racism, we have a problem. Figure 2.2 shows why the blanket ban on arrivals from India is not justified. People from other countries in the chart, whose mortality rates were much higher at the peak of their Covid surge, were coming to Australia in significantly greater numbers.

Of course, the reliability of all mortality statistics from India is suspect amidst such a massive calamity. But there is still no agreed definition and methodology for such key terms as tests, cases and what constitutes a Covid death. PCR and lateral flow tests are known to be very unreliable, with false positives and negatives common. This is why multiple negative tests are required to clear people suspected of having been infected and returning travellers in airport quarantine facilities.

Unlike the common flu, where only those who end up in hospitals are counted as "cases," with Covid, anyone testing positive, including the large numbers of false positives, are commonly recorded as cases. It's only after another year or more that we will be in a position to look at two-year trends and put all-cause deaths during the time of Covid into historical perspective, and then try to estimate how many died from and not just with Covid.

There are several additional features of interest about Figure 2.2. Within the global Covid envelope, India has often stood out as an anomaly, earlier with the puzzling low Covid casualties despite the extremely unfavourable initial conditions with respect to congested living and working conditions, more recently with the anti-seasonal surge of new double and possibly triple mutants.

Countries that experience an exponential growth in numbers killed with Covid always seem to experience a comparable rate of descent as well of their mortality curves, even in second waves. In contrast to all others in the chart, India did not experience an earlier exponential growth of infections, hospitalisations, and deaths. This had bred hubristic complacency and the consequence has been tragic. Assuming Australia and New Zealand cannot close borders permanently to the rest of the world, have they done enough to build up hospital surge capacity to deal with nation-wide exponential growth of some new variant in the future, or have they too succumbed to premature triumphalism?

Figure 2.2 also speaks to the reality that over a year since the declaration of the pandemic, no expert or government is on top of just how the virus behaves and how it is mutating, nor what is the best strategy to check and control it. At least to the point where we can all resume normal lives within an agreed state of endemic equilibrium where a certain level of risk from Covid is accepted.

For that reason, India's current crisis must be placed both in international context and in relation to the totality of health threats to the lives of Indians.

With 1.83mn Covid deaths in the world in 2020, amounting to around 3% of all deaths in the calendar year, the disease is clearly deadly. Nevertheless, there were five killer diseases that were even deadlier: in ascending order, Alzheimer's and dementia, influenza and pneumonia, lung diseases, strokes, and coronary heart disease, with the last causing 9.43mn deaths. This is why policy attention and public resources cannot be monopolised by Covid but must scan the total public health horizon and establish a hierarchy of priorities that reflects the relative gravity of the different threats.

With 20mn total Covid-19 cases and 219,000 total deaths by 3 May, India's numbers are the second and third highest in the world. On the daily new count, India is the worst hit on both key indicators. Yet, on cases and deaths per capita, India still ranks a lowly 114th and 116th (Table 2.2). Even against internal benchmarks, India's average daily death toll is 25,000 from all causes. In the 14 months from 1 March 2020–30 April 2021, with 201,702 deaths Covid was the 13th biggest killer. Suicides numbered 287,435 and lockdowns are both a direct and indirect ("structural') cause of suicides. The annual toll of traffic accidents, low birth weight, diabetes, diarrhoea, and tuberculosis ranged from 397,422 to 559,992.

Table 2.2: Some Covid-19 statistics for selected countries as at 30 April 2021

	Daily deaths/mn	Cumulative DPM	Daily cases/mn
India	1.95	151	222.8
Brazil	11.67	1 900	283.6
EU	4.68	1 548	238.2
UK	0.29	1 882	32.9
USA	2.01	1 740	155.2
World	1.65	408	98.1

Table 2.2 and Figure 2.3 are also graphic evidence of the policy-invariance of Covid-19 with regard to non-pharmaceutical interventions, where the infection, hospitalisation, and mortality curves have followed their own logic and remarkably similar trajectories.

Figure 2.3: Daily new Covid-19 deaths/mn people in Sweden, EU and Czechia

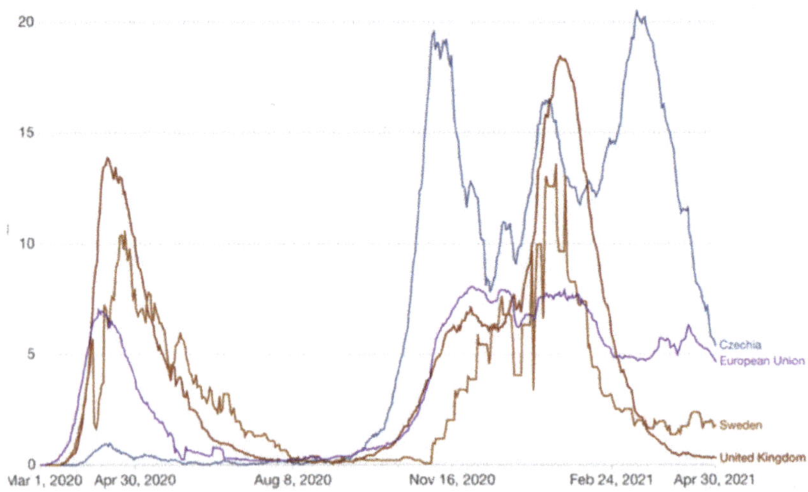

Over a year's worth of actual data therefore have reconfirmed the scientific and policy consensus that existed before 2020, as faithfully summarised in the WHO report in September 2019 and also reaffirmed in the UK national pandemic preparedness plan as late as February 2020. Lockdowns can delay the spread of infections for a short time and this can be critical to ramping up hospital bed capacity and medical supplies, but they do not avoid the virus forever. The American Institute for Economic Research has compiled a list of 35 studies that show lockdowns are ineffective.

If lockdowns worked, Sweden would have a higher death rate than the worst-hit European countries and Florida would be far worse off than locked down California and New York. If anything, data indicate the opposite.

As can be seen in Figure 2.3, the curve of jurisdictions that locked down and those that did not follow a surprisingly similar trajectory. Figure 2.4 shows that US states that did not lock down for the winter are dispersed right across the mortality rates spectrum instead of being concentrated towards the higher end. On a per capita division, of the 2.2mn deaths for the US predicted by Neil Ferguson's model of 16 March 2020 without mitigation, Florida with 6.46% of the US population should have had around 142,000 deaths owing to its lack of mitigation measures. Instead, on 30 April its Covid toll was 35,172.

Where the lockdown states and Florida do differ is in their social, economic, and children's education costs. *Politico* had a memorable headline on 23 December 2020: "Locked-down California runs out of reasons for surprising surge." Experts were similarly puzzled by the failure of any post-holiday surge in Iowa despite dire predictions. In a MSNBC interview on 17 February, President Joe Biden's coronavirus adviser Andy Slavitt visibly struggled to explain similar curves from lockdown California and no-lockdown Florida: "that's just a little beyond our explanation."

Against the questionable benefits of lockdowns, their immediate and lasting harm to health, mental health, livelihoods, social life etc. is immense, especially for the most disadvantaged and poverty-ridden groups and countries. A peer-reviewed article in the *European Journal of Clinical Investigation* by researchers from Stanford University in January 2021 showed that net harms exceed net gains between highly and less restrictive interventions.

Dr Sebastian Rushworth, a practising physician in a Stockholm hospital, reported in his well-regarded blog on a new study by Anna-Mia Ekström and Stefan Swartling Peterson of the Karolinska Institute. Using data from Unicef and Unaids, they show that at least as many people have died as a result of lockdowns as of Covid.

The latter have died mostly in rich countries and been old, while most of those who have died of lockdown were younger people in poor countries who succumbed to malnutrition, lack of vaccination with childhood immunisation programs shut, and treatable diseases like TB and HIV. Considering their respective age-segregated mortality, the number of total years of life lost to lockdown is significantly greater than the number of years of life lost to Covid-19.

Figure 2.4: Total Covid-19 deaths/mn people in US states, as at 16 April 2021

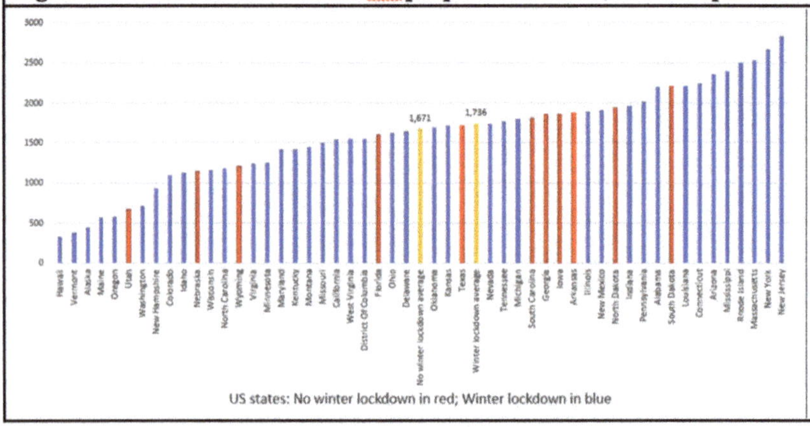

Four medical professors from Harvard, Oxford, and Stanford Universities maintain a very informative website documenting the massive worldwide harm from lockdown measures, called Collateral Global, on physical, mental, and social health, and on education and economy. Not coincidentally, two of the four professors, Jayanta Bhattacharya and Sunetra Gupta, are of Indian origin and therefore have a better idea of conditions in South Asia than most.

For example, lockdowns have forced 500mn children around the world out of school and more than half of them are in India. Pointing this out on the release of a new report, Dr Sunita Narain, Director General of the Centre for Science and Environment, said that similarly, more than half the world's additional 115mn people pushed back into extreme poverty live in South Asia. India, she said, was all set to usher in a 375mn strong "pandemic generation" of children up to age 14 who are likely to suffer long-lasting impacts like increased child mortality, being underweight and stunted, and educational and work-productivity reversals.

Overall, then, the balance of risks and benefits varies between rich and poor countries and between those with good public health infrastructure and those without. Therefore authorities have to work out the best mix of mitigation measures for their own jurisdiction and not fall into the trap of "what's good for Europe is good for India" approach.

One possible explanation for India's sudden vulnerability to the double mutant could be the recommendation to wear masks in public. After all, decades of "settled" science before Covid-19 argued against their general use and it would be surprising to have that overturned so suddenly, especially with no gold-standard randomly controlled trials in the real world and not results from lab experiments using medical masks. Thus the UK's pre-Covid national plan said that, public perceptions on facemasks notwithstanding, "there is in fact very little evidence of widespread benefit from their use" in "the community and household setting."

Figures 2.2–2.4 are good representations of this abiding reality. Under Indian conditions, they may well have been seriously harmful. Photos and TV coverage on any day in different parts of the country show that substantial numbers of Indians are serial violators of critical mask protocols on hygiene practices, before putting them on, while wearing them, and after taking them off: frequent fiddling with masks, lowering them below the chin, touching mouth, nose, eyes and face, single versus multiple use, discarding moist and wet masks, the incentivisation of risky behaviour like dangerously close physical proximity to others from the false sense of security given by masks, reducing distance between people because they cannot hear one another through masks, safe disposal, etc.

All this helps to explain why India has strongly resisted calls for another nationwide shutdown. In a sombre national address on 20 April shorn of his usual bombast and bravado, PM Modi said: "In today's situation, we have to save the country from lockdowns." He explained that current strategies to contain the rapid resurgence in infections were aimed at ensuring the least loss of lives and livelihoods, and appealed to states to consider micro-containment zones rather than lockdowns and encourage migrant workers to remain *in situ* with the assurance they would be vaccinated and not lose their jobs.

On 20 April, just under 10% of Mumbai's 87,443 active cases were in slums and 90% in high rise and other mostly multi-storey buildings. The likely explanation for the tiny infection rate in slums is naturally acquired herd immunity. Conversely, lockdowns compel high-rise dwellers into more prolonged and acute exposure to pathogens than if healthy people were encouraged to spend time outdoors, especially in parks and on beaches, while maintaining physical distance and minimising human contact. Sick people should be told to stay home.

The crux of the problem in India is not the proportion of cases and deaths from Covid. Rather, it is the lack of a fit-for-purpose public health infrastructure and medical supplies of equipment and drugs. The Modi government has been no less negligent in this regard than its predecessors. But where previously the political, bureaucratic, and financial elites have managed to circumvent the public system's inadequacies by going private or abroad, Covid has caught them out with some viciousness.

More than anything else, the humanitarian tragedy blows apart the narrative of strongmen competence based on the pursuit of divisive and polarising policies to expand and consolidate political power.

WHO estimates of India's Covid deaths are highly suspect[13]

On 5 May, the WHO issued a new report estimating global excess deaths at 14.9mn for two years of the pandemic 2020–21 as the true Covid-19 mortality toll, nearly triple the official toll of 5.44mn. "Excess mortality" is the difference between the number of deaths that would be expected in any time period based on data from earlier years, and the number of deaths that have occurred. For countries with robust data surveillance, reporting, and recording systems, this poses no real difficulty. Unfortunately, these conditions are not met in many countries. Therefore their excess mortality can only be estimated and the accuracy is a function of the reliability of the methodology and modelling used in the exercise. Given the overwhelming evidence about the flaws and deficiencies of Covid-related modelling over the last two years, and the damage caused by governments trusting modelling projections over real-world data, this should immediately throw up a forest of red flags about the WHO report.

A second reason to be sceptical is the less than stellar role of the WHO in its well-known Covid-related deference to China, the abandonment of its own summary of the state of the art science on managing pandemics from September 2019, its willingness to manipulate definitions of "herd immunity" in relation to vaccines and natural immunity in order to fit with the experimental pharmaceutical and non-pharmaceutical interventions (NPIs) that came to dominate Covid policy around the world, and its self-interest in expanding its budget, authority, and role in steering global health policies and management by means of a new international treaty.

[13] *The Daily Sceptic*, 8 May 2022, https://dailysceptic.org/2022/05/08/who-estimates-of-indias-covid-deaths-are-highly-suspect/

A third ground for scepticism is they ascribe the total death count to the direct effects of Covid "due to the disease" and indirect effects "due to the pandemic's impact on health systems and society". The first part is questionable because it fails to distinguish between deaths with and from Covid. The second is disingenuous because the indirect toll of the NPIs (lockdowns, masks, induced fear, lost schooling, lost jobs, cancelled screenings and operations, aborted immunisation programs, disruptions to global food production and distribution, etc.) and vaccine-related adverse events will prove to be significantly higher than the indirect effects of the disease *per se*. Any study that fails to disaggregate deaths caused by the disease and by policy interventions to mitigate it lacks credibility.

Like many others including Will Jones on this site, I was especially struck by the new figures for India. The report pushes India up to the very top of the Covid mortality toll with 4.74mn deaths, nearly 10 times more than the count of 481,486 (as of 31 December 2021), almost one-third of the world total. Sorry, but that is simply not credible.

India's geographic diversity, population size and economic conditions make data collection especially challenging. In public lectures in Australia and Canada, to drive home the point about the scale, I usually comment that the entire Australian population is a rounding error in 1.3bn-strong India. It suffers from persistent and widespread mass poverty—India is a country of a few mega-billionaires amidst the world's biggest pool of poor, illiterate and sick people bar none. It might be nuclear-armed, but state capacity when it comes to administration and public and social services is easily the worst of all major economies.

Figure 2.5: India's Covid-19 Deaths, 1 Jan 2020–27 Mar 2022.

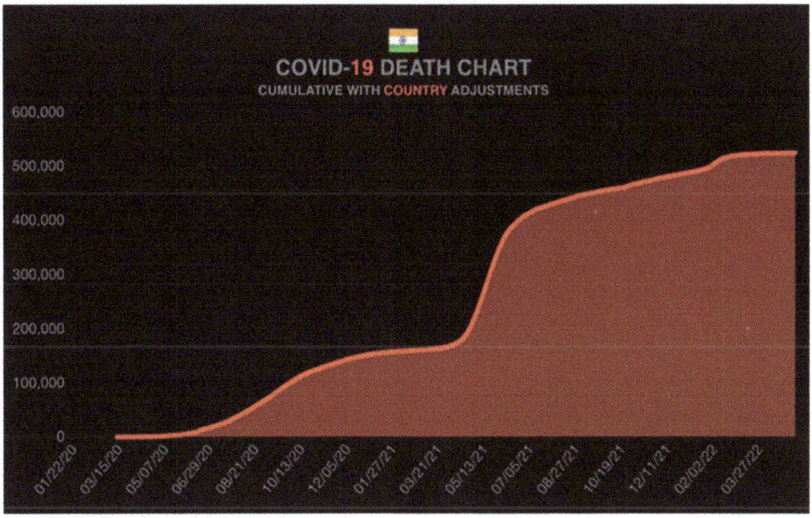

Source: World Life Expectancy, 8 May 2022

The public sector scores high on petty corruption but low on efficiency. The public health service is risible and high quality healthcare is neither accessible nor affordable for ordinary Indians. The best doctors work in the public sector, in medium to large clinics and hospitals in metropolitan centres, and as individual practitioners in most towns and villages. Consequently, health statistics are not all that reliable. But this is a general pathology, not one unique to Covid-19.

From everything I know about India, the WHO estimate does not align with overall death data, historical trends, and Covid death compensation claims on the Indian Government from states. Indian experts believe that official statistics capture over 90% of all deaths. But this also means that about 10% of deaths would have been missed in previous years, yet the WHO's "excess deaths" count uses the official numbers as the baseline against which to estimate the impact of Covid. In a related vein, why would under-reporting be limited to Covid-related deaths and not, say, to suicides with its heavy social stigma and traffic accidents where the operators of overloaded buses and vans would try to drastically reduce actual numbers in order to hide the illegal loads (Figure 2.6)? The WHO estimates are flawed also in relying on 2019 deaths instead of using a five year average 2015–19 to wrinkle out anomalies in any given year.

Figure 2.6: India's top dozen killer diseases (1 March 2020–7 May 2022)

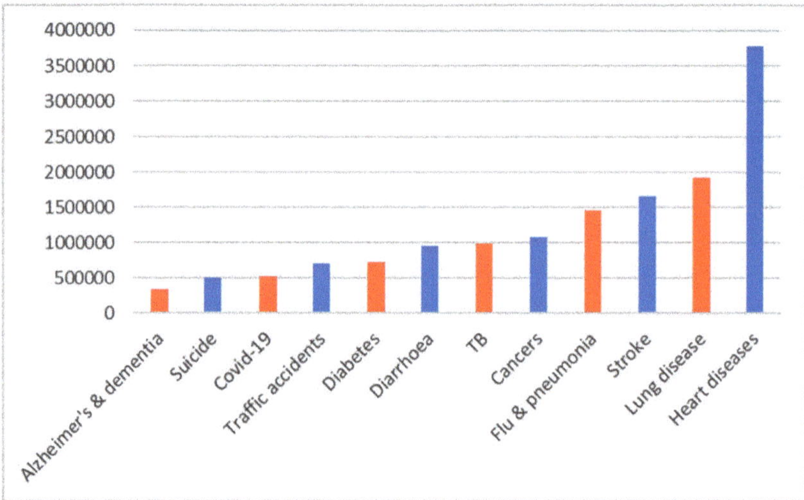

Top six cancers in order: oral, lung, breast, cervical, stomach, colon.

Source: Chart constructed by author drawing on data from World Life Expectancy, 8 May 2022.

Estimates of India's total annual death rate range from 738 per 100,000 people by the World Bank to 1,030 per 100,000 people by World Life Expectancy. The total annual death toll therefore would be somewhere in the 10-13mn range: a very wide range. The WHO estimate of the death rate for 2021 is within the higher range from World Life Expectancy. Simply put, the WHO estimate of all-cause deaths is within any realistic estimate of the margin of error in India's unique circumstances of scale and state capacity.

The caveats to official data notwithstanding, the WHO estimate would mean almost one-quarter additional deaths than normal. In fact it's worse. Looking at the detailed tables, the 4.74mn excess deaths is calculated from a combined excess death rate for 2020–21 of 171 per 100,00 people. This is disaggregated into 60 and 280 per 100,000 people for 2020 and 2021, respectively. That would imply a 38% jump in all cause deaths in 2021. Despite all the horror scenes we saw on TV of corpses lying in the streets and washed ashore on riverbanks, that's just not possible. Perhaps the clue to the error lies in the title of the actual document: "Global excess deaths associated with Covid-19 (*modelled estimates*)" (emphasis added).

Some Daily Sceptic readers had fun with this aspect of the WHO announcement. My favourite exchange was this:

> **BeBopRockSteady**
> Wish I could model. some extra funds into my bank account. Car has stopped on me again.
>
> > **Annie**
> > Get it to identify as the latest model. Models always work.
> >
> > **crisisgarden**
> > I hope no one models rain this afternoon, just hung washing out.

India's own estimates of excess deaths for 2020 compared to 2019 is 480,000, of which Covid-related deaths were just under 150,000. So over 300,000 excess deaths were due to non-Covid causes, which in itself is far more believable because of the impact of the lockdown measures on exacerbating most of the conditions underlying India's leading causes of deaths. By contrast, in 2021 the Covid-related death toll was much higher at 332,492.

Much as I have been critical in the past of official dismissals of international reports on India including weakening democratic practices, in this instance the Government is right to reject the WHO methodology of mathematical modelling based on data on 17 Indian states collected from websites and media reports: "This reflects a statistically unsound and scientifically questionable methodology of data collection for making excess mortality projections in the case of India." As well as defective data collection methodology, the report is marred also by three critically flawed assumptions: that uncounted excess deaths occurred only in 2020–21 and not before; they occurred only for Covid-19 and not other diseases; and Covid-related deaths were due solely to the disease and not caused by policy interventions to control and eradicate it.

The contra example of India's rejection of indemnity for Pfizer[14]

Curiously enough, indirect support for mRNA vaccines driving Covid infections and deaths is also suggested by implication by India's example. Anyone who has followed the Covid story globally will recall the horrific images of bodies being washed ashore on the banks of the Ganga in April–June 2021, and crematoriums unable to cope with the piles of bodies awaiting the last Hindu rites of being put to flame on funeral pyres.

[14] Brownstone Institute, 29 March 2023, https://brownstone.org/articles/indias-rejection-of-indemnity-for-pfizer/

Figure 2.7: 2-dose vaccination and Covid cases in four Western jurisdictions

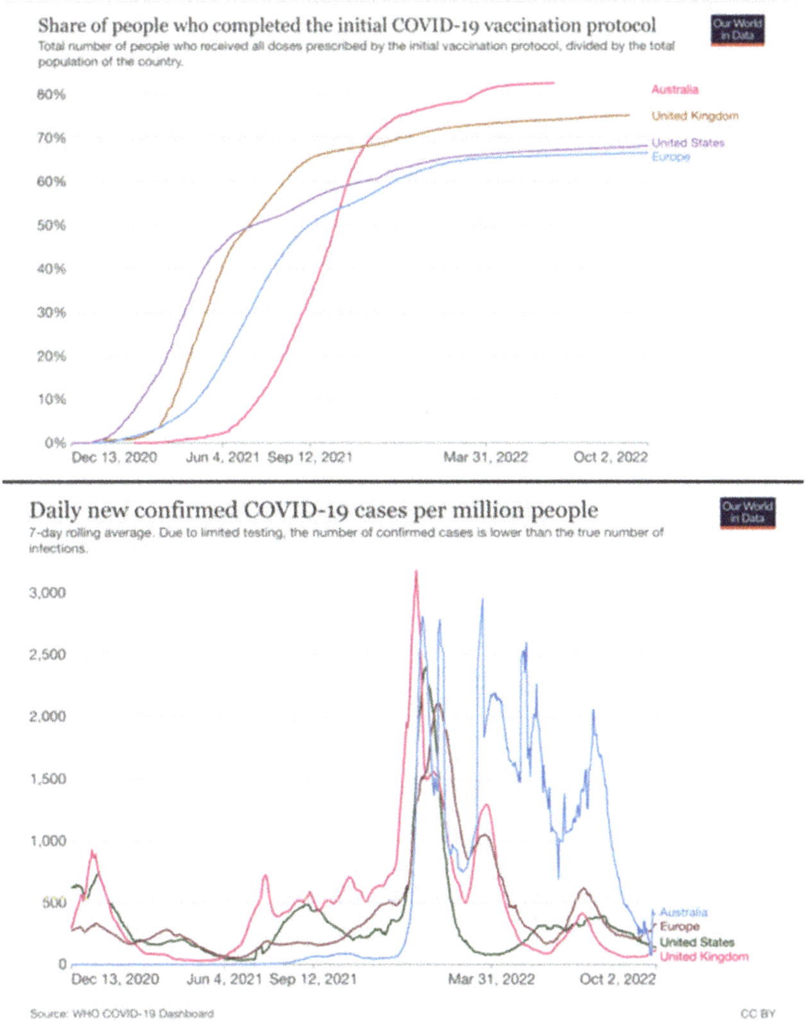

In Figure 2.7, we can see a lagged temporal correlation between vaccine rollout starting in late 2020 and early 2021, and a rise in Covid-19 infections from autumn 2021, in Australia, Europe, the UK, and the US. Had the vaccines proven 95% effective against infection and transmission in the real world, this should not have happened.

Figure 2.8 shows a three-month wave in Covid infections in India in April–June 2021 inclusive, followed by a two-month seasonal winter surge in January–February 2022. There is no correlation with the vaccine rollout.

Figure 2.8: India's 2-dose vaccination and Covid cases

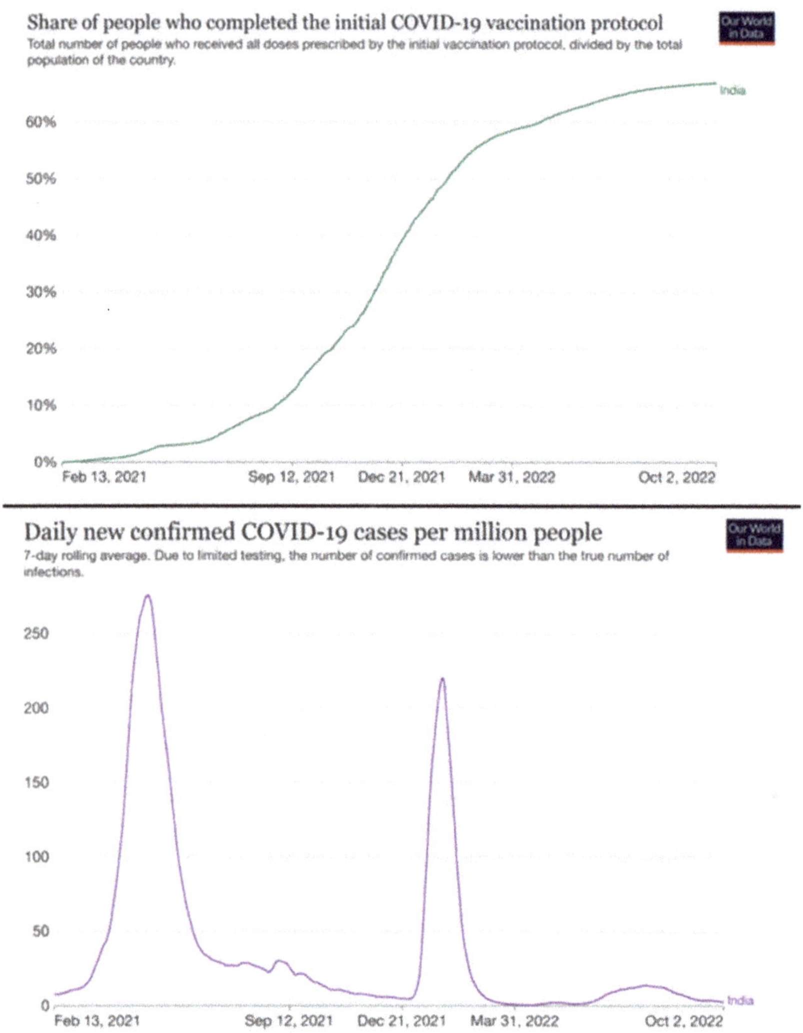

As per Our World in Data, India's daily new Covid death count rose above 1,000 for the first time on 16 April 2021, peaked at 4,190 on 23 May, and fell below 1,000 again on 1 July. It climbed back above 1,000 briefly with a subsequent "ripple" with 1,127 deaths on 5 February 2022. India's double vaccination coverage was only 1.1% on 16 April 2021, still under 3% on 23 May and 4.2% on 1 July. By February 2022 it had reached 50%.

How does this help with the notion that mRNA vaccines might be driving Covid cases and deaths in many Western countries? Because the main vaccine administered in India is a virus-vector type. The Indian government would not agree to demands by Pfizer and Moderna that their approvals elsewhere, based on trial results from overseas, were sufficient to be granted emergency use authorization in India with full legal indemnity.

India's drug regulator, the Central Drugs Standard Control Organisation, said in February 2021 that its experts did not recommend the Pfizer vaccine because side effects reported abroad were still being investigated. It also said Pfizer had not proposed any plan to generate safety and immunogenicity data in India.

In contracts with several European and Latin American countries, Pfizer required the recipient states to acknowledge that long-term effects and efficacy of the vaccine are currently unknown and there may be adverse effects, contradicting both parts of the "safe and effective" mantra drilled into all public messaging.

Instead India administered two main types, neither of which used mRNA technology. Covishield, the AstraZeneca vaccine, is a viral vector vaccine that uses a weakened, non-replicating strain of chimpanzee cold virus (adenovirus) to carry genetic material of the spike protein of SARS-CoV-2 into human cells. This accounted for more than four-fifths of vaccines administered in India by April 2022.

The second was Covaxin that was developed by the local firm Bharat Biotech in partnership with the Indian Council of Medical Research. Covaxin contains an inactivated SARS-CoV-2 virus that has been disabled for replication. All of its 29 proteins are intact and provoke immunity of the host that is closer to the infection-induced natural immunity. Coming out of decades of research in adenovirus-based vaccines, it uses a tried and tested technology platform with an established safety profile that has been used by other vaccines like polio.

As I understand it, Pfizer-BioNTech and Moderna make mRNA vaccines. These give our cells instructions for how to make the spike (S) protein found in the SARS-CoV-2 virus that it uses to enter human cells. After vaccination, muscle cells begin making the S protein pieces which stimulate the body to create antibodies. If infected with SARS-CoV-2, the antibodies will fight the virus.

In a vector vaccine, material from the SARS-CoV-2 virus is placed in a modified version of a different virus (viral vector). The latter gives the cells instructions to make copies of the SARS-CoV-2 S protein. When the cells display the S proteins on their surfaces, the immune system responds by creating antibodies and defensive white blood cells. Upon infection with SARS-CoV-2, the antibodies will fight the virus.

According to a Danish study by Professor Christine Benn and colleagues reviewing randomized controlled trials (RCTs) of mRNA and adenovirus vector vaccines that was published in preprint a year ago, the adenovirus vector vaccines reduce all-cause mortality significantly, compared with the mRNA vaccines that demonstrate no benefit in terms of all-cause mortality. The relative risk of mRNA vaccines compared to the placebo group was 1.03, and that of the adenovirus vector vaccines was 0.37.

Recently Germany's *Die Welt* became the first major mainstream publication to report on the allegations of fraud in Pfizer's clinical trials, with participants who suffered adverse events being unblinded and removed and cover-ups of the death of Pfizer subjects. The *New York Times* has taken the European Commission to court over Commission President Ursula von der Leyen's refusal to release the text messages she exchanged with Pfizer CEO Albert Bourla, in which she personally negotiated the purchase of up to 1.8 billion doses of the BioNTech/Pfizer vaccine. On 15 February Florida issued a health alert on mRNA Covid-19 vaccine safety.

When we add this to the long list of out of court settlements by Pfizer and some convictions, perhaps India did well to dodge this bullet!

In the US, Americans funded the development of Covid vaccines by Pfizer and Moderna, paid for the resulting vaccines, were mandated to take the jabs by governments and many private sector employers, but because of the grant of legal indemnity lost their right to hold commercial entities accountable for neglect and malfeasance.

No one has as yet explained why, if the manufacturers were so convinced that their vaccines were safe and effective, they required legal indemnity against vaccine injuries. Nor have supposedly progressive governments such as New Zealand's, as well as conservative governments like Australia's at the time, attempted to justify the logic behind privatizing the profits but socializing the risks.

Some US states like North Dakota and Arkansas are reportedly considering legislation (1) to prevent mandatory medical treatment if the product manufacturer cannot be held legally liable, or (2) to "make it criminal for pharmaceutical executives to knowingly hide, conceal, or withhold information regarding a medical product's adverse effects if the product results in death or serious injury." This would restore citizens' rights against state-subsidized Big Pharma with its immense lobbying budgets, power, and successes.

Meanwhile India's contra example poses some difficult questions for the drug regulators of countries like Australia. Why is it that local clinical trials were not required before granting emergency use authorization to these experimental vaccines with no established long-term safety profiles? Have they been captured by the very industry they are meant to regulate in order to protect public health?

Do they understand why there is public cynicism that regulators might have morphed from guardians of public health into vaccine enablers, accelerating the approval process by short-circuiting safety trials, yet being noticeably tardy in responding to safety signals and investigating vaccine injuries, as in the case of 24-year-old Amy Sedgwick whose tragic death was featured in *The Weekend Australian* on 25 March ?

In a poignant follow-up Adam Creighton, the paper's US correspondent, pointed out that this story would have been disappeared from the Internet in 2021 owing to the censorship collusion between Big Pharma, Big Tech, and public health authorities.

3: AUSTRALIA AND CANADA DESCEND INTO AUTHORITARIANISM

Among the most shocking developments as the pandemic dragged on for more than two years was the degree of coercion and force used by some of the best known champions of liberal democracy. As someone who is a citizen of three English-speaking countries—Australia, Canada, and New Zealand—I struggled to come to terms with this, and was just as troubled with the compliant acquiescence of the people with the erosion of their freedoms and liberties.

Human rights discarded at the Gates of Hell[15]

Dr Chris Williams, of Public Health Wales, solemnly told the BBC on 29 October: "Every time you stop and talk to someone... then you've just had a potential transmission event." Part of "the problem," he added, is that "we don't see that as a bad activity."

This is beyond "You couldn't make it up." What next—breathing is a potential transmission event and we should all stop it, just stop it?

Six months into the pandemic, on 22 October the president of the Australian Human Rights Commission Rosalind Croucher finally voiced her opinion of lockdowns. Because of the lack of scrutiny

[15] *Spectator Australia*, 7 November 2020, https://www.spectator.com.au/2020/11/human-rights-discarded-at-the-gates-of-hell/

and accountability around lockdowns, she said, Australians have been exposed to "potentially unnecessary restrictions of their rights and freedoms." A good lawyer, Croucher has concerns about process. To be fair, she did point out that the commission's jurisdiction was limited to the federal government's actions and so she was able to voice concern about entry and exit travel rules that prevented families from being reunited.

Still: "potentially unnecessary" infringements? This was her epiphany? Put under 23-hour house arrest, limited to 5km-radius outings for state-approved activities and purposes, mandatory mask requirement, rights to peaceful protest suspended, pervasive police surveillance of social media and public spaces, state control of economic activities, suspension of parliament to rule by executive diktat, instant heavy fines on police officers' whims, martial law masquerading as medical law: how comforting to learn these are all *potential* infringements.

No offence to my many friends in the law professoriate, but I've often wondered about the wisdom of appointing legal academics to positions of human rights chiefs without some broader background and experience. They are, I am sure, supremely qualified in the legal technicalities and niceties. Some training in moral philosophy underpinning Western civilisation would help them to balance competing pulls of the many different streams that make up the total human rights bandwidth.

Human rights claims are claims by citizens on governments. The advocacy, juridical, and enforcement revolutions in human rights led to a rapid expansion of governmental activism on legislation backed by monitoring and compliance machinery. Yet human rights are also abused most systematically, pervasively and widely by governments.

There's also tension between the human rights and anti-discrimination agendas, as in the case of the Queensland University of Technology students. Instead of being given an answer—like me, you don't have to accept the merits of the answer to acknowledge that there is a broad philosophical case for affirmative action—the full weight of the state was brought to bear, in the form of the human rights machinery, to crush the pesky students.

A related tension, and possibly most relevant to the pandemic, is the clash between individual and collective rights. In the name of ensuring the safe health of everyone, governments have trampled willy-nilly on previously inviolate individual rights.

Lockdowns don't destroy the virus. No, they destroy the three "ls" of lives, livelihoods and liberties. Governments have effectively stolen a year of our life. Preemptive press self-censorship has helped to normalise the rise of the surveillance-cum-security state in the name of keeping us safe from terrorists and now from the virus that is so deadly, hundreds of millions must be tested to know they've had it.

On 21 October, despite a modest rise in Covid cases, Sweden lifted all remaining "recommended" restrictions on over-70s. The justification was not economic but emotional health. Health Minister Lena Hallengren explained: "We cannot only think about infection control, we also need to think about public health." Months of social isolation had meant loneliness and misery and a "decline in mental health likely to worsen the longer the recommendations remain in place."

Part of the emotional stress load on the elderly caused by lockdowns results from the destruction of family life. The family is the fundamental unit of human society and the forced separation of loved ones has taken an enormous toll on mental wellbeing, with measurable consequences for physical health. From the UK we've had stories of elderly people refusing to go into rest homes. They'd rather die in pain surrounded by family at home, than face a lonely death cut off completely from family after leaving home. The inscription on The Gates of Hell in Dante's *Inferno*—"Abandon hope, all ye who enter"—was not meant as a forewarning of care homes 700 years later.

The boundary between liberal democracy and draconian dictatorship proved to be virus thin. A Freedom House report concluded that in 80 countries, the pandemic has emboldened governments to engage in abuses of power: "silencing their critics, and weakening or shuttering important institutions, often undermining the very systems of accountability needed to protect public health."

For me the defining image of the pandemic state of siege in Australia will remain the case of Zoe Buhler. The police were actively monitoring social media posts. One Facebook post encouraged people to join a peaceful protest in Ballarat in regional Victoria, a long way away from metropolitan Melbourne as the Covid cluster, while observing all social distancing and mask-wearing guidance. In response cops entered a private house, arrested and handcuffed a pregnant young woman, still in her pyjamas, in the presence of her young child, all the while ignoring her frightened promises to take the post off that she hadn't realised was forbidden.

The episode is the very definition of a police state. Having crossed that Rubicon, how do we walk Australia back? A good start would be criminal prosecution of cops executing dictatorial edicts and of the officers and ministers authorising such action.

"*Potentially unnecessary*" infringements of our most fundamental human rights? Author shakes head as he exits stage left.

Australia's "authoritarian" Covid-19 response[16]

Japan won deserved global plaudits for the 2020 Olympics held under uniquely challenging circumstances. Athletes and national delegations were required to be fully vaccinated, lived in a highly controlled bubble and were tested daily for Covid-19. Australians won 17 gold medals, the sixth best. On completion of the Games, the delegation returned home to two weeks of international border quarantine.

---

[16] *Japan Times*, 20 August 2021, https://www.japantimes.co.jp/opinion/2021/08/19/commentary/world-commentary/australia-authoritarian-covid-19-response/

South Australia's 16 athletes must quarantine for another two weeks—28 days in total—on getting home from Sydney. Commentators have slammed the cruelty of this "Covidiocy." Australian Olympic Committee CEO Matt Carroll said: "While other countries are celebrating the return of their athletes, we are subjecting ours to the most cruel and uncaring treatment."

Vaccines have proven effective in reducing deaths but not so much delta variant infections and hospitalisations. Some of the world's most vaccinated countries are being advised by their scientists—for example Iceland's chief epidemiologist and in the UK, David Livermore, professor of medical microbiology at the University of East Anglia and Professor Sir Andrew Pollard, director of the Oxford Vaccine Group—that breakthrough infections mean herd immunity via vaccines is unattainable. Instead, people must learn to live with the virus as an endemic disease that will keep circulating and mutating over many years. But Australians find themselves mouse-trapped in an endless cycle of lockdowns by governments mesmerised by the cheese of Zero Covid.

Consequently Australia has morphed from being the envy of the world last year for its incredible pandemic management, to international incredulity at the brutality of its authoritarian measures to "crush and kill the virus." The most popular conservative TV host in America, Tucker Carlson, calls Australia a "Covid dictatorship." With unconscious irony, the video clip was removed from YouTube. His colleague Laura Ingraham was incredulous at learning that soldiers and police helicopters were patrolling Sydney's streets and skies to enforce the lockdown: "military in the streets of Australia against their own people"?

The Premier of Australia's largest state said on 14 August, at a time when the Taliban were making lightning advances across Afghanistan in a real war: "This is literally a war". The UK *Telegraph* said in an editorial: "How has it come to the point that Australia needs to call up the military to eradicate a virus that is now endemic in the world?"

China is enjoying schadenfreude. In an article in *Global Times*, the mouthpiece of wolf warrior diplomacy, Lu Xue recalled comments from Foreign Minister Marise Payne critical of China's aggressive pandemic management. "Some countries," she said in June 2020, "are using the pandemic to undermine liberal democracy to promote their own more authoritarian models." Lu added: "Now, quite ironically, it turns out that Canberra plans to send its military personnel to help enforce social lockdown."

The authoritarian streak has seen several instances of cruelty and inhumanity beyond belief. At a time of zero active cases in Canberra, a woman was denied permission to fly to Queensland to see her dying father. A fully vaccinated and thrice-negative-tested Australian, who flew back from the US to say goodbye to a dying father, was let into Queensland, after several days' delay, on a privately chartered plane. A mother from across the border in New South Wales lost her baby after being denied treatment in Brisbane because Queensland hospitals are only for Queenslanders.

In Brisbane, an elderly man on a walk in the Botanical Gardens was arrested by police who refused to believe he couldn't wear a mask because of a heart condition, until he collapsed of a heart attack. Returnees Sarah and Moe Haidar were not allowed to see or touch their 9-week premature baby in a Brisbane hospital, instead relying on FaceTime, until quarantine period was over.

A fully vaccinated Sydney grandmother was denied a permit to go to Melbourne to help care for her grandchildren while her daughter battles advanced breast cancer. In a country town, a pregnant woman posting on Facebook to support a peaceful protest against Victoria's lockdown was handcuffed and arrested in her house in the early morning, still in her pyjamas, in the presence of her family.

Thousands of Australians remain stranded abroad, unable to come home because of government limits on daily arrivals. During the last wave in India, citizens attempting to come home were threatened with hefty fines and imprisonment. Now the government has decreed that Australians who live abroad and came home to spend the last days with a dying parent, must apply for special exemption to fly out again. If you can make sense of that, you have a far better mind than mine.

Yet special arrangements have regularly been approved for billionaires and celebrities to fly in and quarantine at home or in five-star resorts. Athletes and sports officials have also been granted special dispensation. Then there's the sheer perversity, officiousness and anti-scientific idiocy of many of the rules, like mandating a mask while walking outdoors, sitting in a park or driving alone, no matter how far away from anyone else.

Governments have refused to publish the health advice behind edicts that differ from state to state and one month from another. Peta Credlin, chief of staff to Prime Minister Tony Abbott and now a media commentator, concludes in her weekly column in *The Australian*: "Never has this country been more over-governed yet so starved of leadership."

Courts have refused to provide redress no matter how arbitrary, draconian, unscientific and ineffective the regulations. According to one analysis in the *Sydney Morning Herald*, public health measures issued under the enabling emergency powers can only be assessed as a package of measures, not individually, and they could go on indefinitely if the health authorities just declare the emergency still exists. The inability of the judiciary to provide legal relief from the Covid madness has served to deepen public distrust of political, health and police authorities plus the fear-peddling media.

Australia's current daily number of deaths from all causes is around 450. As of 16 August, the total number of Covid-related deaths this year is 57—*about 12% of one day's average number of deaths.* For this we are hollowing out entrenched practices, principles and institutions of democracy and parochial state premiers have heavily diluted Australia as one nation. Sad.

The global media calls out Australia's repressive Covid order[17]

For students of democracy and foreign policy, Australia has been experiencing interesting times in the last two years. All countries devote enormous effort and considerable resources to "public diplomacy." This takes two forms.

The first is positive: the promotion of good news stories highlighting attributes, parts and aspects of life in a country to overseas audiences in order to create, consolidate and expand favourable impressions of and attitudes towards one's country among foreigners. An attempt at this, even though the implementation was embarrassingly wrong in the tag line, was the Scott Morrison-designed marketing slogan "Where the bloody hell are you?" that promoted Australia's lifestyle attractions.

The marketing adage that all publicity is good publicity decidedly does not hold in diplomacy. Instead, the international coverage of the threat to the health of Australia's democracy is truer to the Irish literary great Brendan Behan's bon mot: "All publicity is good, except an obituary notice." The second prong of public diplomacy accordingly is damage control: reacting to bad news stories by countering with broader perspectives, providing context, alleging bias in the messenger, emphasising that authorities are on it, and so on.

A good example is the bad publicity generated in India when Indian students were being attacked and harassed on the streets of Melbourne in 2009 and the Australian government was a bit slow to react but then went into full damage control mode, including by sponsoring trips to Australia by prominent opinion influencers in India: money well spent to protect the lucrative education and tourism market.

---

[17] *Spectator Australia*, 9 September 2021, https://www.spectator.com.au/2021/09/the-global-media-calls-out-australias-repressive-covid-order/

The year 2021 has been marked by a growing series of articles in the world press, many frankly disbelieving, that highlight how easily and comprehensively Australia has slipped back into becoming a remote penal colony. All this is very embarrassing and damaging because it's all so true. What follows is a sample. Follow the links and weep for poor fella, my country.

Australia's Covid response "stands as a warning for how easily core freedoms can erode in even a well-established democracy"—New York Post.

Australia has become a "Covid dictatorship"—Tucker Carlson.

"Up to now one of Earth's freest societies, Australia has become a hermit continent. How long can a country maintain emergency restrictions on its citizens' lives while still calling itself a liberal democracy?"—The Atlantic.

"Heretofore an honourable member of the Free World, Australia has lurched into a bizarre and disturbing netherworld of bureaucratic oppression in the name of public health"—National Review.

Australia is "hollowing out entrenched practices, principles and institutions of democracy and parochial state premiers have heavily diluted Australia as one nation, fragmenting it into several different states and territories that have frequently closed off their borders to other Australians"—Japan Times (disclosure: my own article).

"What's the point of Australia?"—UnHerd.

"How has it come to the point that Australia needs to call up the military to eradicate a virus that is now endemic in the world?"—The Daily Telegraph (UK).

"Canberra plans to send its military personnel to help enforce social lockdown"—Global Times (China).

"If there is one nation that has gone insane with Covid, it's Australia. It's scary because their lockdown protocols mirror what Dr. Anthony Fauci and other Covid panic porn manufacturers want to do here" in the USA—"The risks to Australia's democracy"—Brookings Institution.

"The authoritarian takeover of Australia"—Spiked.

And the last word: "Never has this country been more over-governed yet so starved of leadership"—Peta Credlin, *The Australian*.

All masked up, now for somewhere to go[18]

Dr Clive Dix, former head of Britain's vaccine taskforce, says Covid should be treated as an endemic virus like flu and mass vaccination should end: "We now need to manage disease, not virus spread." Test, trace and isolate programs are akin to keeping a finger in the hole in the dyke after the village is already deep under water.

The Omicron variant rapidly encircled the globe, despite international travel being restricted to fully vaccinated and masked people. Two-thirds of 25 staff at Princess Elisabeth Polar Station, a Belgian scientific research station in Antarctica, caught Covid from a single positive case detected on 14 December. Based in one of the world's remotest regions, all were fully vaccinated, passed multiple PCR tests and were quarantined before entry to the station. Could the utter pointlessness of this theatre of the absurd be any clearer?

Scott Morrison's proposed pandemic pivot is a crucial effort to restore a semblance of sanity to the pandemic rule book and rebuild confidence that we can once again live with one more endemic respiratory virus among the many that circulate continually.

Most governments were panicked by the fast-spreading Covid in 2020. They threw out the existing rule book based on a hundred years of science and real-world experience as conveniently summarised in a WHO document in 2019; conflated "cases" with positive tests using an unreliable test; used the redefined cases as the single metric to drive policy; subordinated all other public policy goals—health, economic,

---

[18] *The Weekend Australian*, 15–16 January 2022, https://www.theaustralian.com.au/inquirer/all-masked-up-now-for-somewhere-to-go/news-story/4853a7d3849b69cb1b730fddf0a2997b

social, educational—to the imperative to crush and kill the virus; treated worst-case modelling scenarios based on flawed assumptions and faulty data as predictions; ignored the exceptionally age-segregated threat of Covid, with people over 75 10,000 times more at risk than those under 15; and silenced dissent and resistance using the full might of the state.

Two years on, actual data clearly prove that, with 5.5mn deaths worldwide, the strategy of defeating Covid via lockdowns for everyone failed to protect the most vulnerable. Scotland's Covid rate has been higher than England's despite tougher restrictions, humiliating "Britain's dismal lockdown establishment" with a collapse of the apocalyptic narrative. After two years of doing it tough, on 11 January 2022, Fortress Australia had 3,405 cases per million people, one of the highest rates in the world, around 50% above the Britain and US.

The harms-benefits balance sheet helps to explain why governments have either refused to conduct or publish cost-benefit analysis using the long-established quality-adjusted life years (QALY) metric that guided public health decisions before 2020.

In a recent review, David Redman and Ari Joffe of Canada show that all 11 studies that used QALY as a common metric concluded that costs of lockdowns exceeded benefits by between 2.5 times at the lowest to 26 times at the highest end of the cost-benefit ratios. Conversely, using Oxford University's Stringency Index as a guide, the level of restrictions does not correlate with Covid mortality for US states or with excess mortality rates in Europe.

Governments then made the mistake of over-promising vaccines as the solution and downplayed its risks, producing a gradual erosion of public trust in leaders, experts, and institutions. UK Health Security Agency data show a 55% majority of England's Omicron cases are double-vaccinated and the triple-vaccinated are 4.5 times more likely to test positive for Omicron than the unvaccinated. On 6 January, the Agency published the weekly vaccine report for the final four weeks of 2021. Around 68% of Covid deaths and 50%

of hospital admissions were the double-vaccinated compared to 28 and 42% unvaccinated. Per capita, however, unvaccinated adults are between four and six times more likely to die with Covid for different age groups and between two and six times more likely to require hospitalisation. Thus vaccines do offer significant protection.

But with infections, among people aged 18-79, the risk of infection for the vaccinated is double and higher. In Novak Djokovic's age group, the infection rate for the double-vaccinated was 2.4 times higher than that for the unvaxxed. The policy conclusion is not that vaccines carry higher risk. Rather, healthy people should worry less about the unvaccinated and more about the infected irrespective of their vaccination status.

In Britain, one-third of patients in hospital are "Covid incidentals"—admitted for another ailment and tested Covid-positive in hospital. With NSW and Victoria admitting to a similar situation, Morrison is right to call for a change from "cases to hospitalisations" as the key metric for policy settings.

We have health, not Covid, ministers. They should take a whole-of-health responsibility for their portfolio and stop neglecting other life-threatening ailments. The cabinet is no less responsible for children's education, people's livelihoods, mental health, and the community's emotional wellbeing. Those of us of advancing age might be the most vulnerable to Covid, but we also have fewer years left in which to enjoy quality time with children and grandchildren.

Omicron spooked NSW Premier Dominic Perrottet into reintroducing mask and check-in mandates that have demonstrably failed to halt transmissions. Omicron is exceptionally infectious but very mild, with only 2383 of 337,818 (0.71%) of NSW's active cases in hospital, 182 (0.05%) in ICU and 60 requiring ventilation on January 12. And it's infecting the low-risk disproportionately while the high-risk elderly are nearly all vaccinated. If, as NSW Health Minister Brad Hazzard claims, every Australian is going to be infected by Omicron, then why persist with testing everyone instead of diagnosing and treating only the sick?

Previous infection adds another protective layer of defence. Noting that population immunity is achieved by the twin routes of vaccination and infection, Queensland chief health officer John Gerrard said the spread of a transmissible but mild virus is necessary to transition from a pandemic to an endemic status.

The unvaccinated have made their choice and are willing to take their chances. It's unconscionable to demonise and exclude from all social and economic activity 99,996 people because four of their cohort are in critical care, while extending full membership to 999,994 vaccinated people even though six of their number are in ICU.

The combination of high transmissibility, mild symptoms, shorter hospital stays, and rapid peaking has sparked speculation among Japanese infectious disease experts that Omicron could signal the endgame as we transition to an endemic. As Steve Brine noted, while he was health minister, 20,000 Britons died of flu in a bad season, "yet it has never been a legal requirement to stay at home if you have flu."

Data from the real world contradicts, as it has from the beginning, the dire warnings of the doomsday modellers and indicates we are now in a good place to be able to get through Omicron with minimal deaths and no more restrictions: just individual precautions based on personal responsibility.

Canada's truckers won't truck it anymore[19]

The Freedom Convoy is the largest, longest, and noisiest honk-fest of a demonstration against a Canadian government in decades. It's laid bare the stark reality that lockdowns are a class war waged by the laptop class on the working class, by the cultural elites on the great unwashed outside urban centres, and by the virtue signallers on independent free thinkers. The world's emoter-in-chief solemnly

---

[19] *Spectator Australia*, 19 February 2022, https://www.spectator.com.au/2022/02/canadas-truckers-wont-truck-it-anymore/

intoned in Parliament on 9 February that the truckies were "trying to blockade our economy, our democracy and our fellow citizens' daily lives." That he himself has been guilty of all three charges for two years testifies to lack of self-awareness.

In 1971, I was living in Canada and visiting family in India. On Boxing Day a friend told me "Your PM Two-door has had a son." That's when I first heard of Justin Trudeau, the epitome of "white privilege." Maybe not two-door but he's given every indication of being two-faced. He wore blackface many times and would have fired any minister before his own history surfaced for the offence, yet champions himself as a warrior against racism. He fired a First Nation woman from cabinet because she showed competence and integrity enough to resist pressures to circumvent the law against a corrupt company in order to save Trudeau's seats in Quebec—google "Jody Wilson-Raybould SNC-Lavalin"—yet fancies himself as a global campaigner for women's rights.

He mouths trite banalities about following the science. On 10 January, with 78% (90%+ of adults with nearly 50% boosted) full vaccination, Canada recorded its highest rate of 1,093 daily new cases per million people (7-day average), almost five times more than the previous high of 229 on 12 April 2021 with 2% vaccination. The double-vaccinated and boosted PM (and Prince Charles) recently tested positive for Covid. Yet still they swear by vaccine passports for stopping transmission.

Trudeau dismisses hard-working truckers and supporters as a fringe minority of far-right racists and misogynists who propagate "unacceptable views." With 85-90% vaccinated and the long hours spent alone in long-haul vehicles, the truckers' defiance is more of a threat to government control than to public health. "Coward-19" went into hiding rather than engage with or face the truckers as they rolled into Ottawa. A fringe minority doesn't raise $10mn dollars within days nor attract thousands of flag-waving supporters along the route on the drive to Ottawa.

The smears thrown at them are so brazen as to be scarcely credible. Politicians, the chattering class, and fund-raising platforms who lined up to take the knee and turn a blind eye to actual and widespread violence by BLM activists, point to rare and isolated examples of relatively harmless words and acts, always with the possibility of complicity by agents provocateurs, to paint the whole movement as beyond the pale.

The convoy has proven to be a galvanising symbol of people power. It has inspired similar protest movements in Australia and New Zealand and may do so in America, once the land of the free and the brave and dozens of other countries. Video footage of thousands of ordinary people lining besides the trans-Canadian highways to cheer on the truckers, braving the bitter Canadian winter and delivering food, supplies and well wishes to the truckers as the people's champions, has fatally undermined the narrative of far right extremists disrupting the lives of everyday Canadians who've done their patriotic duty. The truckers and their cheer squads up and down the country mirror the race, age and gender demographics of modern Canada.

The confrontation has pivoted in public perception to those with lockdown-proof incomes ordering the hardhats to stay in their lane and the latter saying they've had enough and are not going to take it any more. It has also for the first time opened up an honest debate about the science and data behind government diktats. And, perhaps most importantly, it has awakened ordinary Canadians to the realisation that there really are millions of others who share their scepticism, lockdown fatigue, and mounting anger against the inner city scolds and sneers' arrogance and contempt for the deplorables across the country. The result is the wondrous sight of those who self-identify as champions of the little people cowering in fright at a broad-based movement led by real working people.

An especially heartening aspect is how it has demolished the attempt to frame dissent and protest as sedition and insurrection.

The right to dissent is a defining attribute of democracy, neither a negation of nor a threat to it. No commentator seems to have drawn attention to what may well have been the antecedents of the Freedom Convoy. It began in British Columbia, where most Canadian Sikhs are concentrated. Their ancestral home, Punjab, is India's agricultural powerhouse. In September 2020, the Modi government passed by brute force of parliamentary majority three controversial farm reforms. These may well have been merited but the autocratic manner in which they were done, with worried farmers told it was all for their own good, trust us, broke the trust in government, created a backlash and led to a convoy of vehicles that camped just outside Delhi from November 2020 onwards.

The government tried to smear them in every possible way, including linking them to violent secessionists from the 1980s, but in the end Modi backed down a year later and all three laws were repealed. Reasons for the success of the farmers' agitation was they stayed united and peaceful, support for them spread to all parts of the country and their immediate grievances tapped into a much broader menu of resentments against Modi's high-handed approach to governance that seemed to serve the interests of corporate donors against the little people. Sound familiar?

The narrative seems to be collapsing fast inside Canada. Trudeau's own Liberal MPs have begun to attack his confrontational handling of the protests as divisive politics that's pitting Canadians against one another instead of providing a roadmap out of the pandemic. Polls show around half of Canadians expressing sympathy and understanding for the truckers' concerns and supporting an end to all Covid restrictions—even if most don't support the protests. Five provinces have announced a rapid lifting of restrictions like vaccine passports and mask mandates. Developments in Canada might also be influencing other governments to begin dismantling increasingly unpopular restrictions.

Who'd have thought that the country best known for its law-abiding and phlegmatic population would lead the world in trumpeting the message: We are done with Covid restrictions, mandates and government running our lives. While Australians, famed before this for their larrikin, irreverent and authority-defying spirit, would help revive the tired old trope of worthy inheritors of prison guards?

Trudeau's toxic tantrum tyranny[20]

On 8 August 2019, Reuters reported: "Russia freezes bank accounts linked to opposition politician Navalny." On 15 February, the BBC said: "Trudeau vows to freeze anti-mandate protestors' bank accounts." Deputy PM Chrystia Freeland said banks would be asked to freeze personal accounts of anyone linked with the protests with no due process, no appeals process, and no court order necessary. GoFundMe had no problem with BLM crowdfunding the cost of bailing far-left activist Quintez Brown charged with trying to kill a Jewish mayoral candidate in Kentucky. Ottawa's interim police chief Steve Bell warned on 19 February: "If you were involved in this protest we will actively look to identify you and follow up with financial sanctions and criminal charges." Imagine if President Trump had dealt with BLM, Antifa and cat activists as brutally—the mainstream media would have had a meltdown requiring decades-long therapy.

On 22 February, Russian lawmakers authorised President Vladimir Putin to use force to back Ukrainian separatists. The West has framed Russia's actions as a grave threat to democracy and freedom everywhere and responded with swift condemnation and sanctions. The day before, bucking the global trend to ending Covid restrictions, Canada's Parliament voted 185-151 to approve the declaration of emergency and authorise PM Trudeau to use force against anti-mandate protestors. Western leaders responded unanimously with studied silence. If you wish to understand why the non-Western world has

[20] *Spectator Australia*, 5 March 2022, https://www.spectator.com.au/2022/03/trudeaus-toxic-tantrum-tyranny/

turned increasingly cynical about "universal values" proclaimed loftily by Westerners, read this paragraph again.

Trudeau's minority ruling party did this with the support of the New Democratic Party. Trudeau revoked the emergency on the 23rd, proving they weren't needed in the first place. Every MP who voted for it will forever own that stain of infamy. The last time martial law was imposed in Canada was by Pierre Trudeau in 1970. Even though he faced a genuine terrorist threat then, the NDP as the party of workers and the conscience of the nation opposed the measure in principle. By contrast Trudeau junior faced a crisis born of his own arrogance, incompetence and intransigence. With no significant difference in Covid transmissibility between vaxxed and unvaccinated and even the triple-jabbed being susceptible to infection in huge numbers, there is zero medical justification for vaccine mandates. In addition, far from any ethical justification, the mandate is also deeply unethical.

In order to keep essential services flowing for the laptop class of privileged folks typified by Trudeau, truckers kept operating in the high-risk months before vaccines were developed. Their work circumstances rarely bring them into contact with other people. No evidence has been offered to show their risk to others. Their protest was peaceful, good humoured, supported by large numbers of Canadians, and inspired many other countries to take up the cause. Like Poland's Solidarity Movement forty years ago, Canada's truckers have become icons of a larger struggle for freedom and liberty against growing state power that transcends Canada and vaccine mandates.

Truckers sought dialogue and asked to speak to Trudeau but he refused and went into hiding. Martial law should have been invoked as the last resort with willingness to listen and talk as the first to defuse the crisis early. This is why civic associations challenged it in court, alleging it didn't meet the very high threshold of a national emergency. As was the case in Victoria, Illiberal Party and NDP MPs put careers first, the party second, and the country last. Thank goodness

Westminster MPs rebelled last year in sufficient numbers that they thwarted Boris Johnson's instinct to cave to the doomsayers' alarmism that subsequently has been shown to have been BS.

By coincidence, my first academic article was a critical commentary on the declaration of emergency by PM Indira Gandhi in 1975 when I was a PhD student at Queen's University in Canada undertaking research in India. I wrote then that liberty is not a privilege to be granted at the government's whim but an inalienable right held as a claim by citizens against the government. Events around the world in the half century since has firmed that conviction.

Another feature of the crisis of Canadian democracy is Trudeau's multiple hypocrisies. With BLM and climate protests that actually were violent, forget any criticism, jackboots, and freeze on financial transactions. Rather, Trudeau took the knee outside Parliament. He who could find no time to meet the truckers did photo-ops with St Greta of Thunberg. Then there's his history of wearing blackface. And he is fully in tune with celebrities who lecture everyone else on the absolute necessity for sacrifices to our way of life but carry on with their own extravagant lifestyle.

India's Modi government has fine-tuned the defining weapons of populist despotism: smear critics, dissenters and protestors as terrorists, seditionists and insurrectionists in order to deploy the full force of the national security state against them. The targets of Modi's Othering, to be digitally identified and subject to maximum state harassment and excluded from full citizenship, are religiously determined. The targets of the equivalent exercise in Canada are chosen for their vaccination status. Trudeau waded into the domestic Indian controversy on farm reform laws in 2020, declaring: "Canada will always be there to defend the right of peaceful protest." When India protested, Trudeau doubled down and urged "de-escalation and dialogue."

Yet he himself activated emergency powers created to combat terrorism. Justice Minister David Lametti boasted: "We took measures that had been applied to terrorism and applied them to other illegal activity." Social justice warriors have weaponised language to control the discourse in the public square and now governments are broadening this across the board to consolidate control and stamp out dissent. For Trudeau, the ultimate insult is to dismiss protestors as "Trump supporters."

In times of crisis, real leaders step up and those who can't, step down. Trudeau has insulted, stigmatised, wedged and divided Canadians. Rather than defuse the protests, his intolerance and stubbornness inflamed the crisis. Complaints about state overreach and abuse of power were met by still greater abuse of state authority with the power to strip citizens of their money, transport, and even children. Interim opposition leader Candice Bergen gave an incisive and eloquent critique of Trudeau's power grab in the parliamentary debate on the 17th.

Tools of repression like unleashing heavily armed cops on peacefully protesting citizens, once the identifying traits of fascists, communists and tin-pot despots, are becoming uncomfortably familiar on the streets of Western democracies. With Julian Assange, the US successfully pressured financial services companies into terminating WikiLeaks' accounts and tech companies to deny it Internet access. Edward Snowden warned us of the surveillance state and lives in exile. Trudeau's Canada shows how these tactics have become standard operating procedures for Western "democracies" to suppress dissent, punish dissenters, and banish them from participation in social life and the economy.

The Covid horoscope[21]

We've endured two very long years of restrictions to life and liberty as we knew it "once upon a time." I published my first article on the pandemic in March 2020, suggesting that politicians, journalists and

[21] *Spectator Australia*, 9 April 2022, https://www.spectator.com.au/2022/04/the-covid-horoscope/

analysts should substitute sceptical question marks for excitable exclamation marks. The first of many Covid articles for The Spectator was on 17 September 2020 with about another 20 articles in between in the mainstream media and policy blogsites: *Australian Outlook, Lowy Interpreter, Pearls and Irritations, Strategist, ACCORD* (South Africa), *Australian, Daily Sceptic, Japan Times, Times of India.*

The key arguments from day one was that Covid was a once in a decade, not once in a century outbreak, closer to the Asian and Hong Kong flus than the Spanish flu. Even in the West but especially in poorer countries, there were many other deadlier diseases like cancers, heart diseases, TB, diarrhoea, HIV/AIDS. The choice therefore was not lives vs the economy but lives vs lives, although any extended effort to flatten the curve would flatten the economy also and squeeze resources for health. The key policy question was the threshold of risk tolerance for Covid, not pursuit of the fool's gold of eradication. In the long run lockdown could kill millions more than Covid itself which is distinctive for discriminating sharply by age, giving the lie to "we're all in this together."

Policy responses should have focussed all along on protecting the most vulnerable and avoided universal quarantines that amount to mass house arrest of the healthy, not a public health measure for the sick. It's immoral to make children suffer—emotionally, socially, educationally—now and pay the economic price for the rest of their lives to prolong the lives of the elderly by a few months. Lockdowns rejected a century of settled science, driven not by data but by deeply flawed modelling closer to astrological horoscopes than science. Masks are theatre more than science; mRNA vaccines are a potential miracle cure but this is no reason to abandon established protocols for evaluating efficacy, risks and long-term safety; compliance with unethical mask and vaccine mandates was promoted through deliberate fear-mongering that fluffed the threat and hid the costs and risks of policy interventions; the media was fully complicit in the pandemic porn despite "coronaphobia" being deadlier than coronavirus.

The refusal to urgently assess treatment alternatives and the power of natural immunity was suspicious. The demonisation of dissenting voices from the health and medical community was despicable. Covid also revealed weaknesses in the architecture of global health governance. The biggest surprise for me was how easily Westerners surrendered core liberties and freedoms to medical tyranny. The herdlike rush to panicked policies will necessitate a royal commission to learn lessons, establish culpability, and ensure accountability to ensure this never happens again.

Mark Woolhouse, professor of infectious diseases at Edinburgh University and part of the elite Sage group of advisers to the UK government, essentially confirms all of the above in his book *The Year the World Went Mad: A Scientific Memoir*. The book has been widely discussed in the UK media but less so here. On the claim from cabinet minister Michael Gove in March 2020 that the virus didn't discriminate and "everyone is at risk," for example, Woolhouse says to the contrary, "this is a very discriminatory disease." "People over 75 are an astonishing 10,000 times more at risk than those who are under 15." "The result was the worst of all worlds—a reaction that failed sufficiently to protect those who were at risk while imposing hugely damaging lockdowns on those who were not," reported The Telegraph.

Now, I'm not a scientist, epidemiologist or statistician, just a policy analyst who can however see theoretical codswallop when it hits me in the eyes. This begs the question: if the shortcomings of the dominant narrative were obvious to me, why did they escape the attention of the geniuses in charge of public health?

Having puzzled over the question long and hard without a satisfactory answer, I'd like to turn it around, especially as the obverse has in fact been addressed to me a few times. What explains my early conviction that lockdowns embed an inherent imbalance of unclear benefits but proven harms and are racist and elitist in their impacts?

The first and most obvious is my Indian origin and more intimate knowledge of conditions there than most Western analysts who dominate the global policy discourse. People from poor countries are relatively more sensitive to the reality that life presents numerous hazards from the womb onwards; death is inevitable, omnipresent and an everyday reality; and balance, proportionality and policy tradeoffs are essential in navigating the journey with sensible risk management.

Hydroxychloroquine and ivermectin are commonly used drugs throughout the developing world with well-established safety profiles. As well, I was in the Indian hinterland for a month in February–March 2020 and witnessed the Covid-lockdown imbalance of harms to daily wage labourers and interstate migrant workers. Growing up in India also exposes one to the cult-like hold that astrology has in governing people's lives and decisions and the impossibility of countering belief in astrology with facts and science. If a bad prediction doesn't materialise, it's because you followed the astrologer's advice; if it does, you failed to follow the advice precisely as instructed. And vice versa with good predictions.

In my professional work I have postulated that "the national interest" is of limited conceptual utility that leads to flawed analysis and faulty policy prescriptions. Instead, "a balance of interests" better captures the empirical reality of sector-specific interests in continual competition for government attention, resources and prioritisation, for example between airline shareholders, workers and consumers in aviation policy; manufacturers, pharmacies and citizens in drugs policy; the military-industrial-scientific complex, elites and "deplorables" in national security policy, and so on.

The relevance of "a balance of interests" should be self-evident when applied to pandemic policy, viz: the need to balance considerations between different health outcomes for the big killer diseases, not just mouthing the idiotic mantra of even one avoidable Covid death is one too many; physical vs mental health; health vs educational, social and employment objectives; immediate policy interventions vs creation of long term resilience in the public health infrastructure; vaccine nationalism vs national health policy as indivisible from global health policy in a closely interwoven world; state authority vs civil liberties; and state vs individual responsibility for health decisions.

Instead, governments have either refused to do cost-benefit analysis, or else refused to publish the results. No prizes for guessing why.

4: A PANDEMIC OF VACCINES

Many of us were pleasantly surprised at the announcement that they had developed vaccines for Covid-19 within one year using a revolutionary new platform, but still somewhat wary that all the safety and efficacy trials may not have been adequately completed in the accelerated timeframe. We also initially accepted the early claims of efficacy. However, doubts grew with alarming rapidity as all talk of a pandemic of the unvaccinated was increasingly contradicted with real-world data from many countries. Scepticism and opposition to vaccine mandates hardened with barely concealed evidence of gas-lighting on the benefits, denialism on the collateral harms, and refusal either to conduct or else to publish the results of cost-benefit analyses.

The one other significant component of the great vaccine debate was the obstinate refusal to fund and conduct independent and reliable studies of treatment using widely available inexpensive repurposed drugs, in particular hydroxychloroquine and ivermectin (IVM). The latter has been used in the billions and has a long-established safety profile. But if these could be shown to have acceptable levels of efficacy, the legal framework in many countries would make it impossible for regulators to grant emergency use authorisation to Covid vaccines. A study of IVM use in Peru, using excess deaths rather than deaths with Covid as the yardstick, found a 74% mortality reduction in the 30 days after peak deaths in the ten of Peru's 25 states with the most intensive IVM use. Strikingly: "During four months of IVM use in 2020, before a new president of Peru restricted its use, there was a 14-fold reduction in nationwide excess deaths and then a 13-fold increase in the two months following the restriction of IVM use."

Suspicions grew during the Covid years that the financial interests of the pharmaceutical sector might have unduly influenced regulators' decisions in banning the use of ivermectin. These have been strengthened with the removal of the bans: how can a product that was considered safe for decades before 2020 but banned during 2020–22 suddenly become safe once again? In this connection, it is worth noting that the Peru study was published in preprint on 8 March 2021, but it was published as a peer reviewed article in the *Cureus Journal of Medical Science* only on 8 August 2023. The journal says its average time from submission to publication is 33 days. Readers can draw your own conclusions.

On 21 August 2021, reinforcing the message that IVM was a horse de-wormer and not authorized to treat Covid-19, the US Food and Drugs Administration (FDA) tweeted: "You are not a horse. You are not a cow. Seriously, y'all. Stop it." The post went viral. Some IVM-prescribing doctors took the FDA to court. During oral arguments in a US appeals court on 8 August 2023, Ashley Cheung Honold, a Department of Justice lawyer representing the FDA, said the "FDA explicitly recognizes that doctors do have the authority to prescribe ivermectin to treat COVID." Australia's Therapeutic Goods Administration (TGA) had already lifted its restrictions on IVM from 1 June 2023.

The fading case for vaccine passports[22]

Last week, Chief Medical Officer Brendan Murphy said the current surge in NSW infections is due to the Delta variant, not Australia's low vaccine take-up. PM Scott Morrison agreed, pointing to the "nature of the Delta variant" and the "lived experience" of countries with higher vaccination rates. By contrast, during a CNN townhall event on 20 July, President Joe Biden covered all bases. Vaccines, he said in

[22] *Spectator Australia*, 27 July 2021, https://www.spectator.com.au/2021/07/the-fading-case-for-vaccine-passports/

disjointed segments, will ensure you won't get Covid; or if infected, you won't need hospitalisation; and you won't die.

The initial belief in the efficacy of vaccines in breaking the links between infections, hospitalisations, and deaths is being confounded as data begin to accumulate with mass vaccinations. The most embarrassing evidence of Biden's mistake on the first claim is the Texas Democrats who fled to Washington to deny the state legislature a quorum to enact voter reform laws and held highly-publicised meetings with party counterparts in Congress and Vice President Kamala Harris. Despite all being vaccinated, several got infected and then cross-infected people they met in DC.

At a press briefing on 16 July, referencing CDC director Rochelle Walensky's statement that Covid had become the "pandemic of the unvaccinated," White House press secretary Jen Psaki said: "99.5% of people who are in the hospital are people who are unvaccinated." This does not seem credible. If true, the startling claim would put the US on a unique pedestal, showing an efficacy rate well above the claims even of the vaccine manufacturers, which in itself would be a world first—Big Pharma under-claiming.

In England, some confusing data seem to suggest 62% of hospitalisations for the unvaccinated (Chief Scientific Adviser Sir Patrick Vallance had to correct an earlier mistake that attributed 60% of Covid hospitalisations to the doule-jabbed), but 63% of deaths among the vaccinated. Fresh data from Israel for the Pfizer vaccine show efficacy rates against symptomatic illness falling to 41%, and for AstraZeneca in the UK down to 1.5% against infections and 60% against serious illness, from the initial rate of over 90% for both vaccines. The likely explanation is that unlike immunity through natural infection, vaccines do not give mucosal immunity. But it's still 90%+ effective in preventing serious illness. This will lock us into permanent dependency on booster shots.

Malta reached 50% fully vaccinated on 2 June and 75% on 2 July. This has not been enough to avoid a surge in cases and hospitalisations, although deaths have remained flat.

With 50% full vaccination on 24 June (and 74% on 15 July), Iceland lifted domestic and border restrictions on 26 June/1 July but has seen an exponential surge in infections, despite being an isolated island (F0gure 4.1). It recorded 78 new infections, including 52 among the fully-vaccinated, on 21 July. Two further comments on Iceland. Figure 2 shows the gradient of the current surge is as steep as the first two waves last year without vaccines; and, had they been available last year, its advocates would no doubt have credited the steep fall to vaccines.

Figure 4.1: Iceland's Covid-19 infection curve, 4 March 2020–23 July 2021

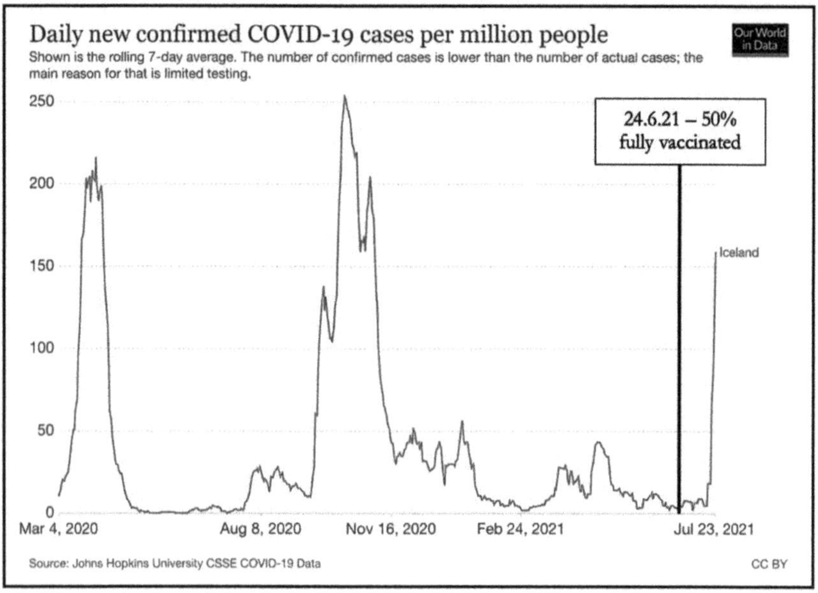

A headline in Scotland's Herald newspaper on 21 July said: "Covid hospital admissions triple in over-60s—and nearly half of patients fully vaccinated." Meanwhile, the weekly all-cause excess mortality in Scotland in mid-July rose to 100, of whom only 38 died with Covid. Scotland's infection, hospitalisation and mortality curves are closely matched for the over-60s (the most vulnerable group). The vaccines are not preventing infection, serious illness or deaths; the modest fall in the mortality metric is likely attributable to the Delta variant being less lethal if more infectious and to better treatment protocols by now. As The Sunday Times notes, "the collateral damage of two national lockdowns" has also begun "to emerge across Scotland."

Meanwhile, Sweden was only 30% fully vaccinated on 25 June and 39% on 22 July. Yet since 30 June, daily new cases have flatlined at between 250-350 and deaths at two or less with no lockdowns, schools and businesses open and masks not even recommended. In sharp contrast to European neighbours preparing for further lockdowns, Sweden is welcoming tourists.

On the harms side of the equation, Dr Rushworth notes, referencing a Lancet article, that patients in the real world experience serious side-effects from drugs four-five times more than reported in trial results from the manufacturers(Covid vaccines were not involved in this study). Rebecca Weisser once again provided a handy summary of adverse reactions to Covid vaccines. The eminent Dr Peter McCullough, in a TV interview with *France Soir* on 28 June, pointed out that the CDC's Vaccine Adverse Events Reporting System (VAERS) normally records about 25 deaths per year from all vaccines. During the Covid pandemic, he said, up to 11 June it had verified 5,993 deaths, 20,737 hospitalisations, 47,837 urgent care visits, 1,538 anaphylaxis cases, and 1,868 cases of Bells Palsy.

Because VAERS is a passive-surveillance system, the general consensus is the numbers are vastly under-reported. McCullough goes on to say this is "a major safety signal … that has exceeded all boundaries of acceptability." Quizzed on the causal link to vaccines, he answered: "it's biologically plausible, temporally associated, internally consistent month by month" and also "externally consistent" with data from the US, Europe and England. "The vaccine is in the causal pathway to death … The majority of these 6,000 Americans, they were healthy enough to walk into a vaccine centre and within 2-4 days they're dead."

How are the Covidians responding to the growing body of evidence about the relatively weak efficacy of vaccines? Essentially, they are doubling down. On 15 July, the University of California published its "final policy" on vaccination policy. "To maintain the health and well-being of the campus community and that of the general public," it says, all employees and students will be required to provide proof of full vaccination "as a condition of their physical access UC facilities, as well as in-person participation in UC programs that may occur off-site." Chillingly, the document adds: "This is a permanent policy. Infectious disease experts anticipate that annual or more frequent boosters will be necessary."

There we have it. Abandon all hope, all ye who seek to enter the Dystopia of the Brave New World in which the Cult of Covidians shall reign supreme and children will be ritually sacrificed on the altar.

Are you sure about that vaccine[23]

Figure 4.2: Vaccination coverage in India and Indonesia

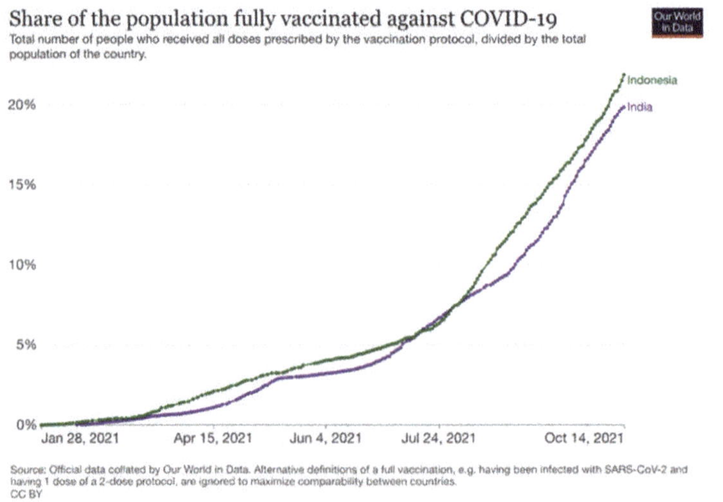

[23] *Spectator Australia*, 19 October 2021, https://www.spectator.com.au/2021/10/are-you-sure-about-that-vaccine/

Figures don't lie, critics insist. Very well, let's look at some figures. I make three arguments here. First, vaccines are not necessary to tame even the highly infections Delta variant of the coronavirus. Figures 4.2 and 4.3 plot the vaccination coverage and cases and mortality in India (where the Delta variant originated) and Indonesia. Several things become immediately apparent. To begin with, the virus infection and mortality curves in both countries follow the familiar bell shape and time duration of 6-10 weeks of growth and a similar period of retreat of the virus that we find just about everywhere. Policy interventions—hard and light lockdowns, timing of lockdowns, mask mandates—make very little difference to the curves going up or coming down. Vaccination coverage in both countries is still very low, around 20%.

Figure 4.3: Covid cases in India and Indonesia

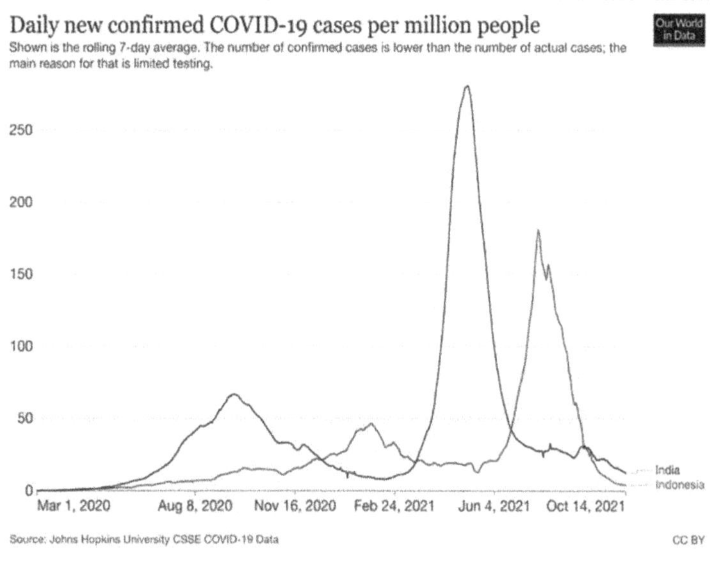

The infection and mortality curves in India peaked and bent downwards at the extremely low full vaccination rate of 2.4% in early May and at 5.7% in Indonesia in mid-July. By the time the cases had come right down (mid-July in India, mid-September in Indonesia), their respective full vaccinations were only 5.7% and 15.5%. So why has the rest of the world shown such little curiosity in finding out what lies behind the non-vaccine driven success of these two populous Asian countries? The question is especially pertinent for Australia as India and Indonesia are within our strategic Indo-Pacific frame of reference. Could the explanation possibly include—whisper it softly—the drug that US authorities have mocked as fit only for equine treatment, that begins with "I"? Say it ain't so, St Fauci.

Second, vaccines are not sufficient. They have proven to be leaky, so much so that, ignoring the moral hazard of further enriching manufacturers for the failures of their claim on efficacy, countries are now into booster jabs and those with two doses in Israel are officially classified a "unvaccinated." Vaccines remain an important tool for significantly reducing hospitalisations and deaths, although the net benefit for under-40s looks negligible.

Third, when it comes to infections, a peculiar anomaly shows up. Vaccines reduce the incidence of infections up to age 29, but thereafter, for every age cohort, they actually increase infections. This is particularly striking for 40-79 year olds, increasing by between 78% (70-79 years) and 109% (40-49 years). For forty-year olds, vaccines more than double the infection rate. Now, either vaccines are dangerous for reducing the pre-existing immunity against infection for adults over 30; or else the testing is, pardon the expression, total crap. Considering the impact of vaccines on severely cutting down hospitalisations and deaths, almost certainly the testing is flawed, and then some. The sooner mass testing is abandoned entirely, the better. It should be restricted for those showing symptoms.

If you don't feel sick, you are not sick. Otherwise, testing is a waste of scarce and costly resources (money, equipment, personnel), and it causes needless stress, anxiety, and lost productivity as people are forced to isolate for no good reason or purpose. A new study published in the *Lancet* on 8 October documents a world-wide increase of more than 129 million cases of major depression (53.2mn) and anxiety

(76.2mn) disorders during the pandemic. The authors attribute this to the combined effects of the pandemic and lockdown measures. Our Chief Health Officers have all callously disregarded this huge toll on mental health. Most masks and mass testing help to maintain the state of fear but are not obviously a good public health tool.

The unresolved debate on Covid vaccines[24]

The latest weekly data from the UK Health Security Agency (UKHSA), covering weeks 40–43 for 2021, confirm the pattern of double and higher rates for the vaccinated compared to the unvaccinated for those aged 40-79 (Figure 4.4). As this began to register with a broader public, it created a controversy among experts and between different agencies. Cambridge University's David Spiegelhalter condemned the statistics as "deeply untrustworthy and completely unacceptable … simply an artefact due to using clearly inappropriate estimates of the population."

Figure 4.4: Infections per 100,000 by age-differentiated vaccination status

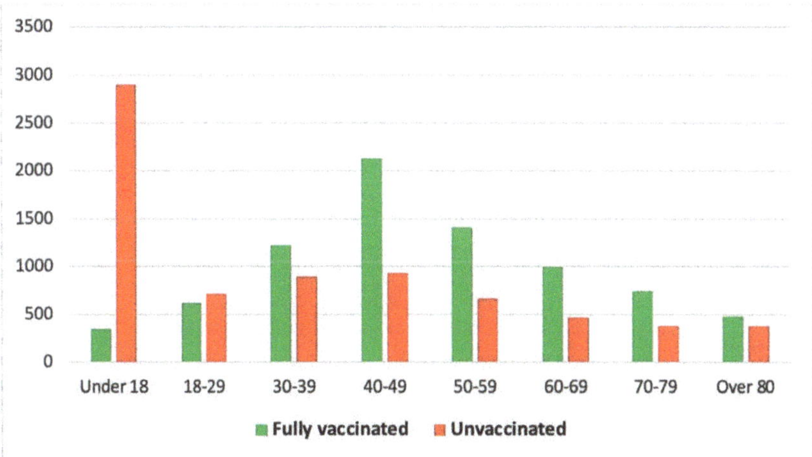

NB: "Fully vaccinated" means 2 doses; hospital admissions and deaths within 28 days of a positive test

---

[24] *Spectator Australia*, 12 November 2021, https://www.spectator.com.au/2021/11/the-unresolved-debate-on-covid-vaccines/

But in a paper on 27 October, a team from Queen Mary University of London "found numerous discrepancies and inconsistencies" in various relevant public government datasets. By reverse-engineering estimates of mortality by age category, and vaccination status, they concluded that official statistics on vaccine effectiveness "may be underestimating the mortality rates for vaccinated people in each age category." Dr Mary Ramsay, head of immunisation at the UKHSA, defended the statistics while noting that differences in risk, behaviour and testing between the vaccinated and unvaccinated should inject caution into inferring vaccine effectiveness from the data.

In late October the UKHSA finally folded and removed the controversial charts in its surveillance report for week 43. Now the Agency monitors but no longer publishes the figures on vaccine effectiveness. Nevertheless, Ed Humpherson, DG for Regulation in the Office for Statistics Regulation, published an open letter to UKHSA CEO Dr Jenny Harries on 1 November, repeating the criticisms of the data that continued to be published in table form.

Data in the tables from week 44 on infections, hospitalisation and mortality trendlines from weeks 36–44 show a faster rise in infections among the vaccinated and a rise in hospitalisation and mortality among the vaccinated alongside a fall in these metrics for the unvaccinated. There are additional reasons for caution against too optimistic a reading of the efficacy of vaccines in reducing hospitalisation and mortality rates. The heavy concentration of Covid dead among people in aged care institutions suffering from multiple comorbidities means that significant numbers of these people would have succumbed within a year or so anyway. Thus the Italian Higher Institute of Health recently adjusted the number of deaths caused by (not with) Covid since February 2020 from over 130,000 to under 4,000.

By contrast post-vaccination illnesses and deaths are not attributed to the vaccines unless investigations confirm a causal link, so the benefits are not assessed against the risks of serious side effects.

Vaccinations also create evolutionary pressure on a virus to mutate into new variants, says the French virologist Prof. Luc Montagnier, the 2008 Nobel Laureate for Medicine.

Figure 4.5: The shifting Covid heat map in the US

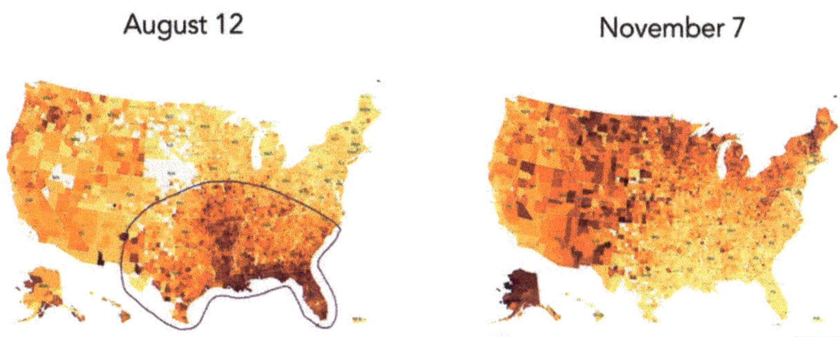

Source: Tom Woods newsletter, 8 November 2021

Meanwhile the case against mandatory vaccines and vaccine passports is greatly boosted by the example of Florida. It currently has the lowest case numbers of all the US states and Figure 4.5, Covid heat maps from the *New York Times* three months apart, depicts the shift in the virus from the southeast to the southwest without any change in behaviour by people in the two regions.

As is the near-universal pattern, Florida's fourth Covid wave collapsed as rapidly as it had ascended despite the lack of regulations. Hospitals weren't overwhelmed at any point and over 90% of the over-65s have voluntarily been vaccinated. But for lockdown fanatics, the upward trajectory was caused by the refusal to mandate restrictions and the collapse was sheer dumb luck.

"A visit to Florida," where 99.8% of people have survived the pandemic without any restrictions, Adam Creighton concluded in *The Australian*, "highlights the gap between the reality of people's lives and the perception of chaos created by mainstream media."

Herding sheeple onto the vaccine treadmill[25]

"We want to see your smiles; masks are optional" read a sign in Adam Creighton's hotel in Miami, Florida. At the height of the fourth "wave" in Florida, Governor Ron DeSantis came under vicious criticism from the Biden administration and the mainstream media for rejecting federal guidelines on vaccine mandates and restrictions. An attack ad in the form of an announcement by the Captain as a flight lands in Florida warned: "You have the right to infect whoever you want whenever with Covid-19." DeSantis politely but firmly explained that the virus sells and recedes on its own logic and this too shall pass. Stay calm and carry on. His new Surgeon-General, the Nigerian-born and Harvard-educated Joseph Ladapo, is the "anti-Fauci" in the consistency of his message and focus on data instead of the career bureaucrat's tendency to tack to the prevailing political and public opinion winds. Stanford epidemiologist Jay Bhattacharya tweeted on 28 September that over 65s had suffered higher Covid mortality rates in locked down California than free Florida.

The illogicality, science-denying and data-defying push for near-universal vaccination of entire populations continues its destructive march through Western societies. According to the approved and one-permitted narrative, the vax keeps us all safe from Covid, which is why we must all get vaccinated. But it doesn't protect us from the unvaccinated, which is why we must implement vaccine passports. Right, got it.

In Australia and New Zealand, it's wrecking families and friendships. PM Jacinda Ardern openly admits to creating a two-tier society divided by vaccination status. Already in the UK the Health Secretary has urged those eligible to take the booster to avoid a return to winter lockdown while eligible travellers who refuse to be triple jabbed could

[25] *Spectator Australia*, 20 November 2021, https://www.spectator.com.au/2021/11/herding-sheeple-onto-the-vaccine-treadmill/

face a return to isolation and testing restrictions. In this Covid-1984 new normal, adults making decisions in the best interests of their body and family are selfish weapons of mass destruction who must be outed, shamed and cancelled; personal health is no longer private; and the vaccine-hesitant—not those granted immunity against legal liability, who push mandates for injecting everyone with a drug cocktail using revolutionary new technology—are immoral and reckless with everyone's health.

Bhattacharya tweeted on 29 September: "Fact: Someone sitting in a room filled with Covid-recovered people faces a lower Covid infection risk than someone sitting in a room of fully vaxxed people who have never had Covid. Lesson: Get the vax especially if vulnerable, but nix the irrational vaccine mandates & passports." Despite his lesson spelt out in black and white in the tweet, Lisa Dresner replied: "So you think that people who have never had Covid should just wait till they get it"? Is it any wonder we despair of detoxicating the cult followers?

Similarly, the "Zero Covid absolutists" of the Scientific Advisory Group on Emergencies (Sage) have the chutzpah to accuse the Joint Committee on Vaccination and Immunisation (JCVI) for being "anti-vax" terrorists who use children as "human shields" to protect adults. Why? Because the JCVI says Covid poses a tiny threat to 12-15 year olds, vaccines also pose the risk of rare but serious side effects, and allowing the virus to circulate naturally could give them strong immunity without the risk of side-effects and also protect adults.

The UK data is backed by an FDA analysis (26 October) that shows that vaccinating one million boys aged 5-11 prevents one Covid death; it prevents 67 ICU stays but adds another 57 ICU stays due to myocarditis/pericarditis; and prevents 203 hospitalisations but adds another 156 hospitalisations from myocarditis/pericarditis. These are hardly compelling figures to support mandates. Moreover, catching Covid in childhood will make them less vulnerable as adults. As a reminder, the JCVI includes some of the UK's most eminent vaccine scientists engaged for sixty years in keeping the country safe by applying the same risk-benefit analysis. Its reasoning is shared by many independent experts, as explained in a peer-reviewed article in *Toxicology Reports* by Ronald Kostoff and colleagues. Meanwhile the Royal College of Paediatrics and Child Health has urged an end to Covid testing in schools because it's forcing very low-risk children to carry the burden of the pandemic and seriously disrupting their education.

On 7 November the Canberra Times had one of the most depressing headlines and stories on this whole sorry saga: "Canberra parents question whether to travel with unvaccinated young children." My question is: who among the politicians, health experts, and media will accept responsibility and be held accountable for the misinformation that has resulted in this level of fear rooted in ignorance in the community?

On 31 October, the twice-vaccinated and double-masked White House Press Secretary Jen Psaki revealed she and members of her family had tested positive for Covid. Did this make her question the "pandemic of the unvaccinated" narrative? Not at all. On the contrary, she gushed: "Thanks to the vaccine, I have only experienced mild symptoms." Cult, much, considering 99% of the infected experience only mild symptoms anyway?

Over 10,000 physicians and medical scientists have signed the Rome Declaration (26 September) which, reaffirming loyalty to the Hippocratic Oath (First Do No Harm), called for no forced vaccination of healthy children, no restrictions or vaccine mandates for unvaccinated Covid-recovered people and sanctity of the doctor-patient relationship.

Jim Barson described as a senior Australian doctor, penned a statement on 25 October that "The facts do not support what has been done in the name of controlling this virus." He notes that even with 909 Covid deaths in Australia last year, the total of deaths from all causes was still 8,001 fewer than in 2019. Of the 909, 695 died in residential care, meaning that the Covid deaths outside residential care were less than from traffic accidents, alcohol and drug abuse, and suicide. In the UK and the US, age-standardised death rates in 2020 were the same as most years before 2008 and 2004, respectively. Even among the elderly, where Covid deaths are heavily concentrated, with the average age of death being above average life expectancy, "over the course of a year you are no more likely to die from Covid-19 than you are to die from anything else." He wryly comments: the "most common symptom of Covid is feeling well." Outside aged care, Australians have a 99.44% chance of surviving Covid infection, notes Luke Massey.

With Covid vaccines, the pharmaceutical firms have managed a unique trifecta in their PR and lobbying. They succeeded in getting authorities to change the definition of a vaccine as the existing wording excluded the new Covid vaccines, in instilling the belief that the failure of their products is due to people who haven't taken them, and persuading governments that the solution is to supplement the two-doses "full vaccination" with booster shots. If you are conspiracy minded, consider this. Australia's total (not just adult) population is around 25 million. On 25 July, PM Morrison boasted that with another 60 and 25 million doses in 2022 and 2023, Australia's total Pfizer doses had increased to 125 million. That's five shots of just Pfizer for every man, woman and child.

What does the government know that it is not telling us, and how long has it known this?

Stop vaccinating children: It's neither medically justified nor ethical[26]

As time passes, Covid policy is proving to be a bigger threat than Covid disease. Promoted as an initial protection measure to buy much-needed time against a once-in-a-century pandemic, it became

---

[26] Brownstone Institute, 12 September 2022, https://brownstone.org/articles/stop-vaccinating-children-its-neither-medically-justified-nor-ethical/

a way of life to which health bureaucrats and autocratically-inclined leaders became addicted and are having trouble letting go.

Yet in the UK: "The effects of lockdown may now be killing more people than are dying of Covid." An editorial in the *Telegraph* emphasised the importance of establishing why a meaningful cost-benefit analysis of Covid policy was not carried out. Australia's vaunted success in controlling the pandemic in 2020–21, meanwhile, looks increasingly hollow in 2022.

The instinct to protect offspring is one of the most powerful in nature across all species, with examples only too common of parents, especially mothers, sacrificing themselves in a desperate effort to save their young. On 4 September, on the edge of the Bandhavgarh Tiger Reserve in central India, Archana Choudhary was working in the fields with her 15-month toddler when a tiger appeared and sunk its teeth into the baby's head. Choudhary grappled the tiger with her bare hands trying to free the baby from its jaws until, hearing her screams, villagers came to her assistance with sticks and stones and the tiger fled. Both Mum and Bub were taken to hospital, with the mother's wounds being the more serious. A real-life Tiger Mom!

The hardwired instinct to protect children might explain why in jurisdictions where vaccines have been approved for children, the take-up, especially for young children, has lagged well behind the adult vaccination rates. The effort to psychologically nudge and politically coerce children's vaccination is abhorrent, distressing and puzzling in equal measures.

Children are at very low risk

Abhorrent, because it's an acute manifestation of the evil that has taken hold following the fear induced in peoples by deliberate psychological campaigns of terror propaganda, aided and abetted by mainstream and social media. Large numbers of people in Western societies have actively colluded with governments in imposing harms on children. Debbie Lerman wrote an excellent account on this site of how instilling and sustaining mass fear was the one unifying theme that explains all the otherwise crazy edicts and policy interventions by the US government.

In almost all Western countries, the average age of Covid deaths has been higher than the average life expectancy and the mortality risk to children is lower by a thousandfold. This is the first occasion in history where children have been made to bear the heaviest costs, with futures mortgaged to massive debts, educational opportunities drastically curtailed and exposure to potentially harmful and even lethal medical interventions, just so the old can cling on to life for a few more months and years. Take two telling examples.

In January Unicef reported on the devastating setbacks to children's education. Robert Jenkins, Unicef Chief of Education, said "we are looking at a nearly insurmountable scale of loss to children's schooling." Large-scale independent studies published in early September documented a two-decade reversal in children's educational progress in the US. Japan experienced a jump in suicides by more than 8,000 between March 2020 and June 2022 compared to pre-pandemic numbers, mostly among women in their teens and 20s.

Unlike the flu, which tends not to discriminate between different age cohorts, coronavirus is very age-specific. The exceptional and extreme age-segregation of Covid deaths was known very early in the pandemic. On April 30, 2020, the *Daily Mail* reported that children under 10 are not transmitters of the disease. Despite more than 26,000 Covid-related deaths in the UK, experts who reviewed the data failed to find a single case of an infected under-10 who had passed on the disease to an adult. The BBC reported on 7 May 2020 that in England and Wales, there were only around 300 deaths in under-45s compared to around 24,000 in over-65s. Older people with pre-existing health conditions were the most at risk, as shown in a visually striking age-adjusted graph from the BBC. For those under 20, the risk is negligible.

On 30 June 2021, Prof. Robert Dingwall, a member of the JCVI, said letting children catch Covid would be better than vaccinating them. Their intrinsically low risk from Covid means they may be "better protected by natural immunity generated through infection than by asking them to take the "possible" risk of a vaccine." In July, Stanford University's Cathrine Axfors and John Ioannidis published their estimate that survivability of infected under-20s is 99.999%, falling to 99.958% for the under-50s..

The persistence of the drive to vaccinate children is puzzling because the lockdown and vaccine narratives are falling apart. One driver of this is the growing realisation that excess death counts from all-cause mortality have risen in many countries, including Australia, Netherlands and the UK. Death is the one statistic that cannot be fudged or subjected to definitional spin. In their analysis of the 50 US states, John Johnson and Denis Raincourt show that if anything, lockdown states have higher all-cause mortality rates than contiguous non-lockdown states. In many cases deaths also seem to track vaccination campaigns in successive doses.

In part the situation reflects the monomaniacal obsession with Covid to the exclusion of other leading killer diseases. *The Telegraph* pointed out that the UK National Health Service is once again on the verge of collapse, this time from "a tsunami of non-Covid patients who were denied treatment during the pandemic."

Lockdown back-pedalling

As noted by Carl Heneghan and Tom Jefferson of Oxford University, prominent practitioners of evidence-based medicine rather than modelling-based projections, the "lockdown back-pedalling race" has begun. In late August, former UK Chancellor Rishi Sunak said it had been a mistake to empower the government's scientific advisory committee Sage, whose analyses and forecasts were dominated by gloom and doom unless stringent restrictions were put in place yesterday.

He added that insufficient attention had been paid to the knock-on effects of lockdowns on health, education, and the economy. The fear messaging had also been wrong and harmful in destroying trust in public institutions. Critics attributed his Damascene conversion to a desperate effort to revive his faltering campaign for leadership of the Conservative Party and hence becoming prime minister of the UK.

I believe this is wrong. By then the writing was clearly on the wall and Sunak, by all accounts a fundamentally decent man, wanted to go on the public record, inwardly accepting that he had already lost, in order to put obstacles in the path of future lockdowns. In that sense Sunak's Spectator interview is more accurately read as the start of the unravelling of the great Covid narrative. Sure enough, he was soon followed by former cabinet colleagues and parliamentarians.

Meanwhile, Denmark has banned vaccines for under-18s and under-50s can get a booster only with a doctor's prescription. The CDC's new guidance acknowledges the "transient" protection from vaccination against infection and transmission and the reality of naturally-acquired immunity through infection. It therefore recommended against any further discrimination by vaccination status for most settings. Yet, again demonstrating bureaucrats' infinite capacity for idiocy, the ban on unvaccinated visitors to the US was maintained and stopped Novak Djokovic from competing in the US Open that was denuded of serious star power in the men's semis and finals.

Vaccines for Australian children

In Israel, as succinctly summarized by Will Jones, public health authorities and the government deliberately covered up serious vaccine side-effects. In September we learnt that several Australian health officials were on a government-sponsored visit as guests of Israel's Ministry of Health.

On 19 July, Australia's Therapeutic Goods Administration (TGA) granted provisional approval to Moderna for administering Spikevax vaccines to children aged 0.5–5 years. Provisional because they are still undergoing clinical trials to assess full safety. The decision is especially strange in light of concerning reports of deaths, adverse events, and long-term side-effects accompanying vaccines. The Therapeutic Goods Regulation (1990) restricts provisional approvals to medicines for "the treatment, prevention or diagnosis of a life-threatening or seriously debilitating condition." This would appear to rule out provisional vaccine approval for children below five, as shown in the data from New South Wales (NSW). The resilience of the under-50s can be seen in Figure 3. In the 14-week period 22 May–27 August, the under-50s made up 27.3% of Covid-related hospitalisation and 19.7% of ICU admissions, but only 1.4% of deaths. In the same period, just 0.11% of all Covid-related deaths in NSW were children and young people up to the age of 19.

On this basis, a group of lawyers is aiming to file a crowd-funded case in the High Court (Australia's equivalent of the US Supreme Court) against the decision. But so far Australian courts have been disappointingly supine toward health edicts.

The TGA's website states that its "regulatory costs are mostly recovered through annual fees and charges levied on the sponsors and manufacturers of therapeutic goods." An article in the *British Medical Journal* by Maryannne Demasi, published on 29 June, documented that a compromising 96% of the TGA's A $170mn 2020–21 budget came from industry sources, higher than the rates (in descending order) for the European, UK, Japanese, US and Canadian counterparts.

This is beyond regulatory capture and closer to the regulator being in the pocket of the regulated. Should we be surprised that the TGA approved nine of every ten applications from drug companies that year? The TGA "firmly denies that its almost exclusive reliance on pharmaceutical industry funding is a conflict of interest," and the TGA is an honourable regulator. Yet the sad reality is the global drug industry has a particularly scandal-ridden record in influencing regulatory decisions via funding with regard, for example, to opioids,

Alzheimer's drugs, influenza antivirals, pelvic mesh, joint prostheses, breast and contraceptive implants, cardiac stents, etc.

In the Declaration for the Protection of Children and Young People from the Covid-19 Response in May 2021, the Pandemics Data and Analytics (PANDA) group said that Covid-19 is "a disease for which they [the young] carry essentially no risk." Therefore vaccinating children is "all risk, no benefit." Are we really going to engage in child sacrifice on the altar of Big Pharma?

Directing attention and resources without age-stratified discrimination—because "everyone is equally at risk"—made no medical or policy sense, unless, as Lerman postulates, the primary goal was to inculcate a self-sustaining state of mass panic. So even the children had to be routinely tested, isolated, deschooled, masked, and vaccinated as part of what Dr Sebastian Rushworth called the "Covid mania" and "collective state of hysteria." Universal vaccines is like the drunk looking for car keys near the light from the street lamp instead of where he lost them.

Against the extremely low serious risk from Covid with a survival rate of 99.99% for 0-19 year olds, the likely greater risk from vaccines, and the completely unknown long-term effects of the new-technology vaccines, if I had young children, I'd resist attempts to jab them, to the death if necessary.

Ordinarily, it would be best to put the whole Covid nightmare behind us and move on. This might be one of the rare exceptions, for accountability for the pain and harms inflicted on individuals and society is the best, and likely the only effective insurance against a repeat. On July 23 the World Health Organization declared monkeypox, which so far has affected few people in a handful of countries, a public health emergency of international concern. David Bell and Emma McArthur warn that the global pandemic industry has no plans for a return to normal. This is why the chief architects of population-wide lockdown and vaccine policies must be identified, put in the dock and made to answer and pay for their misdeeds.

Lest we forget.

The Vaccine narrative is as leaky as the vaccines[27]

Let's start with two simple questions. If regulators had the information available to them of the leakage between Covid-19 vaccine efficacy rates in controlled trials and their effectiveness in the real world, would they still grant emergency use authorization? Would their legal framework permit them to do so?

Remember, all laws serve a dual purpose. On the one hand, they are permissive and enabling, granting powers to do certain things. On the other, they are limiting and restrictive, ring-fencing what may lawfully be done even by the state.

Second, is Denmark being ruled by an anti-vaxxer government and health authority? From 1 July Denmark, which has an excellent health infrastructure including data collection, banned under-18s from being vaccinated and in mid-September the ban was extended to boosters for under-50s, other than in exceptional circumstances for immunocompromised and high-risk individuals in both cases.

The explanation offered by the health authorities is interesting both for what they said and what they did not say. They anticipate a rise in Covid-19 infections over autumn and winter and "aim to prevent serious illness, hospitalisation and death." This risk applies to 50-year olds and above and not those younger. Because the vaccines are not meant to prevent infection, they will no longer be offered to the under-50s.

However, governments don't ban products merely because they are not beneficial. Bans apply only to products that inflict harms. So the unstated reality is the benefit: harm ratio is no longer favourable. The really interesting question therefore is: why don't they say so? The empirical data from around the world demonstrates negligible to negative vaccine effectiveness for healthy under-50s and greater

---

[27] Brownstone Institute, 22 September 2022, https://brownstone.org/articles/the-vaccine-narrative-is-as-leaky-as-the-vaccines/

risk of serious adverse events. Denmark's decision marks official if implicit acknowledgment that harms are greater than benefits.

India's experience: Vaccines are not necessary for beating back Covid

Figure 4.6: India's Covid-19 deaths/mn people, 16 March–16 Sep. 2022

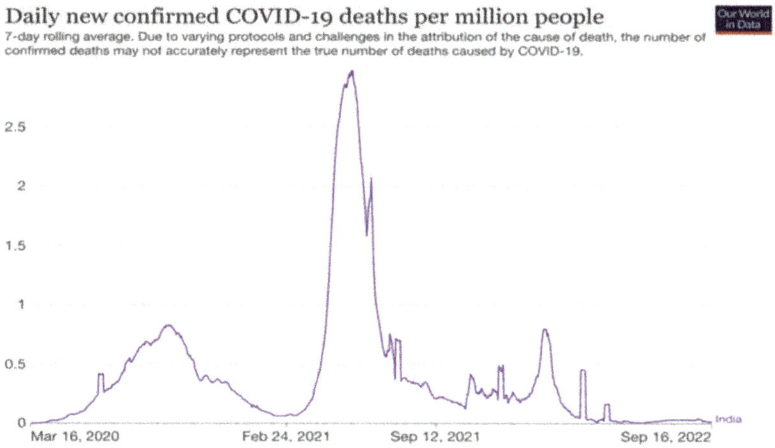

India's experience in mid-2021 proved that vaccines are not necessary for rapid mass recovery from a virulent Covid wave. The mortality gradient was broadly similar during the curve's ascent and descent, with the death rate reaching 1.06 per million people on 20 April, peaking at 2.98 on May 21 and 23 and falling back to 1.00 on 24 June (Figure 4.6). On those three dates India's full vaccination coverage was 1.26%, 2.96% and 3.53% of the population, respectively.

People questioned the reliability of the data, openly asserting a vast undercount in order to cushion the political embarrassment. Knowing something of India, I disagree and noted more than a hint of racism in the coverage. No matter. Even if the authorities deliberately suppressed the rising numbers of dead, it would be absurd to suggest they did the same with the downward numbers. The symmetrical rise and fall is consistent with the experience of most countries with successive waves of the virus.

Whatever else might explain the fall, it certainly wasn't high vaccination coverage. Herd immunity to the then-dominant Delta variant through a mix of uncontrolled infections and modest vaccination, possibly. Another contender for the explanation is the widespread use of ivermectin. Mid-crisis in May last year, the state government of Uttar Pradesh (India's most populous state with 200 million people!), boasted it had been the first to authorize large-scale prophylactic and therapeutic use of ivermectin against Covid-19 in May–June 2020. Studies were confirming that "the drug helped the state to maintain a lower fatality and positivity rate as compared to other states."

A meta-analysis by Andrew Bryant and Tess Lawrie in the *American Journal of Therapeutics* of 24 randomised control trials (RCTs) in 15 countries (one of which was subsequently pulled as possibly fraudulent) concluded that ivermectin significantly helps to prevent and treat Covid-19 and, with a 62% mortality reduction, can potentially save millions of lives. They published a follow-up analysis in the same journal that removed the suspect study and the results still showed robust ivermectin efficacy.

An analysis of seven RCTs, covering 1,327 patients, by Swedish physician Sebastian Rushworth found "a 62% reduction in the relative risk of dying among Covid patients treated with ivermectin." A large-scale study from Brazil published on 31 August found that, compared to regular users, non-use of ivermectin increased the risk of Covid-related mortality by 12.5 times and dying from Covid by seven times.

Yet for some strange reason, Western health bureaucracies would neither recommend ivermectin—a low cost, off patent and no profit drug for Big Pharma—nor fund a rigorous but fair (that is, not designed to fail) clinical assessment of its efficacy against Covid. It had morphed into Voldermectin: the drug that must not be named.

Global experience: Vaccines are not sufficient to beat back covid

My earlier articles show why Australia's Covid numbers this year demonstrate that vaccines are not sufficient to prevent mass infections, hospitalization and deaths either. Steve Kirsch alerted his Substack subscribers on September 17 to an internal report for the governing Liberal Party of Canada back in June. It makes for depressing reading that will come as no surprise to all of us who have grown increasingly cynical about public health authorities and governing elites. The report draws on official Ontario data, is informed by wide international scholarship and emphasizes that the empirical results are in line with trends in other Canadian provinces and countries.

The fully vaccinated show rise in hospital admissions within 5-6 months; the boosted, within two weeks and rising thereafter for several months. Immunity through natural infection can last up to 20 months. Vaccination shows considerable benefits to over-70s and some benefit to over-60s but virtually no benefit to under-60s with respect to hospitalization and mortality rates. By contrast, adverse events are concentrated in the 18–69 age groups, and especially, in order of most to least, in the 40–49, 50–59 and 30–39 age groups.

Because the "abundance of data" demonstrates that vaccines do not prevent infection, transmission, hospitalisation, and deaths for the under-60s, "public health policy tools such as, mass vaccination campaigns, mandates, passports and travel restrictions need to be re-evaluated for relevance." Factoring in also "known adverse events and unknown long-term effects," the "empirical evidence investigated in this report … does not support continuing mass vaccination programs, mandates, passports and travel bans for all age groups."

Meanwhile there continues to be very little evidence in the real world that countries with high rates of multiple vaccine doses suffer correspondingly lower rates of Covid-19 mortality. For example,

Chile has very high booster rollout and Covid-related death rate per capita, while India has very low booster coverage and mortality rate.

A study of almost 900,000 5-11-year-old children in North Carolina, published in the *New England Journal of Medicine*, adds to concerns that vaccines don't just lose their effectiveness in just a few months; they also destroy natural immunity against reinfection severe enough to put them in hospital. Three conclusions follow:

- The risk of severe outcomes for children from infection by current Covid variants is low;
- The risk of severe adverse reactions from vaccines is higher, meaning vaccination is a net harm for young children—exactly why Denmark has banned them for children;
- Exposing healthy children to the risk of infection may be better for both individual and herd immunity than mass vaccinating them.

The FDA is not likely to restore its credibility as the US regulator with the widely ridiculed revelation that the new bivalent boosters were authorized on the basis of trial results from eight mice. Professor Marty Makary from the Johns Hopkins School of Public Health tweeted his concerns about this and also about the announcement of an annual Covid vaccine that is not data-driven and ignores natural immunity as well as the risks of immune imprinting (where the immune system remembers its initial response to infection or vaccination in a way that usually, but not always, weakens the response to future variants of the same pathogen) from a multi-dose vaccination strategy.

From mRNA vaccine hesitant to anti-vaxxer

The *Financial Times*—as mainstream establishment as they come—recently warned that the US decision to roll out new booster shots without clinical testing on humans—already dubbed the mouse vaccine by some—risks undermining public trust and deepening vaccine hesitancy. "We already have a trust problem in this country and we don't need to make it worse," Eric Topol, founder and director of the Scripps Research Translational Institute, said. Yet, even while bemoaning the loss of public trust in health experts and institutions, Topol just couldn't help himself and smeared the Covid vaccine hesitants and sceptics as "anti-vaxxers, anti-science" people.

He thereby demonstrates precisely the pathology so beautifully described by Julie Sladden in an article in *Spectator Australia* on September 8. The Tasmanian doctor, "Having probably received more vaccines than most, given I am both a doctor and fairly well travelled," used to begin her apology for refusing the Covid jab with "'I'm no anti-vaxxer!'" However, after two years of "government-endorsed segregation and dehumanisation of those who exercised their right to refuse the jab," she has changed her mind:

> *If an "anti-vaxxer" is someone who cannot give informed consent to a "vaccine" that fails to prevent infection or transmission, has alarming safety signals, must be taken to earn back the right to live and work in society, for a disease that has a greater-than 99% survivability rate, then "yes," I'm an anti-vaxxer... My government made it so.*

To this we should add the very high likelihood of crossover vaccine hesitancy to other vaccines. In my own case before the pandemic I have dutifully gone in for the annual flu shot strongly recommended for my age demographic. Not any more. The Covid experience killed my trust in the medical and public health establishment and, having done my own research, I now politely decline the annual pre-winter flu shot.

Is the vaccination emperor as naked as his lockdown cousin?[28]

In my article in *The Spectator Australia* on 13 July, on discrepancies between models that predicted a reduction and data that showed a surge in coronavirus cases following the rollout of vaccines, I noted the reality of the decoupling between numbers and severity of infections following vaccination. This would likely reduce Covid-related hospitalisations and deaths.

In response, a reader suggested I look at the pre and post-vaccination mortality data from the European Union. Many readers in Australia and other Western countries might not be all that impressed by the examples of Bhutan, Seychelles, India and Malta because of dodgy data or small numbers, but will find it far more challenging to question the reliability of the data from the EU, he wrote.

Figure 4.7: Covid-19 deaths in the European Union, 1 March 2020–21 July 2021

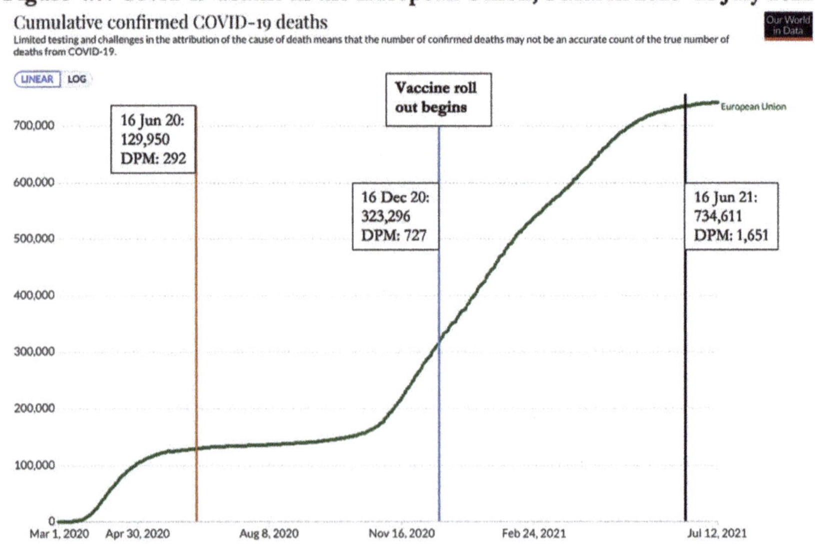

[28] *Spectator Australia*, 15 July 2021, https://spectator.com.au/2021/07/is-the-vaccination-emperor-as-naked-as-his-lockdown-cousin/

He has a point. The EU's vaccination campaign began on 16 December. By 16 June 2021, 46% of people had received at least one dose of the Covid vaccine and 26% were fully vaccinated. As this extremely informative chart shows (Figure 4.7), the EU's total number of Covid deaths in the 6 months before vaccinations began was 193,346, during which period the cumulative deaths per million people increased from 292 to 727. The total number of Covid deaths in the 6 months after vaccination rose steeply to 411,315 and the deaths per million increased from 727 to 1,651.

In other words, the total number of Covid-19 related deaths more than doubled in the six months following vaccination compared to the six months before vaccination in the European Union. Has anyone offered a convincing, or even a plausible explanation? To be fair, the 7-day rolling average of daily new deaths per million people was 0.59 on 6 June 2020, 7.82 on 6 December, and 1.37 on 6 June 2021, respectively. The steep decline began on 13 April, was down to 0.36 on 12 July, and has not yet changed direction again. So it is entirely possible that the good that vaccines do will show through in the total mortality statistics from now on, several months after the campaign got under way.

However, a nagging suspicion remains that the epidemiological and public health experts still have not got on top of the virus and are making it up as they go along, wanting to appear tough and decisive. No one really seems to know why, where, when, and with how much ferocity the virus, and its always mutating variants, will return. A new wave seems to surge, crest, crash and retreat spent and exhausted. In no country has it continued to grow exponentially forever, which is why 'Do the maths' glib comment was always fatuous and science-illiterate.

The downward slope of daily deaths per million people that inevitably follows the upwards slope is almost always equally steep, regardless of what measures are in place and not in place. In addition, variants are often more infectious but far less virulent. The so-called "harvesting" effect, which kills off the pool of the most vulnerable cohorts in the initial waves, also helps to break the link between infections and hospitalisation, ICU admissions and deaths.

In sum, the true measure of the effectiveness of vaccines will not be known until after the 2021–2022 'flu' season.

Explaining vaccine hesitancy[29]

According to the Department of Health's current report on vaccination status, in the last six months, only 3.5% of 18-to-64-year-old Australians had received the Covid-19 booster. Our vaccine hesitancy is in line with global trends. Unicef reported last year that public perceptions of the importance of childhood vaccines fell in 52 countries, by as much as 44% in some cases. Vaccination coverage had dipped in 112 countries and 67 million children had missed out on at least one vaccination between 2020 and 2023 because of disruptions caused by the lockdowns and diminished confidence in vaccines, producing "the largest sustained backslide in childhood immunisation in 30 years."

Vaccination rates against measles have fallen in Europe with a 45-fold annual rise in measles cases, according to the World Health Organisation, and also in the UK. While some of this might be the lingering effect of lockdown-era disruptions of immunisation services, in part it also arises from falling trust in public health edicts and institutions that has spilled over into a more generalised vaccine hesitancy. Unicef warns that, "the confluence of several factors suggest the threat of vaccine hesitancy may be growing," including, "uncertainty about the response to the pandemic… declining trust in expertise and political polarisation."

I offer five Covid-management-related policies as likely explanations for the rising vaccine hesitancy.

---

[29] *The Spectator Australia*, 18 May 2024, https://www.spectator.com.au/2024/05/explaining-vaccine-hesitancy/

First, the benefits were over-hyped. In July 2021, President Joe Biden said vaccines will ensure you won't get Covid; or if infected, you won't need hospitalisation; and you won't die. At a 2021 press briefing, referencing CDC director Rochelle Walensky's statement that Covid had become the "pandemic of the unvaccinated," White House press secretary Jen Psaki said, "99.5% of people who are in the hospital are people who are unvaccinated." Once a senior Pfizer official admitted that they had never tested Covid vaccines for transmissibility, the entire vaccine passport requirement was shown to have been built on a conspiracy of lies.

The initial belief in the efficacy of vaccines in breaking the links between infections, hospitalisations and deaths was confounded as data accumulated with mass vaccinations that vaccine efficacy was short-lived and very modest indeed against escape variants like Omicron. On 20 June 2023, Stanford Medical School's Dr Jay Bhattacharya tweeted that emails from Walensky, newly released under freedom of information access, showed that she, head of the National Institutes of Health Francis Collins, and Anthony Fauci were all aware a month after the vaccination campaign began, of the reality of breakthrough infections. Yet they continued to push vaccine mandates anyway. Fauci said in a CBS interview in May 2021 that, "when you get vaccinated, you not only protect your own health… you become a dead end to the virus."

Second, governments and health bureaucracies went to extraordinary lengths to censor, suppress and deny information about the many serious side-effects of Covid-19 vaccines. Cases of adverse side-effects from Covid-19 vaccines include anaphylaxis, Guillain-Barré Syndrome, myocarditis, pericarditis and thrombosis with thrombocytopenia syndrome. Some doctors have begun to identify vaccines as "the leading cause of coincidence" in deaths. Unsurprisingly, not only has this failed to keep the truth of vaccine injuries hidden, it has in fact created growing distrust of pharmaceutical giants, governments, health authorities and the media that have colluded to hide and disguise the truth.

Third, the durable protective benefits of natural immunity acquired from viral infection, that has been known to physicians since the Athenian plague, was memory-holed for three years with respect to Covid before being rediscovered. Those who issued reminders of the reality and powers of natural immunity were simply ignored. On 30 June 2021, Professor Robert Dingwall, a member of UK's Joint Committee on Vaccination and Immunisation, said letting children catch Covid would be better than vaccinating them. Their intrinsically low risk from Covid means they may be "better protected by natural immunity generated through infection than by asking them to take the "possible" risk of a vaccine." A study of almost 900,000 5-to-11-year-old children in North Carolina, published in the *New England Journal of Medicine*, added to concerns that vaccines don't merely lose their effectiveness in just a few months; they also destroy natural immunity against reinfection severe enough to put them in hospital. Vaccination should have focused on the uninfected and unvaccinated and natural immunity could and should have been accepted as vaccination-equivalent, but few countries and institutions did this.

Fourth, vaccine mandates came under sustained assault with respect both to medical justification and ethical underpinnings, especially for healthy children, adolescents and young adults. Their risk of seriously bad health outcomes from catching Covid was modest and lower than the risk of serious side-effects from the vaccine. The collateral harms inflicted on school- and university-age pupils made the mandate deeply unethical. Another medical question was the impact of mandates on staffing levels in healthcare institutions at a time when they were already stretched, with accompanying social and economic impacts that extended to the families of those dismissed. By the northern autumn of 2022, with the widespread emergence of Omicron as an escape variant, both the personal protective benefits and reductions in transmission had become insubstantial. A

2022 study in the *New England Journal of Medicine* showed comparable rates of viral shedding for vaccinated and unvaccinated people with Covid-19. Denying entry into public spaces to the unvaccinated was unethical when vaccination status could not separate those who could spread the disease from those who could not.

Finally, even eminent epidemiologists and medical scientists who voiced responsible cautionary notes about the questionable efficacy being claimed and the harms being ignored were censored and silenced. The difference between conspiracy theories and facts turned out to be six to 12 months. But government officials were never held to the same standard for pro-vaccine claims.

In September 2022, FDA Commissioner Dr Robert Califf tweeted that the updated Bivalent Wuhan-Omicron BA.4/5 booster "increases your chances of being in attendance at upcoming gatherings with family and friends."

Dr Vinay Prasad and Dr Alyson Haslam note wryly, "Had the company said this, the FDA could fine them for false and misleading statements."

Covid Vaccines: Savior or Killer Shot?[30]

It's interesting that the esteemed editor of this site has concluded, after more than four years of cogitation, that mRNA technology-based vaccines were a solution in search of a problem in the minds of a health-cum-national security elite, that SARS-CoV-2 was the answer to their prayers, and that lockdowns, masks, school restrictions, and rejection of alternative treatment options were necessary to prevent the achievement of herd immunity via infections before vaccines could be mass manufactured and rolled out to the whole world.

---

[30] Brownstone Institute, 25 May 2024, https://brownstone.org/articles/covid-vaccines-savior-or-killer-shot/

Unfortunately, Jeffrey Tucker points out, their preferred solution "failed spectacularly." Instead, what we have "unfolding here is the biggest and most destructive flop in the history of public health." Others go further, arguing that mRNA vaccines in particular have correlated so strongly with rising all-cause excess mortality that causation must be a strong presumption.

Yet, not everyone buys the overarching judgment of spectacular failure. The holdout proponents of the success of public health intervention's point to the gravity and universality of the threat from Covid, on the one hand, and the public health benefits of the vaccines, on the other. On the first, for example, a year ago the World Health Organisation published estimates that in the two years 2020 and 2021, nearly 15 million people had died with Covid, or almost three times the official estimates.

A study published in the journal *Lancet Infectious Disease* in June 2022 estimated that Covid-19 vaccines saved 19.8 million lives in the first year of their availability, helping to reduce the global death toll by 63%. The study used a "mathematical model of Covid-19 transmission and vaccination." Another modelling study concluded that in two years, vaccines had saved around three million US lives. A paper by two US researchers in March this year, from the University of Colorado and University of California Los Angeles, calculated that 800,000 American lives were saved by lockdowns, social distancing, and vaccines.

A computer simulation modelling from Monash University in Melbourne estimated that vaccination prevented nearly 18,000 deaths in New South Wales alone in the one-year period from August 2021 to July 2022, reducing the death toll to one-sixth of what might have been expected otherwise. Unvaccinated 50 year olds and over had twelve times higher mortality rates than their boosted counterparts.

These are tall claims, in both senses of the word. It's impressive how many still try to bamboozle health reporters and the public with abstract mathematical models to claim spectacular success for Covid-19 vaccines. Assumptions are made about infection and case fatality rates and about the efficacy of vaccines to produce such favourable estimates. Several also assume that no immunity existed from natural infection at any point. Voluntary modifications of individual behaviour to reduce risks as awareness of the pandemic spread is totally discounted. The variability in transmissibility and lethality of successive variants as the virus mutated is ignored.

The public health clerisy and vaccine manufacturers self-servingly classify everyone until two or three weeks after the second dose as "unvaccinated," when empirically the more useful binary data classification would be into the ever- and never-vaccinated.

There is the problem of coding errors in data collection, including wide variations in recording deaths as Covid-related. The difference between dying with and from Covid may well be impossible to disentangle by now. That doesn't mean it is trivial. Covid as the sole or chief cause of deaths could amount to anything between 10-50% of the seven million total number of Covid-related deaths as of 21 May, as per Worldometers.

Then too, it is both indisputable and largely conceded by now that vaccine efficacy declines rapidly, and particularly so with successive booster doses, so that the date of data measurement also becomes critical. The healthy vaccinee effect is yet another confounding factor.

The most critical consideration is this: few studies promoting vaccines take care to separate the protection conferred by vaccines from that of naturally acquired immunity from prior infection. In a pithy summary on 20 May, Alex Berenson observed: "*Science* brought us an epidemic. *Nature* saved us."

Figure 4.8: Relationship between Covid vaccination and mortality rates for Australia, Canada, New Zealand, and the US

Figure 1: Relationship between Covid vaccination and mortality rates for Australia, Canada, New Zealand, and the US

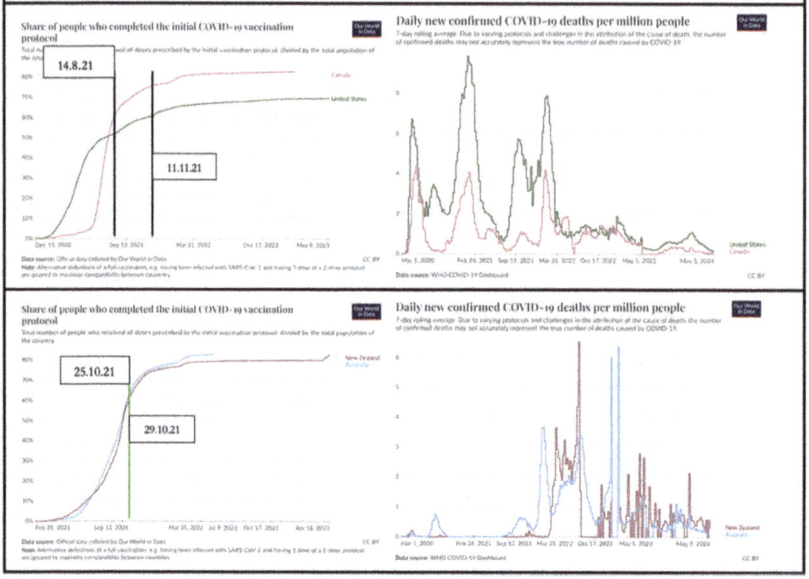

Consider two pairs of neighbouring countries in the northern and southern hemisphere: Canada and the US, and Australia and New Zealand (Figure 4.8). Because the US achieved 70% full (that is, two doses) vaccination quite late, I have chosen the arbitrary threshold of 60% for present comparative purposes. Canada and the US crossed the threshold in August and November 2021, while the Australasians did so in October.

Next, look at the dates on which the four countries recorded their highest daily mortality rates (7-day rolling averages) (Table 4.1). In the North American pair, this happened well before getting to 60% vaccination; in Australasia, well after.

Table 4.1: The timing of peak Covid mortality rates

	US	Canada*	Australia	New Zealand
Date	21 Jan 2021	15 May 2020	8 Feb 2023	25 Jul 2022
Deaths per mn	9.84	4.36	6.34	6.50

* Unusually among the four countries under consideration, Canada experienced three broadly comparable peaks. The other two occurred on 28 January 2021, with a deaths per million rate of 4.05, and on 1 February 2022, 4.15 deaths per million people.

Source: Our World in Data

Canada hit 60% full vaccination on 14 August 2021, fifteen months after its peak daily Covid mortality rate and seven months after a mini-peak in January 2021. The United States hit 60% full vaccination on 11 November 2021, ten months after its highest daily Covid mortality rate. In other words, mortality rates had fallen in both these North American countries well before vaccination coverage got to 60%.

By contrast, Australia and New Zealand achieved 60% full vaccination on 25 and 29 October 2021, respectively and their Covid mortality peaked well afterwards: 16 months later for Australia and nine months later for New Zealand.

This is even better captured in the total number of cumulative Covid-related deaths.

For the United States, 63% of Covid-related deaths until May 2024 were recorded before 60% full vaccination, which is why public health and administration officials could not resist the temptation to conflate correlation and causation in the post-vaccination fall in deaths. This is less obvious for Canada, with 51.4% of its total deaths being recorded after 60% vaccination.

In Australia's case, an astonishing 93% of the deaths were after 60% full vaccination. For New Zealand, the share is a staggering

99.3%. How anyone could claim this as vaccine success with a straight face is beyond comprehension. If correlation is to be posited as causation, therefore, clearly vaccines were driving Covid cases and deaths that had been remarkably low before vaccines began to be rolled out. But obviously, the same vaccines could not be driving Covid cases and mortality down in the US but causing a surge in Australasia.

In any case, even without equating correlation and causation, the two Australasian examples are sufficient to falsify the general claim of vaccine effectiveness. Unless, of course, the vaccine faithful would like to argue that there is some mysterious force that corrupts the vaccines as they cross the equator.

There is an alternative explanation that covers the four countries rather better. This points to the key role of natural immunity from prior infection. As shown in Figure 4.9, owing to the combination of summer in the southern hemisphere when the pandemic broke, geographical location, and international border closures, Australia and New Zealand succeeded in quarantining their populations from the virus for two years. As of 31 December 2021, the cumulative cases (defined as a positive test irrespective of feeling well or ill) per million people was 2,686 for New Zealand and 25,068 for Australia, but 56,907 for Canada and a whopping 161,373 for the United States. Thus huge numbers of Canadians and (especially) Americans had acquired natural immunity by then.

Figure 4.9: Cumulative Covid cases per million people, 1 Mar 2020–1 Apr 2022

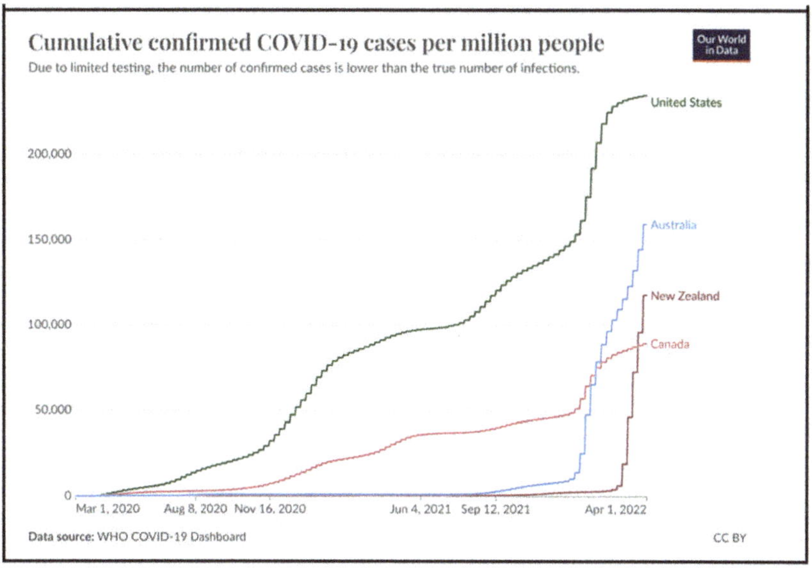

But this meant that over two years of isolation, unless the vaccines were highly efficacious and sustained their immunity for long timeframes, Australia and (especially) New Zealand had created immunologically naïve populations. Unless they intended to close off their borders to the outside world permanently, therefore, which was never even a possibility, their peoples were highly vulnerable to fresh waves of the virus once they reopened and until they acquired immunity that was both more robust and more durable.

In sum, therefore, looked at together, the two pairs of examples from North America and Australasia indicate weak to negligible role of vaccines and the critical role of infection-acquired immunity in ending the pandemic. It's called re-learning the same lessons all over again.

Dr Fauci: welcome to the sunny side of Freedom Street[31]

Writing for Flat White on August 13, 2021 arguing against the idea of vaccination certificates, I noted that vaccines don't stop either transmission or hospitalisation. But because they can reduce the severity of the illness and mortality rates for target groups, I said: "Vaccines should be made available to all, strongly recommended for all vulnerable groups, but not made mandatory for anyone. Embrace personal choice and individual responsibility as the core elements of Covid risk management as we all learn to live with it as individuals and a nation.'

Guess what? In an interview with Jon Karl of the US ABC TV on September 10, Dr Anthony "Call me Mr Science" Fauci was asked who should get Covid boosters. The question was prompted by a spike in cases and hospitalisations and the consciousness that this will intensify as the country heads into the northern winter. Fauci replied he believes that, "We should give the choice to people that are not in the high-risk groups, to have the vaccine available for them." Even high-risk people, he added, should be given the choice but not compelled to get vaccinated: "Make [the vaccine] available to everyone, but certainly recommend it to high-risk people.'

Fauci also highlighted the level of immunity in the population is high owing to people who have been vaccinated, boosted, and infected. In other words, he is now also acknowledging naturally acquired immunity from prior infection.

Writing in the *Washington Examiner*, Jon Miltimore comments that the use of words like "choice" and "recommend" even for high-risk people is "a stunning reversal" from Fauci's earlier support for mandates. He attributes the change of position to a string of legal defeats in the courts of various vaccine mandates and to the rising legal costs

[31] *Spectator Australia*, 23 November 2023, https://www.spectator.com.au/2023/11/dr-fauci-welcome-to-the-sunny-side-of-freedom-street/

of the Department of Health and Services defending a flood of legal suits from the vaccine injured.

How about an apology from him, from the public health institutions and authorities, from all the vaccine mandate pushers in the media, and from the social media fact-checkers to all of us who were smeared, vilified, shadow-banned, and de-platformed? Crickets?

And isn't it about time Australian courts began to hold our health officials to account and provided relief to all those who lost their jobs because of their principled refusal to be vaccinated and compensation to those who were injured by the vaccines?

As the great economist, social theorist, and political philosopher Thomas Sowell said: "The most basic question is not what is best, but who shall decide what is best." Or, to put it another way. It's not that people will make the right choice for themselves. Rather, people have the right to make the choice for themselves.

5: VACCINES—AUSTRALASIA

Gradually, I began to focus more directly on the vaccine landscape in Australia, and in particular New South Wales which is the most populous Australian state and also published the best data for much of the time. It is also the state where I live.

All deaths are equal, but some are more equal than others[32]

From the start, those sceptical of lockdowns for managing the coronavirus pandemic have offered three complementary lines of argument. First, a respiratory virus will never be eradicated and as it becomes endemic, the public health goal should be to protect against severe illness. Second, we said science and experience showed that lockdowns might work as a temporary measure to delay the spread and "flatten the curve," but cannot contain or avoid the disease indefinitely. Third, they produce collateral harms that accumulate as lockdowns persist and will afflict societies for years and decades to come.

The first is becoming clear around the world, the second is being experienced in Australia and the third is starting to show up here and elsewhere. Yet for some incomprehensible reason, governments have focussed single-mindedly on avoiding Covid deaths on their watch even while oblivious to short and long-term deaths caused by

[32] *Spectator Australia*, Part 1, 4 August 2021, https://www.spectator.com.au/2021/08/all-deaths-are-equal-but-some-are-more-equal-than-others/

harsh society-wide shutdowns. To paraphrase one of George Orwell's most-quoted sentences, all deaths are equal, but a Covid death is more equal than all others.

By now there's a wealth of studies establishing the ineffectiveness of lockdowns, many of which I have referenced in earlier articles in *The Spectator Australia*, and some that purport to show their effectiveness. Writing in our British parent publication, statistician Professor Simon Wood showed that new infections peaked and fell before lockdown on all three occasions in England.

The indifferent results of lockdowns can be seen in Covid-19 deaths per million people (DPM) of several countries from around the world. While non-lockdown Brazil is at the higher end of the scale, Sweden is in the middle of the European pack (24/48) with a sub-European mortality rate. The same pattern can be seen with US states, where Texas and Florida have the 25th and 26th highest DPM of 50 US states, below the national average, but South Dakota ranks 10th.

As is well-known but hushed in a conspiracy of silence by the mainstream media, Florida, Georgia and Texas—The States That Must Never Be Named—lifted all restrictions and, despite model-based grim warnings of becoming death traps, suffered no visible exit waves. The ripples of new cases of the Delta variant in these states follow the same curves as those in states with restrictions. Florida Governor Ron DeSantis is holding firm, insisting that "We're going to lift people up. We're not locking people down." Are any Australian leaders listening?

The worldwide Covid deaths in the eight months from 1 March to 31 October 2020 were 1,279,085. In the next eight months from 1 November 2020 to 30 June 2021, the total was 2,678,166. That is, there were more than double the number of Covid-related deaths in the second eight months, when most of Europe, North America and

South America—the three continents with the most severe outbreaks of the disease—were implementing hard lockdowns, than in the first eight months. This is not evidence in support of the effectiveness of lockdown interventions.

There is no question that Covid-19 has exacted a terrible toll for 18 months and counting, even with the caveat of not distinguishing dying with and from Covid. The number of deaths from all causes worldwide was 59.23mn in 2020. For the pandemic period from 1 March 2020 to 26 July 2021, it was 93.7mn.

However, Covid was not the only and not even the world's leading killer in that period. Several other diseases like coronary diseases, cancers, strokes and lung diseases, have killed more people. Some of these other tolls were worsened with attention, resources and health services redirected to deal with Covid. Western governments behaved in herd-like fashion to repurpose the existing health system to focus disproportionately on Covid to the neglect of all other illnesses, including the big killer diseases. But they proved curiously reluctant to promote repurposed existing drugs for outpatient and early treatment of Covid.

In the UK, owing to lockdowns, three million cancer screenings were missed, heart attack and accident and emergency attendances dropped by 50% and emergency heart surgery dropped by 38% in London in the second half of March. Around 5.3 million people are awaiting routine operations. Up to 60,000 Britons could die of flu next winter because lockdowns have reduced immunity. Health Secretary Sajid Javid said on 6 July that about 7mn people didn't come forward for help during the pandemic for illnesses including cancer, heart disease and mental health and this could rise to 13mn. "As Health Secretary I can't just be thinking about Covid alone, I have to think about all the other health problems that are out there and have a plan to deal with those," he said.

According to a Statistics Canada summary of data published on 7 July, from the end of March 2020 to the beginning of April 2021, an estimated 62,203 Canadians up to age 64 died. This represents an age-adjusted excess mortality of 5,535. Of these, 1,380 were Covid-19 related deaths and 4,155 may be "related to other factors." In other words, three times as many Canadians under the age of 65 appear to have died from lockdown-related causes as with Covid.

Part two, 5 August 2021[33]

The Australian response has not been science-driven, not unified, not sensible, and neither consistent nor coherent. Figure 5.1 gives the statistics on leading causes of deaths, with Covid coming in at 26th. In the calendar year 2021 to date, Covid deaths are just 15. But our politicians, health bureaucrats and media remain spooked by the deadly waves that have swept through other parts of the world. At least the self-congratulatory smugness at being the envy of the world has abated and there is dawning recognition that instead, we are becoming the laughing stock with our fixation on "cases," even as others recognise the silliness of using this unreliable measure based on often wildly inaccurate test results.

[33] *Spectator Australia*, 5 August 2021, https://www.spectator.com.au/2021/08/all-deaths-are-equal-but-some-are-more-equal-than-others-part-two/

Figure 5.1: Four date-stamped snapshots of Australia's leading causes of death, 1.3.20–23.6.23

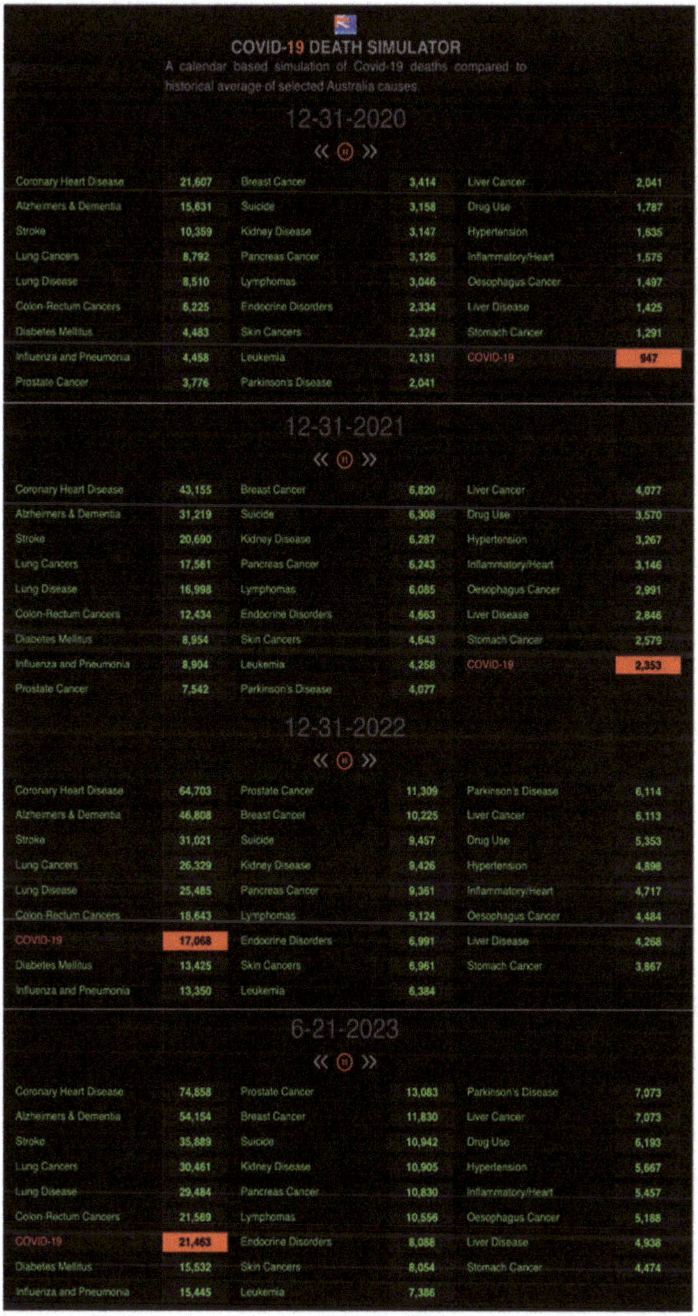

COVID-19 DEATH SIMULATOR

A calendar based simulation of Covid-19 deaths compared to historical average of selected Australia causes.

12-31-2020

Coronary Heart Disease	21,607	Breast Cancer	3,414	Liver Cancer	2,041
Alzheimers & Dementia	15,631	Suicide	3,158	Drug Use	1,787
Stroke	10,359	Kidney Disease	3,147	Hypertension	1,635
Lung Cancers	8,792	Pancreas Cancer	3,126	Inflammatory/Heart	1,575
Lung Disease	8,510	Lymphomas	3,046	Oesophagus Cancer	1,497
Colon-Rectum Cancers	6,225	Endocrine Disorders	2,334	Liver Disease	1,425
Diabetes Mellitus	4,483	Skin Cancers	2,324	Stomach Cancer	1,291
Influenza and Pneumonia	4,458	Leukemia	2,131	COVID-19	947
Prostate Cancer	3,776	Parkinson's Disease	2,041		

12-31-2021

Coronary Heart Disease	43,155	Breast Cancer	6,820	Liver Cancer	4,077
Alzheimers & Dementia	31,219	Suicide	6,308	Drug Use	3,570
Stroke	20,690	Kidney Disease	6,287	Hypertension	3,267
Lung Cancers	17,561	Pancreas Cancer	6,243	Inflammatory/Heart	3,146
Lung Disease	16,998	Lymphomas	6,085	Oesophagus Cancer	2,991
Colon-Rectum Cancers	12,434	Endocrine Disorders	4,663	Liver Disease	2,846
Diabetes Mellitus	8,954	Skin Cancers	4,643	Stomach Cancer	2,579
Influenza and Pneumonia	8,904	Leukemia	4,258	COVID-19	2,353
Prostate Cancer	7,542	Parkinson's Disease	4,077		

12-31-2022

Coronary Heart Disease	64,703	Prostate Cancer	11,309	Parkinson's Disease	6,114
Alzheimers & Dementia	46,808	Breast Cancer	10,225	Liver Cancer	6,113
Stroke	31,021	Suicide	9,457	Drug Use	5,353
Lung Cancers	26,329	Kidney Disease	9,426	Hypertension	4,898
Lung Disease	25,485	Pancreas Cancer	9,361	Inflammatory/Heart	4,717
Colon-Rectum Cancers	18,643	Lymphomas	9,124	Oesophagus Cancer	4,484
COVID-19	17,068	Endocrine Disorders	6,991	Liver Disease	4,268
Diabetes Mellitus	13,425	Skin Cancers	6,961	Stomach Cancer	3,867
Influenza and Pneumonia	13,350	Leukemia	6,384		

6-21-2023

Coronary Heart Disease	74,858	Prostate Cancer	13,083	Parkinson's Disease	7,073
Alzheimers & Dementia	54,154	Breast Cancer	11,830	Liver Cancer	7,073
Stroke	35,889	Suicide	10,942	Drug Use	6,193
Lung Cancers	30,461	Kidney Disease	10,905	Hypertension	5,667
Lung Disease	29,484	Pancreas Cancer	10,830	Inflammatory/Heart	5,457
Colon-Rectum Cancers	21,569	Lymphomas	10,556	Oesophagus Cancer	5,188
COVID-19	21,463	Endocrine Disorders	8,086	Liver Disease	4,938
Diabetes Mellitus	15,532	Skin Cancers	8,054	Stomach Cancer	4,474
Influenza and Pneumonia	15,445	Leukemia	7,386		

Source: World Life Expectancy (updated since original publication)

By the end of 2021, 75.5% of all Australians (meaning around 90% of all adults) were double vaccinated. Even then, Covid-19, with a cumulative total of under 1,000 deaths, was well down on the list of the leading causes of death. Yet it is after that date that Covid-related mortality really hit Australia and at the end of 2022, and until June 2023, Covid was in the top ten causes of death (Figure 5.1).

Figure 5.2: Excess deaths from all causes, Nov 2020–June 2021, Australia and Sweden. Based on data from the Australian Bureau of Statistics, Our World in Data

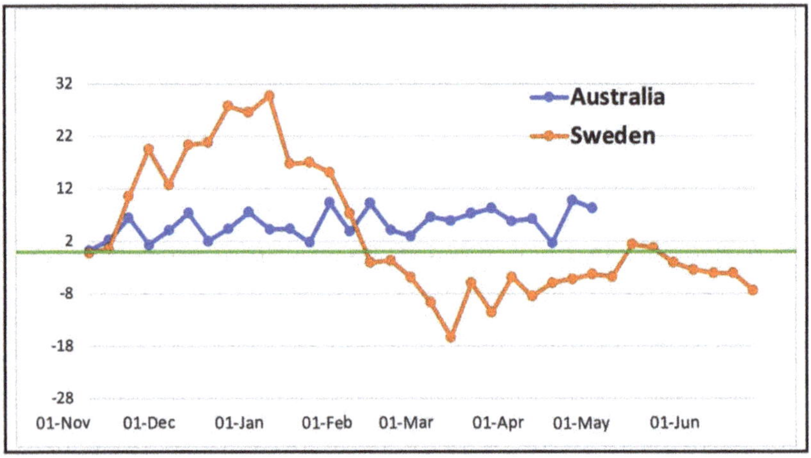

What is yet to register on the public, media and political consciousness is the rising numbers of all-causes excess deaths (Figure 5.2). There is still radio silence in the mainstream media about Australia's excess deaths. For reasons beyond comprehension, Covid deaths are to be avoided at all costs, including causing more deaths from other causes by measures implemented to minimise Covid deaths. The collateral harms to other health outcomes, mental health, the economy and liberties are simply brushed aside as not worthy of consideration.

Australia's estimated deaths in 2020 were 169,000, or about a daily average of 463; and for the pandemic period 1 March 2020 to 26 July 2021, 267,000. The total number of Covid deaths in 2020 thus amounted to just two days of all-causes deaths. The total number of all deaths from 1 January to 30 April this year was 44,407 (ABS release on 29 July 2021). Within this, there were 2,427 (5.6%) excess deaths to 30 April—7,382 annualised and more per day on average than the total Covid deaths this year so far.

The ABS says in the summary of key statistics: "Counts of deaths were above historical averages for each month of 2021." In fact, the tables of weekly deaths show that the count has been above average for every single week since 1 November 2020. Cancer deaths were up by 780 (5.1%), diabetes by 113 (8.4%) and dementia by 742 (18.5%). All three are among the list one would include in the likely areas of damage from the neglect of regular health services, screenings and treatments.

By contrast, Sweden's excess deaths have been below the five-yearly average for every week since 7 February, except for a fortnight in May. The country of course is legendary for rejecting lockdown advice and pressure.

Is it any wonder that people are starting to take to the streets to protest against the serial imposition of lockdowns by Australia's one-trick pony state governments? As for banning the protests, it's worth repeating this sentence from The New York Times on 11 May 2021: "There is not a single documented Covid infection anywhere in the world from casual outdoor interactions, such as walking past someone on a street or eating at a nearby table." In a matching report, on 5 July NSW Health confirmed that throughout the entire pandemic, not a single confirmed case of Covid transmission had occurred outdoors.

If mass rallies are indeed super-spreaders of the virus, why did we fail to see surges in infections after the Black Lives Matter protests last year in the US, UK and Australia? How easily we have ignored the confirmed reality that the biggest super-spreader in Australia was Victoria's hotel quarantine system last year, for which of course no one has been held accountable.

Vaccination certificates: an idea whose time must never come[34]

Chris Richardson of Deloitte Access Economics wrote in the *Australian Financial Review* on 10 August: "Delta is so infectious that the vaccination rates we need are at least as high as those already achieved by the likes of Canada, the United Kingdom, Israel and Italy." He argued that timidity is proving costly and will end badly. Instead, the government needs to bite the bullet, make vaccination certificates mandatory for all wishing to return to active life in society and the economy, and shield businesses imposing no jab, no job policies with a firm legislative framework.

On 9 August, the spread of fully vaccinated was from 55.7% (Italy), 58.3% (UK), Canada (62.2%) to 62.4% (Israel). The Covid-19 daily new infections and deaths per million people for these countries on that date was: Canada (40/0.27), UK (407/1.32), Israel (442/1.19), Italy (99/0.36).

Let's look at some selected countries in a bit more detail. Iceland is currently 75% fully vaccinated. Chief Epidemiologist Þórólfur Guðnason says vaccination has not led to the herd immunity that experts hoped for. In recent weeks, as the Delta variant outstripped all others in Iceland, it became clear that vaccinated people can easily contract it as well as spread it to others. He said in a briefing on 3 August: "the Covid-19 pandemic is not close to being over and will not be over until it's over everywhere." On 8 August, he conceded the goal cannot be to eradicate the virus from the community. Instead, he now believes it is necessary to try to achieve herd immunity by allowing the virus to spread throughout the community, but to try to prevent serious illness by protecting vulnerable groups (Google translation). Looking at Iceland (75% vaccinated) and Australia (18%

[34] *Spectator Australia*, 13 August 2021, https://www.spectator.com.au/2021/08/vaccination-certificates-an-idea-whose-time-must-never-come/

vaccinated) together (Figure 5.4), why would we think vaccination is our golden key out of the Covid nightmare?

Figure 5.3: Covid cases in Australia and Iceland

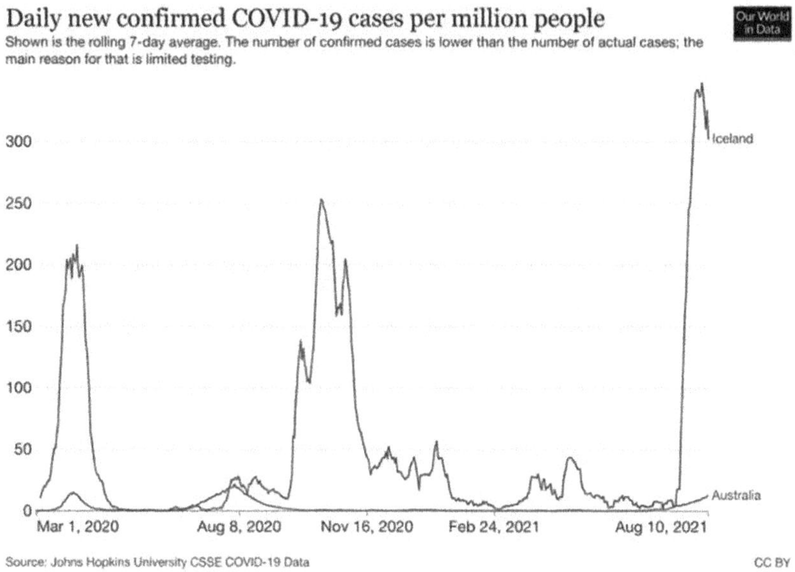

The waning efficacy of vaccines is also seen in Israel, including some who have been thrice-jabbed. In a locality in Jerusalem where only 42.9% of the population has been fully vaccinated, 85-90% of all hospitalised patients were fully vaccinated. According to a report in Arutz Sheva on 13 July citing health ministry data, only 72 of the 835,792 Covid-recovered Israelis had been reinfected, compared to over 3,000 of the 5,193,499 vaccinated Israelis. Referencing these statistics, Martin Kulldorff from Harvard Medical School tweeted: "Vaccinated people were 6.72 times more likely to get infected than those with natural immunity from prior" Covid disease. And Dr Marty Makary of Johns Hopkins University declared: "The pandemic of the unvaccinated is a misnomer. It's a pandemic of the non-immune."

In other words if we ignore models—and I wish we had done so from the very beginning, they've proven so thoroughly unreliable and dangerous in their impacts—the recommendation for vaccination certificates flies in the face of massive actual data from the real world. This is even without bringing up the case of India itself where this damn Delta variant first made its appearance at scale. India's steep infections curve crossed 50,000 daily new cases on 26 March 2021 with 0.6% fully vaccinated, peaked on 8 May with 391,000 cases with a mere 2.5% of people fully vaccinated, and came down to 50,000 on 26 June with only 4% full vaccination (Figure 4.10 in the previous chapter).

On 30 July, the US Centers for Disease Control and Prevention announced that the Delta variant was showing similarly high viral loads among unvaccinated and vaccinated cases. This suggests "an increased risk of transmission and raised concern that, unlike with other variants, vaccinated people infected with Delta can transmit the virus." A similar conclusion was reached by Public Health England on 6 August: "levels of virus in those who become infected with Delta having already been vaccinated may be similar to levels found in unvaccinated people. This may have implications for people's infectiousness, whether they have been vaccinated or not," meaning that vaccines will not suppress the virus spread as much as had been hoped.

Public Health England's Technical Briefing 20 in early August showed that while vaccination does reduce mortality in the over-50s by more than threefold, for those under 50, the fatality rate among the vaccinated is 57% greater than in the unvaccinated. On 10 August, a panel of experts, including most importantly the head of the Oxford vaccine team, called for an end to mass testing in Britain because the Delta variant has destroyed any chance of herd immunity through vaccination. The scientists believe it's time to accept there's no way of stopping the virus spreading through the entire population and monitoring people with mild symptoms is no longer helpful.

Confirming that history does irony, this development came on the same day that the Australian Parliament condemned George Christensen MP for conveying pretty much the same message: "Covid-19 is going to be with us forever, just like the flu and just like the flu, we will have to live with it, not in constant fear of it." PM Scott Morrison and Coalition MPs voted in support of the Labor censure motion, simply ignoring the substantial scientific literature to support Christensen's assertions on the questionable efficacy and collateral harms of masks and lockdowns.

In other words, having tried lockdowns and vaccinations, some of the most highly vaccinated countries are coming round to the view of the Great Barrington Declaration of October 2020—which itself was a restatement of the official WHO position of September 2019—of focussing protection efforts on the most vulnerable. Maybe instead of targeting Christensen, our media, public health experts and political leaders should rethink their entire approach? Because vaccinations do not prevent infection or transmission, they cannot stop the spread of the virus. Because they do reduce the severity of the illness and mortality rates, they remain important. Putting the two together, vaccines should be made available to all, strongly recommended for all vulnerable groups but not made mandatory for anyone. Embrace personal choice and individual responsibility as the core elements of Covid risk management as we all learn to live with it as individuals and a nation.

Is this what "success" looks like?[35]

As someone who has been looking at Covid-related data since the outbreak of the pandemic and a resident of the ACT until the end of last year, my curiosity got the better of me and I checked the Covid situation on the *Canberra Times* online on Sunday.

---

[35] *Spectator Australia*, 26 May 2022, https://www.spectator.com.au/2022/05/is-this-what-success-looks-like/

The opening sentence was memorable: "Covid hospitalisation in the ACT has risen above 90 for first time and hit a record high for the fourth day in a row." There were 92 Covid patients in hospital on Saturday night, including three in intensive care and two on ventilators. In the preceding 24 hours, 758 new Covid cases had been reported in the territory. Meanwhile, the number of influenza cases was also higher than pre-pandemic levels. Strikingly, however, the paper failed to report on the breakdown between vaccinated and unvaccinated Covid cases and hospitalisations.

My curiosity was piqued by the cynic in me. Could it be that Australia's Covid story has morphed into a pandemic of the vaccinated? So I checked out the Commonwealth Department of Health's coronavirus website, but it too, while providing all manner of details on Covid statistics by age, sex, states etc, was conspicuously silent on the relationship between Covid cases, hospitalisations and deaths on the one hand, and vaccination status (unvaccinated, single dose, double dose, boosters) on the other.

My next stop on the journey was the trusty Our World in Data. At the end of 2021, 77% of all Australians and 75% of all Kiwis had been double vaccinated. Vaccination coverage of adults therefore would be above 90% in both countries by January 1, this year.

From the start of the coronavirus pandemic in early March 2020 until the end of 2021, a grand total of 2,253 Australians and 51 Kiwis had died with Covid. As at 20 May 2022, the total Covid-related death count had climbed steeply to 8,076 in Australia and 997 in New Zealand. In other words, in less than five months so far this year, despite world-leading vaccination rates, their respective Covid mortality tolls were 2.6 times higher for Australia and 18.5 times higher for NZ than in the 22 months until the end of last year.

If this is vaccine success, what would failure look like?

With this to hand, I tracked down the data for my new state of residence. The NSW Respiratory Surveillance Report for the week ending

14 May offered the answers I was looking for. In this "epidemiological week 19," there were 570 Covid cases admitted to hospital, 58 in ICU and 90 deaths. Fully 82% of all Covid-related deaths in the state in this week were at least double vaccinated, including 64% who had received boosters.

And still the conspiracy of silence continues among all state and federal governments about this disappointing failure of vaccine efficacy and lack of justification for vaccine mandates and passports.

There never was any ethical justification for vaccine coercion to begin with. And clearly the regulators, health authorities and governments are stubbornly refusing to entertain, let alone scrutinise, the current data coming in for the pandemic, either by accelerated loss of efficacy or by weakening natural immunity with successive doses.

Also, given the massive budget blowouts, why are the authorities even recommending universal vaccination instead of targeting the high-risk group of elderly and people with underlying conditions, just like with flu every year?

Let people make their own informed decisions—now there's a revolutionary thought.

Yet more "vaccine success"[36]

I recently received a communication from my GP's surgery: "Influenza is spiking early. Our GPs report that those with 2022 flu have a rapid onset of illness with high fevers, dry cough, body aches, and headache. They are generally more unwell than those with a Covid infection. We recommend everyone receive a flu vaccine."

This was followed by the same advice on a second Covid booster (that is, fourth vaccine). When will the penny drop? Perhaps more pertinently, what—if anything—will make the penny drop?

---

[36] *Spectator Australia*, 10 June 2022, https://spectator.com.au/2022/06/yet-more-vaccine-success/

Some of us have been arguing for some time that we must learn to live with the virus as we live with the flu, including (maybe) an annual vaccine, provided it has better efficacy and less concerning safety signals. Lo and behold, in an editorial on May 30, The Economist turned this around and suggested that maybe governments should begin to treat flu like Covid, with active monitoring, surveillance, home testing, working from home, and vaccines—of course.

Describing this as a "thought experiment," the magazine noted: "Epidemiologists worry that two years of low exposure to flu may have caused immunity to wane to low levels. That may result in an extraordinary number of cases this winter, at a point when huge waiting lists will still clog up the National Health Service (NHS)."

An alternative twofold conclusion from this is that it proves the NHS is no longer fit for purpose, should be abandoned and a new system built from scratch; and that prolonged lockdowns that drastically reduce mass exposure to the perennially circulating pathogens to interfere with the build-up of natural immunity are perhaps not such a good idea?

Reduced immunity may be one explanation, along with the collateral harms from widely predicted warnings that lockdowns would lead to increased deaths down the line from preventable diseases that were no longer caught in time because of cancelled screenings, etc. According to a study published this month from the National Bureau of Economic Research, between April 2020 and December 2021, "Americans died from non-Covid causes at an average annual rate 97,000 in excess of previous trends," including 32,000 from hypertension and heart disease, and 12,000-15,000 each from diabetes, obesity, drug abuse, and alcohol abuse.

Meanwhile, a Swedish study published in The *Lancet* on February 4 based on 1.69mn individuals, divided equally between vaccinated and unvaccinated "found progressively waning vaccine effectiveness against SARS-CoV-2 infection of any severity across all subgroups." This, of course, is the question I had raised in my last *Flat White* article on 26 May.

Figure 5.4: Covid-19 daily new cases per million people

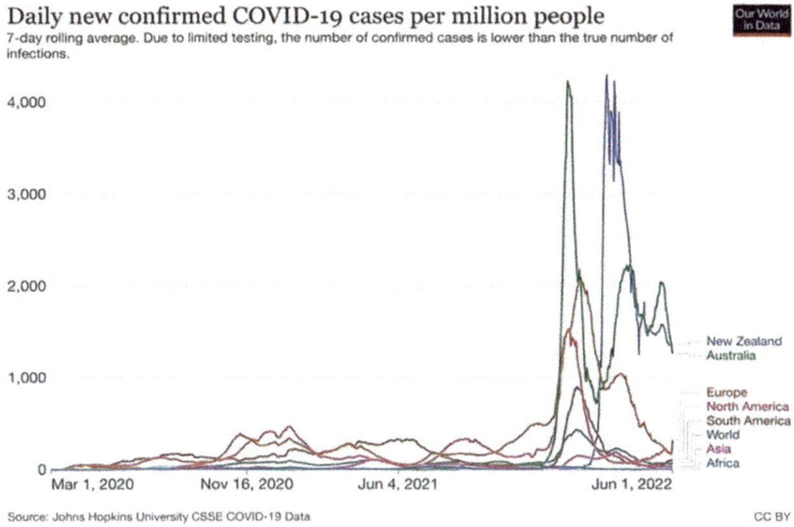

Figure 5.5: Covid-19 daily new deaths per million people

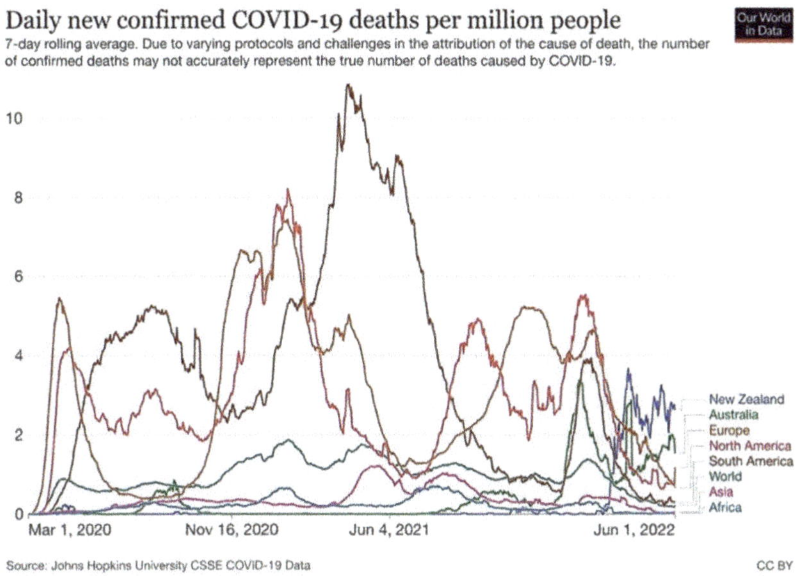

The one thing I had neglected to do is to put the Australian and New Zealand experience in global context. Figures 5.4 and 5.5 rectify that neglect. For the last two months, Australasian Covid cases per million people have been dramatically higher than African, Asian, European, North and South American, and world averages *at any time throughout the pandemic*. The current Covid mortality rates in Australasia too are higher than elsewhere.

I ask again: if this is vaccine success, what would vaccine failure look like?

Coronavirus has become endemic, making Australia's policy settings obsolete[37]

A major study from the National Bureau of Economic Research in June, based on all-causes mortality data from 44 countries and all US states, concluded that earlier and longer lockdowns do not reduce deaths and if anything, lockdowns may increase deaths. Consistent with the NBER and several other studies confirming that lockdown restrictions are ineffectual for virus control, on Friday, weeks into the state's 7th—or is it 8th?—lockdown, Victoria announced 510 new cases. Meanwhile on the same day, five weeks into a lockdown imposed after one case and with 55% full vaccination, the ACT recorded 30 new cases, bringing the total of active cases to 245 and another 341 recovered.

We know the virus doesn't keep climbing and growing exponentially. That hasn't happened anywhere in the world. Sooner or later, the curve will bend and head down. The strategy seems to be to wait for that peak, claim proof of success for restrictions and begin lifting them. Otherwise the doubling down on lockdowns despite daily evidence of how completely ineffectual they are makes no sense whatsoever.

Even more depressingly, most journalists and people seem to accept that transparent but flawed logic and credit their government

[37] *Spectator Australia*, 20 September 2021, https://www.spectator.com.au/2021/09/coronavirus-has-become-endemic-making-australias-policy-settings-obsolete/

with successful Covid management, despite clear evidence—both locally and globally—that policy interventions enforce coercive control on human behaviour without materially altering virus behaviour.

Unused to sceptical and aggressive questioning—remember the good old days when this was the norm for journalists worth the name in interactions with politicians and officials?—ACT Chief Minister turned testy when grilled by Sky News reporter Tom Connell last Wednesday. On Friday Barr warned of "thousands of cases and an overwhelmed health system" if the ACT opens up at 70% full vaccination.

The closest approximation to a petri dish for studying the infectiousness and lethality of SARS-CoV-2 was the cruise ship *Diamond Princess*, site of the largest early outbreak outside China in February 2020. Outbreaks seed easily on cruise ships because of the high numbers of susceptible elderly passengers living and socialising in confined quarters. Yet even under the worst possible conditions, only a small proportion of the entire captive population was infected, a small number of the infected died and 98.2% recovered. Consistent with this, of the world's current 18.7mn active cases, only 0.5% are "serious or critical."

Table 5.1: Covid-19 metrics/mn people, Israel and the UK, 2020 and 2021

Date	*Israel*			*UK*		
	Cases	Weekly hospital admissions*	Deaths	Cases	Weekly hospital admissions*	Deaths
14 Sep 20	428	112	2.0	44	14	0.2
14 Sep 21	1254	156	3.8	477	99	2.0

* 6 Sep 20 and 5 Sep 2021

Source: Our World in Data.

This is useful background for debating vaccines. In September 2020 vaccines had not yet been developed. On 13 September 2021, 63% and 65% of the Israeli and British populations were fully vaccinated. Yet the infections, hospitalisation and mortality rates are higher than a year ago by orders of magnitude in both countries (Table 5.1). We can but wonder: What would these statistics be if the vaccines were not so highly efficacious in reducing Covid infections, hospitalisations and deaths? Of course, the mischievous question aside, the obvious riposte is that the last wave was caused by the much more transmissible Delta variant.

In the UK, based on the risks of Covid and the benefits of vaccines, the Joint Committee on Vaccination and Immunisation (JCVI) recommended against vaccinating 12-15 year olds. A group of 26 Tory MPs warned on 10 September that overruling expert advice from the JCVI risks "dissolving the bond of trust" between the public and the government. But because the government had already decided to do so, it tasked the chef medical officers to formulate a recommendation based on broader considerations than just the science. Surprise, surprise—they recommended vaccination, including overruling parental decisions because a child is deemed to be fit and able to offer informed consent on its own, to offset the mental health stress of students caused by—wait for it—lockdowns! Even more surprise—the government promptly acted on their advice.

Thus a 12-year old without the legal capacity to vote or drive is mature enough to inject itself with a vaccine using a revolutionary new technology after a fast-tracked approval process for emergency use before all short and long-term safety trials have been completed. Taking children's welfare decisions away from parents and vesting it in the state as the arbiter of the family was something we've previously associated only with communist regimes. A nominally Conservative government has undermined parental authority, and that too against the best judgment if its own scientific experts.

The coronavirus pandemic has been the biggest and most successful power grab by self-aggrandising medicine men—sorry, health experts and officials—in Western history. Careerist politicians simply rolled over and then discovered that actually, spreading mass fear and hysteria through pandemic porn is a pretty effective way to dismantle all checks on the exercise of power and to win re-elections with massive mandates. The media has failed to do its job and hold the government's feet to the fire.

It's beyond belief and very dispiriting that we can all be locked up on the whim of a state or federal chief medico with no health advice published, against the mounting data from around the world that the pre-Covid consensus on the futility-cum-long term harms from lockdowns was correct.

Mandatory vaccine passports would be justified if:

- The disease was exceptionally severe, highly transmissible and lethal;
- There was clear and compelling evidence of efficacy;
- There was extremely low risk of serious side effects; and
- Alternative treatment options were lacking.

Every one of these is questionable on good scientific and observational data grounds. As I have argued in previous articles, the efficacy of vaccines is more limited than initial claims for infections, hospitalisations, and transmission.

Figure 5.6: Infections among unvaccinated and fully vaccinated Israelis

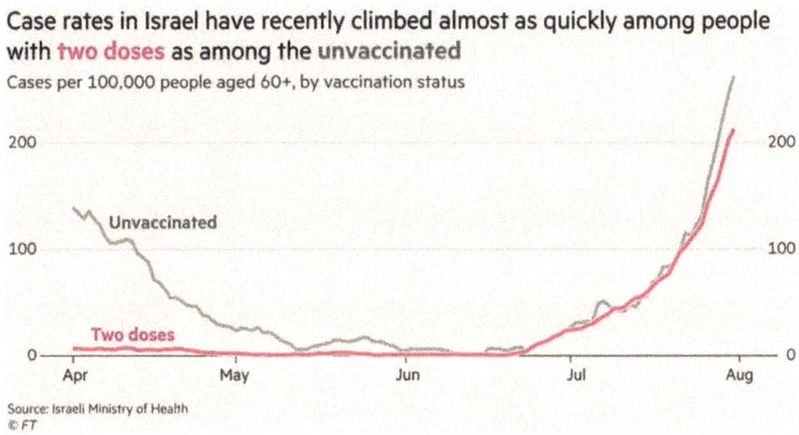

The known, immediate harms are greater than for existing approved mass vaccines. In some cases, as in Israel, there is also a curious positive correlation between vaccine doses and infection curves (Figure 5.6). Moreover, the risk, efficacy and harms equation changes dramatically by age groups because Covid is so exceptionally age-segregated. Thus a senior pharmaceutical executive, using JCVI data, notes that with 12-15-year-olds, one vaccination dose is expected to prevent seven children and two doses will prevent just eight kids from ending up in the paediatric ICU. On the harms side of the equation, between 9-54 children will likely suffer vaccine-induced myocarditis following one dose and 38-108 after two doses.

Alternatives have not been explored rigorously with any sense of urgency. Instead, they've been summarily dismissed. The most contested of these today is ivermectin. The signals from three parallel tracks—observational data, meta-analyses and randomised controlled trials—are suggestive but not conclusive in pointing to its potential efficacy both for preventing and for treating Covid.

Consider, for example, the case of India. After all, that is where the Delta variant originated and we all remember—or should remember—the conscience-shocking footage of corpses washing ashore on the banks of the Ganges and people dying on the streets like fish out of water gasping for air. Both the infections and mortality curves in India are more or less bell-shaped, with a slight hiccup in the mortality curve. But the steep descent in both cases began when just 2.45-3.0% of Indians had been fully vaccinated, and were completed with the full vaccination coverage still under 7%. Vaccines therefore could, at best, have played only a minor part in ending the surge.

Figure 5.7: Ivermectin use in Delhi and Uttar Pradesh, India, 2021

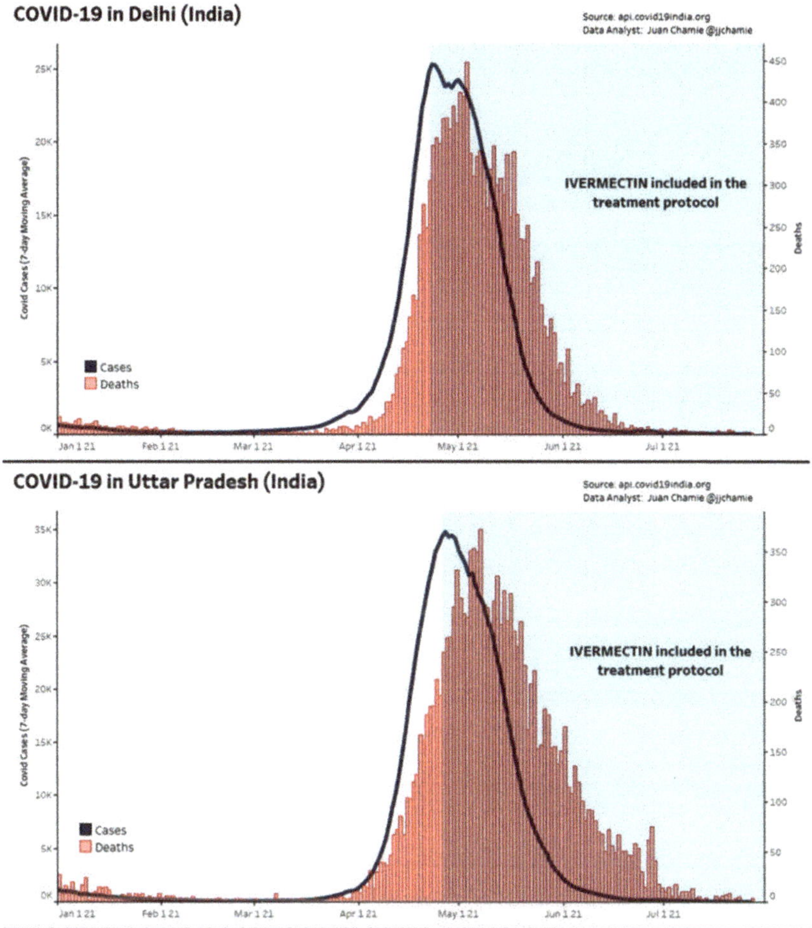

Source: Front Line COVID-19 Critical Care Alliance

A more plausible explanation is that Delta, while ferociously transmissible, is not in fact so deadly. And, in contrast to the reigning scepticism among Australia's all-powerful health bureaucrats, another likely candidate is the widespread adoption of ivermectin to treat the disease by several states, including Delhi and Uttar Pradesh (population 200 million!) (Figure 5.7).

Unaware that he was being broadcast live to the nation on a TV station with a microphone still switched on, Israeli health minister Nitzan Horowitz admitted on 12 September that vaccine passports were primarily about putting pressure on a hesitant public to get vaccinated and not for medical reasons. Meanwhile, who would have expected Sweden, which never imposed a hard lockdown but is 61% fully vaccinated, to ban travellers from Israel? There's a turn for the books.

There is no medical or ethical justification for vaccine compulsion and coercion because both groups can be infected and transmit the virus. To survive Covid-19, infected people must have mounted an effective immune response. The goal of vaccination is to generate memory cells that can recognise the virus and rapidly mount an effective immune response. As a group of doctors from Arkansas note in the British Medical Journal, "There is now a growing body of literature supporting the conclusion that natural immunity not only confers robust, durable, and high-level protection against Covid-19, but also better than vaccine induced immunity." Ignoring this reality instead of developing policy around it has seriously damaging real-world consequences, especially for poor countries.

With many infectious diseases, naturally-acquired immunity through infection is more powerful than vaccine-induced immunity and also lasts a lifetime. Several studies show stronger and more durable natural than vaccine-induced immunity against Covid-19. In August, for example, Israeli researchers published the largest real-world observational study to date comparing natural and vaccine-induced immunity using the 2.5 million strong database of Maccabi Healthcare Services. The team conducted two analyses to show that uninfected but vaccinated Israelis were 6-13 times more likely to get infected than the naturally immune through prior infection; their risk of symptomatic infection was 27 times higher; and their risk of hospitalisation was eight times more.

We seem to be in the gloaming phase of the dystopian night of a technology-enabled takeover of our lives by big business and government. It's time to "ditch-'n-switch" as a pathway out of the nightmare.

The phone is an instrument for my convenience, not a tool of control and coercion for the convenience of governments. The use of facial recognition AI technology by China to control the Uyghurs is one frightening example of the potential. Given how quickly Western governments seem to be moving towards China's social credit system in "keeping us safe" from Covid, there can be little confidence that China doesn't also offer a foretaste of what to expect as the surveillance state tightens its grip on our lives. In fact the first step has already been taken with South Australia's Covid app, as Alex Antic wrote here last week.

Almost all Australian governments, captured by "worrywart epidemiologists" (thank you, Judith Sloan), seem obsessed with test and trace as the silver bullet to virus eradication. It's expensive, intrusive and of limited utility in managing the disease, but it does keep alive the fear and paranoia and elevates stress and anxiety in society.

It's long past time to acknowledge that SARS-CoV-2 is already endemic in the world and will keep circulating, mutating and escaping variant-specific vaccines; abandon mass testing and contact tracing of the asymptomatic; return to treating symptomatic cases only; encourage vaccine take-up through persuasion of its beneficial protective effects for individuals without vilifying the unvaccinated who pose no greater risk to others than the vaccinated; and lift all remaining restrictions on people's lives and business activities.

Panic merchants, be gone... Covid is just another virus[38]

From the very start of the pandemic, a small but critical minority of us has argued that irrespective of the paths taken to get there, the end state will be living with Covid-19 as an endemic virus. The key

---

[38] *The Weekend Australian*, 19–20 February 2022, https://www.theaustralian.com.au/inquirer/panic-merchants-be-gone-covid-is-just-another-virus/news-story/8b350a03acbc0061c7162e207789df36

question was never: how do we eradicate this virus? Rather: what is the level of risk that we are prepared to accept and live with?

Unfortunately, like cascading dominoes, governments all over the world engaged in herd behaviour to lock down their countries based on apocalyptic modelling projections.

Models are neither science nor data but a set of assumptions that generate their own tautological conclusions. The Spectator UK has a brutal set of charts showing the wildly inaccurate projections of most models by various British teams that vastly over-estimated the harms with regard to cases, hospitalisations, ICU occupancy and deaths.

The actual data was massively better than the best-case scenarios of the original Doherty Institute modelling of March 2020.

The serial parties in No. 10 suggest the people at the very top of the British government knew the risks were low but terrified the populace into blind compliance with draconian curtailments of liberties just because they could.

At best, non-pharmaceutical interventions so beloved by governments keen to indulge their inner bossiness have had only a modest effect on the life cycle of each outbreak. Successive waves powered by new variants seem to rise and fall according to similar patterns—independent of the timing and duration of restrictions.

Last month, a major meta-analysis of 24 international studies from Johns Hopkins University by US and Scandinavian researchers found that "ill-founded" lockdowns reduced Covid-19 mortality only by between 0.2 and 2.9%, but at considerable economic cost and health and social harms. Therefore "lockdowns should be rejected out of hand as a pandemic policy instrument".

Another study on February 1 by a nine-strong team of American, British and Canadian researchers concluded that vaccine mandates, passports and segregated lockdowns can cause more harm than good. "While Covid-19 vaccines have had a profound impact on decreasing global morbidity and mortality burdens," "population-wide mandatory vaccine policies" impinge "on human rights, promote stigma and social polarisation, and adversely affect health and wellbeing," and could have detrimental impacts on future public health measures including immunisation programs.

From March 1, 2020, to January 31, 2022, the average total deaths would be around 307,000. The total number of Covid-related deaths in that period, whether "with" or "of" Covid, is 3,835 or 1.2% of all deaths. As always, Australia's big killers remain cancers, heart diseases, Alzheimer's and dementia, and strokes. Improved diet and more exercise would have given us better health returns as a country. Instead, locking people in their homes for prolonged periods, restricting exercise, curtailing social interactions, increasing weight gain, stress, loneliness and alcohol dependency, forcing families apart, stopping the bonding and healing rituals of birthdays, weddings and funerals, denying quality time with children, grandchildren, parents and grandparents, creating a backlog of health demands, and depriving children of friends and education, all as the pathway to better public health, indicate just how unhinged some "experts" are.

Less acutely in Australia than elsewhere, the public health system was saved but, sadly, tens of thousands of patients died and many more suffered neglect and delays. No country can improve long-term public health and human wellbeing by making itself poorer. In the 23 months to February 1, Australia's recorded number of suicides was 73% more than Covid deaths.

The "hygiene hypothesis'" suggests that long-term normalisation of extreme hygiene practices like "masking, deep cleaning, distancing and isolation can be harmful to health, especially for children, precisely because it reduces exposure to microbes," says Dr Eran Bendavid from the Stanford School of Medicine. By impeding the development of natural immunity, vaccines may make the vaccinated more vulnerable to virus variants.

Despite 76% and rising full vaccination since 1 November, more Australians have died with Covid in the past three months than in the 20 months before. In the US, this is more politically charged as Covid deaths under Joe Biden exceed those under Donald Trump and case rates are currently highest in the most vaccinated states.

Closer to home, consider Kiribati. As of 18 January, its total number of Covid cases since the pandemic started was just two. By 15 February, the numbers had exploded to 2,665 (and eight deaths). The virus came in on a flight from Fiji on 15 January. All 54 passengers were fully vaccinated, had tested negative three times prior to departure, been quarantined for a fortnight before departure and again after arrival, and were masked during the flight. Despite the stringent precautions, 36 tested positive on arrival and the virus then spread quickly through the tiny Pacific island despite lockdown since 22 January.

Vaccines continue to show strong protective benefits for the elderly and vulnerable groups. But governments overhyped claims about vaccines ending the contagion by checking infection, exaggerated universal vaccination as the key to freedom from restrictions thereby blaming the failures of the product on those who didn't take them, causing the stigmatisation of the unvaxxed.

More than a war on the virus, lockdowns proved to be a war on the poor to protect the laptop class. The loudest calls for lockdowns have come from those with secure incomes in lockdown-proof jobs. Yet sceptical voices from the beginning pointed to the existing data, experiences and plans developed over a century that emphasised the futility and collateral harms of prolonged society-wide lockdowns, on the one hand. On the other, noting the pronounced age-segregated severe effects of Covid-19, they recommended targeted policy interventions to protect the most vulnerable while keeping the rest of society functioning. And third, they dismissed the search for the holy grail of Zero Covid and insisted that the destination, as with all such disease outbreaks, would be endemic Covid.

Like Churchill's bon mot about the Americans, having tried everything else, will governments now do the right thing? Denmark and Sweden have already ended all restrictions, England has abandoned mandatory vaccination for health and social care workers and about another 10 European countries look set to follow.

Florida surgeon-general Dr Joseph Ladapo's prescription for managing Covid is: "Keep shutdowns short, keep the economy going, keep schools in session, keep jobs intact, and focus single-mindedly on building the capacity we need to survive this into our healthcare system." The experts who have held sway for two years are mostly research scientists in thrall to abstract models or public health experts with a bias towards controlling all of society. The minority of lockdown sceptics among medics, on the other hand, are concentrated among those engaged in clinical practice on the Covid frontline.

We neither require mandatory testing nor encourage universal vaccination for the annual flu, vaccines for which are even less efficacious than for Covid. Dr Arnold Monto from Michigan University's School of Public Health recommends managing endemic Covid like flu: make vaccines (bi)annually based on best-guess estimates of dominant variants, target the elderly and vulnerable populations for free recommended vaccination, make it available at cost to anyone wanting it, and learn to live with Covid as we've learnt to live with flu.

New Zealand: Mugged by Covid reality[39]

Initially, New Zealand attained extraordinarily successful results in keeping Covid under control and was widely lauded—by Anthony Fauci, ABC in Australia, the *Guardian*, NPR, the *New York Times*—as a model for hardline policy under decisive leadership (read: in contrast to Bad Orange Man who lived in a white house somewhere in Washington, DC).

With the passage of time, as evidence mounted of the folly of Zero Covid policy and the accumulating harms it was causing, the

[39] Brownstone Institute, 13 August 2022, https://brownstone.org/articles/new-zealand-mugged-by-covid-reality/

New Zealand government was trapped in a prison of its own construction and found it difficult to change course, even after the futility of the entire program became obvious in the data.

In truth the initial success owed much more to several fortuitous advantages attaching to New Zealand. When the first big wave of Covid swept across the world in February–March 2020, it was the height of summer in the Southern Hemisphere. While Covid can infect people in all seasons, it is mostly a winter virus and this gave New Zealand much more of a warning time than was available to Europe and North America.

New Zealand is also a small country of two inhabited islands, which makes border controls much easier to police and enforce, especially with most international passenger traffic coming through one terminal at one airport in Auckland. It is geographically distant from the world's major international traffic hubs and population centres.

Figure 5.8: New Zealand's cumulative Covid-19 deaths, Mar. 2020–Aug. 2022

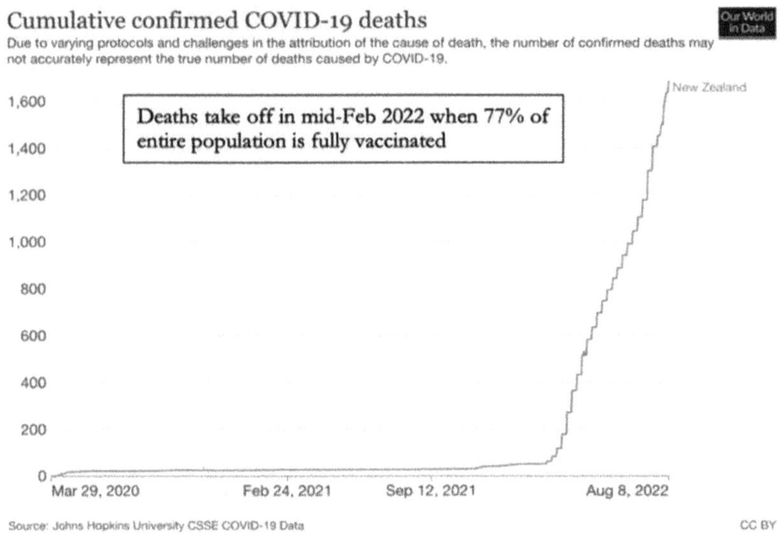

In combination with domestic isolation requirements, the prolonged strict border control measures kept New Zealand's Covid mortality down to around fifty until the end of 2021 (Figure 5.8). But by this time Covid was deeply seeded in the world's major population centres. Accordingly, unless New Zealand were to shut itself off permanently from the rest of the world, an impossible stipulation, the eradication strategy was already doomed.

New Zealand's strategy had bet the house on stringent measures until vaccines were developed and then the attainment of herd immunity through mass immunization. The bet seemed to have paid off with the development of Covid vaccines in December 2020.

But then the initial efficacy rates of the vaccines, which were granted emergency use authorisation long before the standard period for completion of safety as well as efficacy trials, proved to be of exceptionally short duration, necessitating boosters whose efficacy waned even faster.

This meant that the best pathway to herd immunity was through the combination of more robust and longer-lasting natural immunity from prior infection, and vaccines. It also meant that countries that had avoided mass infection through strict isolation measures had built up an immunity debt that left their populations more vulnerable to globally circulating pathogens once they did open up.

And the adverse eventual outcome would only be worsened if, as some epidemiologists had warned, contrary to the professional consensus, a mass vaccination campaign in the middle of a pandemic gave an evolutionary advantage to mutations of the virus with greater vaccine escape properties.

When the far more infectious if less lethal Omicron variant struck New Zealand, therefore, the vaccines developed to combat the original Wuhan strain proved unfit for the purpose of controlling the spread. New Zealand's cases and deaths really took off in mid-February 2022, despite a vaccination coverage of 77% of the entire population by then. In addition, the greater vulnerability of its population to new viral strains produced some sort of a catching-up effect in the Covid-related case, hospitalisation, ICU and death numbers.

By August 2022, New Zealand's cumulative Covid-19 cases per million people had surpassed the US and was on track to catch up with the UK and EU. Australia was ahead of all of them. To be fair, though, by this date Australia still had a Covid death toll only about one-fifth to one-sixth, and New Zealand between one-seventh to one-ninth, of the European, British and American figures.

Finally, the little matter of vaccine effectiveness. By August 2022, 80% of Kiwis were fully vaccinated, yet 85.5% of the total death toll was of people vaccinated with 2-4 doses. According to official data from the Ministry of Health (the infamous single source of truth), as at 9 August 2022, the country's total Covid deaths since February 2020 were 2,413.

People aged over 60 accounted for 91.5% of the total. Covid-19 was officially coded as the underlying cause in 44% of the total deaths, and as a contributory factor in another 24.2%.

As late as mid-March this year, the narrative of a pandemic of the unvaccinated was still plausible, as they comprised more than twice the number of Covid dead compared to their share in the general population, while the boosted dead were only around 40% of their population share. But in just three months there was a dramatic switch in their proportions. By now the unvaccinated are broadly the same share in the general population and among the Covid dead, while the boosted are overrepresented by almost 20% among the Covid dead compared to their population share.

According to Jennifer Margulis and Joe Wang writing in *The Epoch Times*, a couple of recent studies conclude that successive doses of mRNA vaccines can habituate and desensitize the body and in essence, teach it to become more coronavirus spike protein-tolerant. That is, the vaccines convert the body's natural immune response from protecting the body by attacking the spike protein, to tolerating it as non-threatening.

Yet another explanation of the turnaround since mid-March could be that with mass infections and the resulting naturally-acquired immunity, the vaccinated have lost their "competitive advantage" over the unvaccinated.

Whatever the explanation, as with the case of the state of New South Wales in Australia that was discussed in an earlier article, can we fairly talk of the pandemic of the vaccine-boosted in New Zealand?

For over two years, the Australian Human Rights Commission has been essentially missing in action insofar as the wide-ranging assault on civil rights and political freedoms are concerned. The same seems to have been true of the vast human rights machinery that has grown up in every democratic society that kept prudently quiet rather than confront the unchecked power of the administrative state as it rode roughshod over long-established individual rights vis-à-vis the state.

Recently, however, Australian Human Rights Commissioner Lorraine Finlay wrote in *The Australian* calling for a re-examination. "The failure to embed human rights considerations into pandemic planning," she wrote, resulted in "Covid-19 response measures that did not give sufficient weight to human rights concerns." Human rights considerations, she concludes, must be incorporated into future emergency planning "as a priority. Even in the middle of an emergency—perhaps especially in the middle of an emergency—human rights matter."

Yes!

Biggest mistake wasn't extra portfolios—it was this[40]

Scott Morrison finds himself in the eye of a growing storm for five additional portfolios he assumed, mostly without the knowledge of the cabinet and minister concerned. Most of these powers were never triggered and only one was possibly abused to overrule the resources minister to cancel a politically unpopular offshore gas drilling project.

---

[40] *Weekend Australian*, 20–21 August 2022, https://www.theaustralian.com.au/inquirer/uncertain-science-blighted-pandemic-management/news-story/74fc01d56c2f56676f328cc8da4e94e6

The justification for all this was the realisation that the declaration of a biosecurity emergency transforms the health minister into a de facto dictator. The other four portfolios will further cement the former prime minister's reputation for secretiveness and deception (of cabinet colleagues and the nation).

In the health portfolio, however, the problem lies with the law that grants such sweeping power to one person. Morrison was acting prudently to put in place guardrails against abuse. The secrecy betrayed his penchant for controlling behaviour. Instead, he should have openly explained the dangers and committed to amending the law.

The biggest mistake was to hand over control of the Covid agenda, in the false belief of following the science, to chief health officers (CHOs) who tend to be bureaucrats more than leading scientists engaged in cutting edge medical research. In the blink of an eye, they morphed from obscure officials to all-powerful chief executives. Australian authorities in effect copied New Zealand Prime Minister Jacinda Ardern's doctrine of the health ministry as the "single source of truth" on coronavirus. The unavoidable consequence of this was attempts, with legacy and social media help, to marginalise and silence all dissenting voices. The more the latter's warnings come true, the greater is the loss of trust in experts, institutions and ministers.

On 13 August 13 the Australian Medical Professionals Society published a wide-ranging letter addressed to all Australian colleges and associations of health, medicine and science. Along with the attached report by Dr Phillip Altman, the letter is an extraordinary yet authoritative catalogue of mistakes made in Australia's pandemic management and the many harms resulting from it, the uncertain science behind it, the limitations of vaccines, and the efforts of regulators to come between doctors and patients.

The Covid report from NSW Health for the week of 10–16 July says: "The minority of the overall population who have not been vaccinated are significantly over-represented among patients in hospitals and ICUs with Covid-19." Just two pages later the same report gives the number of unvaccinated people admitted to hospital and intensive care units as zero. The sentence is repeated verbatim in the latest weekly report for 31 July–6 August, with the number of unvaccinated people admitted to hospital at zero and to ICU just one.

Even by the standards of public health authorities across the world gaslighting the people to nudge them into docile—and often performative—compliance with official edicts, this level of internal contradiction of narrative with data is breathtaking.

Not a single Covid death under 40 was reported in the week to 6 August. The total number of boosted people who died with Covid was 71.3% of the 1,281 Covid deaths whose vaccination status was known, slightly above the "more than 68%" of eligible people who have been boosted. Thus the effectiveness of boosters in preventing death lasts only a short time.

People who have received two to four doses made up over 95% of the over-16s and 98.1, 95.8, and 82.6% of Covid hospital admissions, ICU admissions and deaths, respectively. In the 11 weeks from 22 May 22 to 6 August, the unvaccinated comprised 0.2%, 1.8% and 13.1% of all NSW Covid-related hospital admissions, ICU admissions and deaths, respectively. The double vaccinated and boosted made up 98.1%, 95.4% and 85% of the same respective totals. Just the boosted added up to 73.3%, 73.4% and 69.9%.

We are no longer in the realm of a pandemic of the unvaccinated. Despite major protective benefits, Covid vaccines are undeniably leaky. Their real-world effectiveness lasts a disappointingly short time.

Australia's relative success in 2020–21 was helped by fortuitous circumstances. Being an isolated island country, geographically distant from major international traffic hubs and population centres, made border controls easier to police and enforce. The international and domestic restrictions on travel, movement and activities kept Covid-related deaths to around 1,000 until September last year: an impressive accomplishment by global standards.

Then they exploded. In 2020–21, the government's response to the harsh international spotlight on the curtailment of many freedoms was to point to results. By now the performance-based international comparison has lost lustre. On 14 August, Australia's rate of 378,475 cumulative Covid cases per million people had surpassed the US (275,750), Britain (349,425) and EU (361,870) rates.

To be fair, though, the death toll is still only about one-fifth to one-sixth of the European, British and American figures, and we are in winter, when the virus is at its most virulent. Both case and mortality figures track the rise in the boosted from 1.51mn to 14.16mn in the period from mid-December to mid-August.

The best pathway to herd immunity was through the combination of natural immunity from prior infection and vaccines. Countries that avoided mass infection through strict isolation measures built up an immunity debt that left their populations more vulnerable to globally circulating pathogens once they reopened. When the highly infectious if less lethal Omicron variant struck, vaccines developed to combat the original Wuhan strain proved inadequate to controlling the spread.

Bowing to the growing body of studies and the weight of accumulating data, on 11 August the globally influential US Centres for Disease Control and Prevention issued new guidance. It marks a quiet yet major retreat from previous Covid management, based on the triple acknowledgment of "transient" protection from vaccination and boosters against infection and transmission, breakthrough infections among vaccinated, and naturally acquired immunity through infection. It also quietly dropped the false claim that the mRNA and spike protein "do not last long in the body."

The guidelines have moved sharply away from social distancing, quarantining, track-and-tracing, asymptomatic testing, and even vaccine requirements, abolishing the distinction by vaccination status for most settings. Their net threefold effect is to transfer much of the responsibility for risk reduction from institutions to individuals, to prioritise preventing severe illness over slowing transmission, and to switch from sweeping population-wide precautions to targeted advice for vulnerable populations.

If this looks similar to the much-reviled Great Barrington Declaration of October 2020 that merely restated the pre-Covid-19 medical-scientific consensus, that's because it is.

Ivermectin makes a comeback[41]

Writing for the Brownstone Institute, Debbie Lerman asked a provocative question: "What If There Had Been No Covid Coup" and the leading US public health agencies had been left in charge of the pandemic response? Instead, it was taken over by the National Security Council and the departments of defense and homeland security. The prevailing assumption being, of course, that the same set of responses would have unfolded over the next two to three years. She refutes this and explains with great clarity and considerable plausibility why the national security elite had to take over and what the implications are.

For one thing, the existing national and World Health Organisation guidelines would have been followed, to wit: don't panic, treat serious cases on presentation, keep society functioning as close to normality as possible, and look for inexpensive and widely available early treatment options to reduce the risk of serious illness. With national security agencies taking over, the new pandemic response paradigm became that of biowarfare: shut down society, institute medical countermeasures, and develop and roll out vaccines at warp speed. Designed to counter biowarfare and bioterrorism, they upended the scientific underpinnings and ethical principles of existing public health-based interventions. Propaganda, censorship and silencing of critical and dissenting voices were essential and therefore integral to the new normal.

---

[41] *Spectator Australia*, 2 September 2023, https://www.spectator.com.au/2023/09/ivermectin-makes-a-comeback/

In a complementary article, also for Brownstone, Dr Meryl Nass speculates that "maybe the vaccines were not made for the pandemic, and instead the pandemic was made to roll out the vaccines." As part of the evidence, she notes that Australia, the EU and the US were purchasing 8 to 10 vaccine doses per capita in mid-2021, despite unresolved doubts over their safety and prophylactic efficacy in infection and transmission. Because these were unresolved, the Covid vaccines could only be granted "emergency use authorisation" after a public health emergency had been declared in order, says the US Food and Drug Administration (FDA), to "prevent serious or life-threatening diseases or conditions when certain statutory criteria have been met, including that there are no adequate, approved, and available alternatives." In sum, fear porn was necessary to convince the public of the gravity and urgency of a public health emergency, which was then used to justify cutting corners in the development, manufacture and rollout of vaccines. But this could not be done if an alternative treatment was available. It therefore became necessary to reject any role for cheap, widely available and potentially lifesaving drugs like hydroxychloroquine and ivermectin, repurposed to treat Covid-19, and doctors were banned from recommending them for prophylaxis and early outpatient treatment.

With around four billion pills sold around the world over several decades, ivermectin's safety profile was well established. There were three parallel tracks along which to assess ivermectin efficacy and risks: randomised control trials, observational data and meta-analysis. The signals from all three indicated moderately positive outcomes. These included observational data from Brazil and states in Peru and India, plus meta-analyses supported by the WHO, Stockholm-based physician Sebastian Rushworth, and biostatistician Andrew Bryant and medical doctor and researcher Tess Lawrie. These showed between 56% and 62% mortality reduction associated with ivermectin use. However, although suggestive, these were not conclusive enough to establish ivermectin's efficacy in preventing and treating Covid.

A study of ivermectin (IVM) use in Peru, using excess deaths rather than deaths with Covid as the yardstick, found a 74% mortality reduction in the 30 days after peak deaths in the ten of Peru's 25 states with the most intensive IVM use. Strikingly: "During four months of IVM use in 2020, before a new president of Peru restricted its use, there was a 14-fold reduction in nationwide excess deaths and then a 13-fold increase in the two months following the restriction of IVM use."

Unfortunately, pharmaceutical companies frown on cheap generic drugs like ivermectin and few regulators of rich Western countries were able to escape industry capture. On 4 February 2021, Merck—which makes patent-free low profit Ivermectin and has been selling it for years—questioned its safety. In August 2021, the FDA warned Americans against taking ivermectin, a medicine used to deworm livestock: "You are not a horse. You are not a cow. Seriously, y'all. Stop it." The next month, Australia's TGA banned GPs from prescribing ivermectin for preventing or treating Covid-19, citing "a number of significant public health risks associated with taking ivermectin in an attempt to prevent Covid-19 infection rather than getting vaccinated." In other words the ivermectin ban was meant to promote vaccination.

The August 2021 tweet from the FDA, reinforcing the message that ivermectin was a horse de-wormer and not authorised to treat Covid-19, went viral. In response, some ivermectin-prescribing doctors took the FDA to court. During oral arguments in a US appeals court on 8 August 2023, Ashley Cheung Honold, a Department of Justice lawyer representing the FDA, said the "FDA explicitly recognises that doctors do have the authority to prescribe ivermectin to treat Covid." Australia's TGA had already lifted its restrictions on IVM from 1 June 2023. Suspicions grew that the financial interests of the pharmaceutical sector might have unduly influenced regulators' decisions in banning the use of ivermectin. These have been strengthened with the removal of the bans: how can a product that was considered safe for decades before 2020 but banned during 2020-22 suddenly become safe once again?

In this connection, it is worth noting that the Peru study was published in preprint on 8 March 2021, yet it was not published as a peer-reviewed article in the *Cureus Journal of Medical Science* until 8 August 2023. The journal says its average time from submission to publication is 33 days. Readers can draw their own conclusions.

On 12 May, Governor Ron DeSantis signed four laws aiming to give Florida the strongest protection of medical freedoms in America. The package protects citizens against testing, mask and vaccine mandates by government, business and educational institutions. It also protects medical professionals' freedom of speech and their right to prescribe alternative treatments to their patients.

Writing in the *Federalist* on 21 August, Jay Bhattacharya and Martin Kulldorff, two of the three authors of the Great Barrington Declaration, argue that after the litany of lies, abuses of power and conflicts of interests exposed during the Covid years, the US Congress must enact structural reforms of the National Institutes of Health.

Could we please copy both initiatives?

They Profiled Citizens According to Their Degree of Compliance[42]

There has been an unexpected validation of the title of *Our Enemy, the Government* (Brownstone, 2023). In a stunning indictment of the state of governance in the Australian state of Victoria, an unidentified senior bureaucrat classified citizens according to their compliance with the government's Covid diktats. This is the state whose capital Melbourne suffered through the world's longest lockdown (267 days!).

Yet, according to the Australian Bureau of Statistics Victoria had the worst overall Covid mortality outcome between March 2020 and

[42] Brownstone Institute, 12 December 2023, https://brownstone.org/articles/they-profiled-citizens-according-to-their-degree-of-compliance/

the end of September 2023, with a standardised death rate of 16.1 per 100,000 people compared to the national average of 12.4. New South Wales was the second worst with a rate of 13.5 and Western Australia the best with 7.7 deaths per 100,000 people. But rather than concern about mismanagement of the pandemic, peoples' compliance score (Figure 5.9) was of more interest to the government than investigating the scientific validity, factual basis, collateral harms and the net cost-benefit equation of their Covid interventions.

Figure 5.9: Five classes of Victorians based on lockdown compliance, 2022

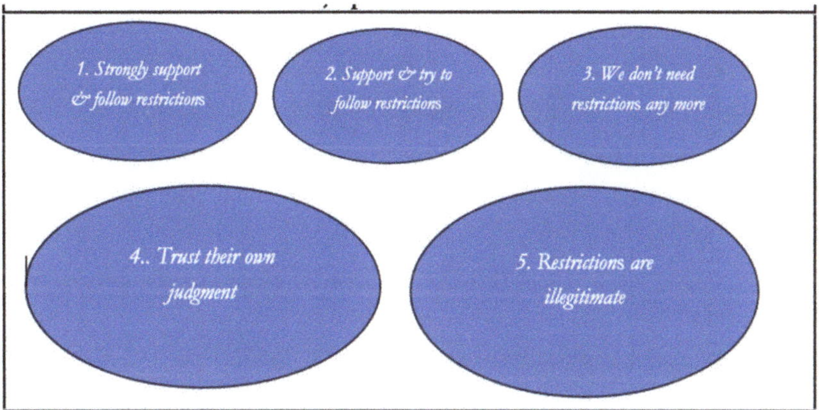

Source: *The Australian*, 12 December 2023, https://www.theaustralian.com.au/nation/politics/official-in-lockdown-profiling-of-victorian-citizens/news-story/a33645ca047d598df4c9c8998d5ce450

The Australian reported on 12 December that those most critical of and strongly opposed to the volley of pandemic triggered restrictions on individual and commercial activities and personal freedoms, who had the critical faculty and temerity to believe that the threat of Covid was exaggerated, "tyrannical government is the enemy," prioritised individual over collective rights, didn't accept the authority of the government to "tell them what to do," believed the restrictions to be "illegitimate" and to be followed only under coercion, and were all too likely to embrace "fantastical conspiracy theories."

Unfortunately, Premier Dan Andrews' shadowy political intelligence and strategy from QDOS Research conceded, this small share of the total population still covered a "lot of people." The report was sent to the government on 6 April 2022. It was only recently released to the *Australian* under a Freedom of Information request.

At the opposite end of the five-band spectrum (Figure 1) were the most compliant people who trusted the authorities to act in the best interests of the community, were inclined to "strongly support and follow restrictions" as the right thing to do for the family and the community, didn't want to catch Covid or pass it on, and did not consider the restrictions to be "overly onerous."

Thus the government was using taxpayer money to commission research from a private consultancy into grading people according to their Covid compliance score, in order to devise a strategy to persuade them into following government directives and obey government orders. Addressed chiefly as a public health matter, the primary concern would have been the health and safety of the people. Instead the primary motivation was clearly political control and moulding public opinion for partisan advantage.

Unfortunately, once collective welfare is allowed to override individual rights, the government acquires unlimited unchecked power. Whole societies ended up with every aspect of their lives micromanaged by bureaucrats and technocrats with no philosophical grounding in public health ethics. Several governments will have been delighted at the success of the trial run in demonstrating just how weak and narrow the pushback was. Even now, it would be a check on future abuse and thus a deterrent if the name of the top bureaucrat(s) were to be published.

The optimists in us might hope that the next time, the noncompliant group 5 will be substantially bigger and stronger, even though most of them are likely to have fled Victoria as soon as they could. The pessimists will feel vindicated by a new poll in the UK showing support for the reintroduction of mandatory facemask in public transport, if required on health grounds, by 41-46% of people depending on age (those above 40 being the most supportive), one-third of people backing closures of nightclubs, and one-fifth being prepared to support confinement in homes again except for essential activities. If this is how people feel now absent any sense of a health emergency, they would appear to be ripe for serial repeats of the restrictions of 2020–22 if accompanied by fearmongering by the medical-public health-industrial complex.

Carbon Insights: Foreshadowing a social credit system?

Meanwhile a friend alerted me to a sneaky item from the Commonwealth Bank of Australia. The CBA, originally government owned but privatised in 1996, is one of Australia's big four banks. It operates something called the "Carbon Insights" program. The site helpfully says: "We're helping our customers understand their environmental impact by providing insights through a personalised carbon footprint based on spending transactions and tips that promote sustainable living."

The website explains that customers' carbon footprint is measured by considering the spending transactions made on their personal CommBank accounts, including transactions, credit cards and digital payments, against averaged industry carbon emissions data for the fashion and transport sectors. Meaning collecting my data for any fashion products and travel tickets purchased by credit cards, payment for which is linked to my CBA account.

Understanding individuals' carbon footprint is the first step in learning about how to become more environmentally conscious. The feature records information on how customers' emissions are associated with personal spending habits and additional insights on the relevant categories that contribute to a personalised footprint output.

This sounds suspiciously like the necessary first step in designing and then implementing a social credit system, the end point of which will be to reward and punish based on government defined social good. We agreed that, as far as we could recall, that none of us had been asked to consent to this. So next I followed their advice on learning how they handle personal information by checking out their Privacy Policy here. There is nothing about carbon footprint or the Carbon Insights program here.

Puzzled as well as worried, as I have a neuralgic aversion to being tracked online, I read the details again, this time slowly and more deliberately, I registered the sentence: "The Carbon Insights feature is now available in the CommBank app." Since, despite what seems like weekly enticements I have refused to download the app, I breathed a sigh of relief.

Even so, to use the environmental activists' language, another dispiriting sign that we may be very close to the tipping point for entry into the brave new world.

Perrottet's Covid apology is not good enough[43]

Former New South Wales Premier, Dominic Perrottet, came out yesterday and declared that Covid vaccine mandates enforced by his government were "wrong."

It's all well and good for Mr Perrottet to come clean now, during a valedictory speech, as he retires from politics.

There are no consequences for his admission, no risk to his political future, and therefore no bravery or credit which I am prepared to offer him.

At the time the mandates were discussed, Mr Perrottet was the one man in NSW with the power to protect people from dangerous, insufficiently tested, and unsatisfactorily trialled vaccines. He, alone, was the person with the elected power to protect the rights of every New South Welshman and allow them to *choose* what to put into their body and what sort of health risk they were prepared to take.

[43] Flat White, *Spectator Australia*, 7 August 2024, https://www.spectator.com.au/2024/08/perrottets-covid-apology-is-not-good-enough/

He could have kept people employed and put an end to idiotic and patently false health messaging. As Premier, that was his job.

I have always said that the government should not be allowed to mandate a citizen drink a glass of water, let alone inject a product from pharmaceutical companies who are protected—by law—from damages. We are people, not common lab rats.

As far as I am concerned, it is not good enough for Mr Perrottet to insist the government was acting with "the right intentions," especially when the government was told—in the pages of this magazine—that what they were doing was wrong.

The vaccine handbook, which has been with us for a long time, made it clear that Mr Perrottet's decision, and that of Gladys Berejiklian before him, was wrong and that the advice from the Health Minister was in violation of the basic liberties we expect to enjoy as a civilised people. A Health Minister, I might add, who ignored mountains of evidence that contradicted their assertions.

None of this is news to Mr Perrottet, who seemed as uncomfortable with what he was saying at the time.

What he lacked was not a conscience, but a spine—a spine tough enough to stand up to the peer pressure of power-hungry Labor Premiers and the Liberal Prime Minister, Scott Morrison, who looked down the barrel of the camera and declared that there was no such thing as a vaccine mandate while tens of thousands were marched out of their jobs. Most of them never got their jobs back. Many of them sit idle today, broken by what they have lost.

Mr Perrottet's valedictory speech is weaker than the headline trending on social media: "If the impact of vaccines on transmission was limited at best, as is now mostly accepted, the law should have left more room for respect of freedom. Vaccines saved lives, but ultimately, mandates were wrong. People's personal choices shouldn't have cost them their jobs."

Mr Perrottet, these Covid vaccines killed people and left many more seriously injured.

A state mandate—a mandate put out by the Liberal government—not only robbed people of their liberty, but of their lives. This is inexcusable.

> *When I became premier, we removed [vaccine mandates] or the ones we actually could, but this should have happened faster. If a pandemic comes again, we need to get a better balance encouraging people to take action whilst at the same time protecting people's fundamental liberty.*

No, Mr Perrottet.

We need to urgently reverse the expanded emergency powers that premiers—in particular Victoria's Daniel Andrews—gifted themselves. We need legislation to prohibit politicians taking advantage of a public health situation and ensure that every single emergency decision has a non-negotiable sunset clause coupled with an extremely high bar of physical data before they can be implemented. None of this, "Oh well, if the premier *thinks* there's a risk of a pandemic, we can do…'

Pharmaceutical companies need to have their immunity stripped and ensure that the public and the State (on behalf of the public) remain free to seek damages for faulty, dangerous, or non-functioning drugs. We never want to see another situation where hundreds of billions of public money is spent on foreign drug companies for a mandated vaccine only for large quantities of it to be thrown in landfill. Who is responsible for this hideous waste of money? Mr Morrison? He's toddled off. Mr Albanese? He's washed his hands of Covid.

Most importantly, we need to have some kind of severe punishment for the behaviour of our premiers, prime ministers, health ministers, and media class (who took marketing money from vaccine companies) for the deliberate crucible of wall-to-wall fear propaganda that was created to manipulate the public perception of Covid and encourage them to take risks with their health they never would have done in a sane environment.

There remains no excuse for daily press conferences with death tolls posted in the corner without context, the constant creation of petty and unscientific health orders, the deployment of police and army personnel onto the street, the invention of digital stalking apps, the assignment of "ticks" and "crosses" to gatekeep the economy based on vaccine status, the setting up of "dobbing" websites to encourage neighbours to spy on each other—I could go on… Those who partook in and set up the framework for this abusive behaviour must face personal punishment or they will do it again.

Australians cannot like a post of Facebook without police knocking on the door, and yet every level of our government engaged in crimes against our humanity—what is their punishment? Cushy jobs and juicy retirement packages.

> *'If we established Australia today, no one in their right mind would set up the federation the way it is. We currently have federal and state health systems that don't even work alongside each other. Rather, they actively work against each other.*
>
> *If we can't reform the federal health system after a one in 100-year pandemic, we never will.'*

These are nonsense excuses, none of which absolve Mr Perrottet of his part in this sorry story. As Premier, he was elected to protect us—and he didn't. He threw us to the wolves and bent over at the first strike.

Are you too frightened to go outside? Are you "up to date" with Covid boosters? Why not? There is a 33% increase in Covid and serious flu infections. People are filling hospitals and plenty are dying.

Australia is not gripped by fear because the political swamp and the media class aren't up there on the screen telling everyone to be afraid. There's no political traction in peddling fear—so they're not doing it. They've moved on to the trillions of dollars waiting to be distributed on their new favourite headline—Climate Change.

I will never stop being angry about what happened to us during the Covid years but the least those in power could do is punish those who abused their position or—through inaction and cowardice—failed to act.

Hell, I'd settle for all of them having their pensions stripped. What do you think?

6: HEALTH INTERVENTIONS, PUBLIC MORALISM AND SILENCING DISSENT

As the weeks and months passed, and lockdowns turned into mask and then vaccine mandates in repeating cycles, with no end in sight, many wondered at the continuing public support. An important explanation seemed to be a belief that compliance was the right thing to do for the sake of the community, despite individual reservations.

Lockdowns could kill more people than Covid-19[44]

There has been a remarkable lack of observed statistical difference in the rates of death for countries, and for US states, that have and have not locked down. An assessment of the models used to project different scenarios must be evaluated relative to the lived reality.

There are strongly divergent views among software engineers, epidemiologists, medical scientists, physicists, chemists, and statisticians over the quality of the computer code behind the original Imperial College London model of 16 March, the reliability of modelling, the infection fatality rate (IFR), the evolutionary curve of the virus, the proportions and infectiousness of asymptomatic cases, its controllability by severity and timing of lockdowns, the threshold at which herd immunity is achieved, and if there is any

[44] *Australian Outlook*, 12 June 2020, http://www.internationalaffairs.org.au/australianoutlook/lockdowns-could-kill-more-people-than-covid-19/

realistic alternative to herd immunity. Some experts now believe there is cross immunity from people's exposure to the existing endemic coronaviruses, or natural T-cell immunity in certain genetic populations, while the WHO said most recently that it's very rare for asymptomatic cases to infect others.

There is little observational data that the reproduction rate has shot up alarmingly in places that have opened up. Instead the trend remains downward at broadly comparable rates logarithmically, providing mathematical confirmation of the observed reality. As people like Karl Friston, one of the world's topmost statisticians, Sunetra Gupta, John Ioannidis, and Michael Levitt have been predicting in opposition to the modellers from the beginning, the pandemic is as fast burning out in Europe and the US as it did in China.

It's hard to see much evidence in India either of the effectiveness of a stringent lockdown after two-and-a-half months, or of a self-flattening curve. On 30 May, India reported a record daily rise in coronavirus cases by almost 8,000 for a total of over 180,000 cases and 5,000 deaths. Yet, on that very day, India announced a substantial easing of lockdown restrictions. By 9 June its total death tally was 7,750. The explanation for the lifting of lockdown measures despite the continuing high numbers of infections and deaths is simple: the rise in deaths and misery caused by the lockdown, well beyond the capacity of India's health and transport networks and social safety nets to support, had become a huge national shame and scandal. India is not alone. *The Wall Street Journal* reported that many poor countries have shifted to easing lockdown restrictions despite rising infections and deaths because they've concluded that the cost in lives, livelihoods, and destitution are just too high.

On 29 May, Zaria Gorvett reported for the BBC Future program that most Covid-19 deaths will be not from the virus but from the collateral damage inflicted by the various lockdown measures. "Across the globe, patients have reported being denied cancer care, kidney dialysis and urgent transplant surgeries, with sometimes fatal results," she said. Reports from reputable bodies like Oxfam, the UN, and the Johns Hopkins School of Public Health have contained mutually reinforcing warnings that the severity of the lockdown measures could reverse a decade's worth of gains in infant and child mortality with over a million additional deaths, exacerbate health, hunger, and misery insecurities, and push another half billion people into poverty. There are some impassioned attacks on the immoral and callous indifference of epidemiologists to the deadly consequences of their prescriptions for millions of lives and livelihoods around the world.

Unfortunately, this isn't just a "Third World" worry. Australia's top mental health experts warn that a lockdown-induced 50% jump in suicides could kill ten times as many as the virus. With elective surgeries and routine screenings suspended, many cancers and heart diseases that are treatable if caught in time will dramatically elevate the death toll. An analysis of the official UK data from the Office for National Statistics concluded that of the excess deaths in England and Wales this year over last year's data to the week ending 1 May, only one-third can be explained by Covid-19. David Spiegelhalter, chair of the Winton Centre for Risk and Evidence Communication at Cambridge University, said on 12 May that, of the "staggering burden" of 30,000 more deaths than would normally be expected, only 10,000 have had Covid-19 specified on the death certificate.

Meanwhile Germany is in damage control after a leaked report challenged the established narrative. Its main conclusions are that the lethality of Covid-19 was overestimated compared to the normal flu level. The report highlights the grave, manifold, and heavy consequences of the measures to fight the virus and warns that more people are dying because of state-imposed mitigation measures than are being killed by the virus. Initially, the government dismissed the report as the work of one employee. But it turns out the 93-page report was drafted by a scientific panel that included medical experts from several German universities. Its authors issued a joint press release on 11 May criticising the government for ignoring expert advice. The

German government has not yet reacted, but on 23 May authorities confirmed that 52,000 cancer operations had been delayed.

Politicising science

The lack of robust science behind epidemiological modelling suggests that the policy has been transformed from a scientific to a political mission. Boris Jonson's top adviser, the by-now notorious Dominic Cummings who made a questionable 260-mile roundtrip to Durham during the lockdown, is said by Bloomberg news to have pressed the independent scientific advisers to recommend lockdown measures. On the excessive two-metre distancing rule, Professor Robert Dingwall is reported in *The Telegraph* on 7 May to have said a senior public health specialist told him "we knew it was one metre but we doubled it to two because we did not think the British population would understand what one metre was." So "we doubled it to be on the safe side."

In the UK, the Scientific Advisory Group for Emergencies (Sage) provides scientific and technical advice to support government decision makers during emergencies. Under pressure from a legal challenge from aviation tycoon Simon Dolan, on 29 May the government released the minutes of Sage meetings from the period leading up to the lockdown announcement on 23 March. Lawyer Paul Chaplin went through the minutes. On 18 March, Sage advised that "the measures already announced should have a significant effect," and additional measures might be needed only "if compliance rates are low." At no point before 23 March did Sage recommend anything resembling a full lockdown. Instead, at a meeting on 10 March, the group noted that banning public gatherings would have little effect since most viral transmission occurred in confined spaces, such as within households. Based on the earlier broad summaries provided, Christopher Snowdon from the Institute of Economic Affairs concluded: "the strategy which preceded the lockdown… was based on science whereas the decision to go into lockdown was political."

A scandal is brewing in Denmark because of a leaked email to the *Politiken* newspaper. The head of the health ministry told the head of the Health Authority to suspend his professionalism as a public servant, and instead adopt an "extreme precautionary principle" when giving political advice based on a deliberately inflated reproduction number (2.6, not 2.1). Prime Minister Mette Frederiksen then proceeded to mislead the public, it's alleged, by implying that her decision to impose a strict lockdown on the country was based on advice from the health agency. Queensland's Chief Health Officer Jeanette Young's logic on school closures is also primarily political. She accepts the evidence that schools are not a high-risk environment for the spread of the virus but closing them helps to convince people how grave the situation is. "So sometimes it's more than just the science and the health, it's about the messaging."

We need a Royal Commission to look back so we can go forward

All countries should undertake brutally honest retrospective analyses of the modelling used to design and implement mitigation, suppression, and elimination strategies in order to answer basic questions: how many deaths did lockdowns forestall; how many more could have been avoided by earlier hard lockdowns; how many excess deaths were caused by the direct and indirect effects of lockdowns? Typically, the models project various scenarios based on different policy interventions, from doing nothing to a growing list of mitigation measures as the best-case outcome. Yet the wide disparity between the predicted figures of deaths in Sweden and the observed reality as it played out is significant.

Figure 6.1: Australia's Covid-19 new cases vs recoveries

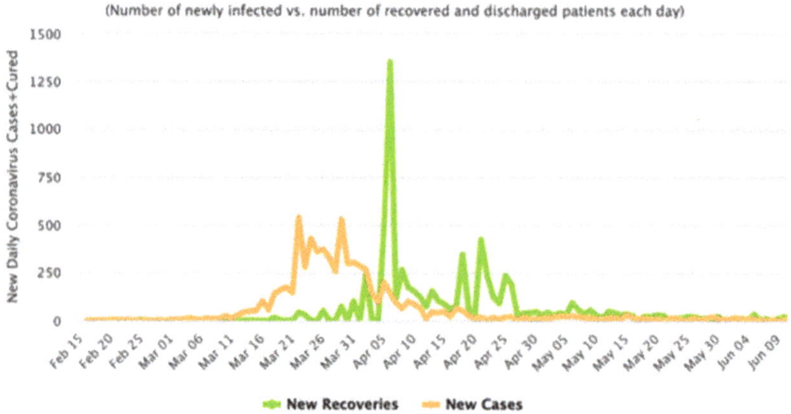

Source: Worldometers, 11 June 2020

The same would appear to be true of the Australian modelling released on 7 April. Here too the reproduction rate (R) had fallen below 1 and the number of recoveries had begun to exceed the number of new cases when stage 4 restrictions were imposed at the end of March (Figure 6.1). This then provides an independent and objective check against real data of the predictive utility of the models. Only that can give confidence about their predicted mortality tolls without the hard lockdowns. Governments that refuse to publish the modelling they based their decisions on back in March almost certainly are trying to hide their embarrassment. In Australia, on 5 June, a 29-strong group of economic and political figures called for the public release of modelling used by governments to make decisions on health emergencies and for governments to rely on broader sources of advice than just epidemiologists and public health experts.

As things stand, there are too many holes in the dominant narratives being peddled by governments, many of them inconsistent with one another. The federal government is unlikely to face significant backlash even if the inquiry concludes that the tough lockdown measures were not necessary and may have caused more harm than good.

Most people recognise that the situation looked fearful at the time and the authorities acted with the best motives for the collective interest. Citizens treated with respect as adults will reciprocate, provided mistakes are acknowledged and learned from. New institutions and procedures are needed to better prepare for future crises and move forward instead of being stuck in the past.

On 27 May, Norway's Prime Minister Erna Solberg went on television to confess she had panicked at the start of the pandemic and introduced the tough measures unnecessarily. In particular, closing of schools was not just unnecessary, but counterproductive. Margrethe Greve-Isdahl, the Norwegian Institute of Public Health (NIPH) expert on infections in schools, told the UK's Sunday Telegraph that if schools had stayed open, they could have played a role in informing people in badly hit immigrant communities of hygiene and social distancing rules. It's important to admit the truth, NIPH Director-General Camilla Stoltenberg said, because if the infection levels were to rise again, or a second wave hit Norway next winter, the country needed to be brutally honest about the effectiveness of lockdown.

Just so.

Maskerade: To wear not to wear?[45]

On the day of his inauguration, President Joe Biden signed a slew of executive orders, one of which mandated masks in all federal buildings. That evening he was spotted at the Lincoln Memorial *sans* mask. Press Secretary Jen Psaki explained that Biden was "celebrating an evening of a historic day" and there are "bigger issues to worry about at this moment in time." Biden thus began his presidency by joining a long list of officials who flout the rules they impose on all others, including Dr Anthony Fauci, director of the National Institute of Allergy and Infectious Diseases.

---

[45] *Spectator Australia*, 6 February 2021, https://www.spectator.com.au/2021/02/maskerade/

Masks are dehumanising and a potent force for stoking mass fear. Facial expressions are crucial in social interactions, including for babies. Compulsory masking for everyone in all settings is a gross violation of fundamental human rights. It can be justified only if the evidence for their efficacy in community protection is compelling and the risk of harms is negligible. Instead mask mandates have been heavy on fear-mongering and virtue-signalling but light on data and science, overturning, in a couple of months, cumulative scientific consensus built over decades. The empirical data from around the world last year mostly validates the previous consensus. Rather than protect communities, masks have given politicians delusions of omnipotence and liberated some cops to indulge their inner thugs against peaceful dissenters, as we saw in Melbourne.

In March, Fauci told people not to walk around with masks. It might make them feel better but doesn't provide perfect protection and people keep fiddling with it and touching their face. In July, after calling for everyone to wear masks, Fauci defended his original advice: "in the context of the time, it was correct" because we had "a serious problem with the lack" of personal protective equipment for healthcare workers. On 15 September he said a "national mandate probably would not work." But in a CNN interview on 23 October he called for a nationwide universal mask mandate.

Roger Koops explains how in the general population, masks confer no benefit and pose a net transmission risk to the wearer and others by trapping the virus on the inside and through surface contamination. Fauci's earlier comment accurately stated the existing consensus on benefits versus harms. This can be found in:

- The UK's Pandemic Preparedness Strategy (2011), reaffirmed on 27 February and by Deputy Chief Medical Officer Professor Jonathan Van Tam on 3 April;
- The state-of-the-art WHO report in September 2019, repeated by top WHO doctors Mike Ryan and Maria Van Kerkhove on

31 March 2020 and softened only slightly in the updated guidance on 5 June;

- An article in the prestigious New England Journal of Medicine;
- A large Danish study, based on the only randomised controlled trial anywhere (lab studies are useless in predicting real-life outcomes) published in the top-three medical journal *Annals of Internal Medicine*;
- A note from Oxford University's Centre for Evidence-Based Medicine.;
- An Australian Department of Health document in July 2020.

In the US, most randomised trials of community or household masking show mask-wearing has negligible effect on virus transmission. The Centers for Disease Control and Prevention (CDC) said 85% of coronavirus-infected Americans reported wearing masks always/often in the two weeks before their Covid illness. On 4 November, a team of US-based researchers withdrew their paper because of increased rates of Covid-19 cases in areas analysed in the study. They'd forgotten that respiratory infections decline in summer and climb again in autumn. In country after country and US states, caseloads surged in autumn/winter despite universal mask mandates—and did not surge as sharply in Denmark and Norway without mask mandates. When Sweden modified its anti-mask policy in mid-December, it was to recommend masks in public transport during rush hour.

The CNN said on 19 October: "Masks made Czech Republic the envy of Europe. Now they've blown it." On 26 January Czechia's deaths per million (DPM) was 1,441, a third higher than Sweden. Or consider New York and Florida with comparable populations. Florida is better on population density, warmth and sunshine, but has an older population. It's had open borders, parks, restaurants and schools for months. New York cancelled these simple pleasures and essentials of life with a stringent lockdown, including a statewide mask mandate from 17 April for anyone in a public place. Florida let individual counties decide. As of 26 January, Florida's mortality rate was half new York's: 1,185-2,189 DPM. Among Florida counties, 22 that had mask mandates for some time had 230 daily cases per million people in mid-December, and the 45 that never imposed a mask mandate had 220.

While useful as a psychological crutch against fear, masks can cause a range of potential harms as listed by the WHO. Many engage in riskier behaviour believing in the protective efficacy of masks. A German study published on 5 January noted a range of impairments experienced by 68% of children and adolescents wearing masks.

Government directives have been riddled with scientific illiteracy. There's no need for masks inside a car, for a family playing in a park or on the beach separated from others, or for a solitary farmer on his tractor in a lonely paddock in country Victoria. A Wisconsin state agency ordered its employees to be masked during Zoom meetings when home alone. Washington state mandated masks for youth sports whenever playing outside including in rain, even though a wet mask is useless. Proving history does irony, banks that once feared masked robbers now fear mask-free customers.

Covid "science," lockdowns and flat-earthers[46]

As we hurtle towards medical apartheid with ethically-challenged vaccine passports following anti-science lockdowns, answer me this: have you ever known any government refuse to publish expert analysis that supports its policy? Me neither.

Sweden famously framed policy in line with settled science and worldwide experience gained over a century. Florida flirted with the panic-driven mass flight from science, but only briefly. Settled science doesn't flip overnight. It wasn't a sudden scientific Eureka moment that resulted in lockdowns but being impressed by China's elimination

[46] *Spectator Australia*, 16 October 2021, https://www.spectator.com.au/2021/10/covid-science-lockdowns-and-flat-earthers/

of the outbreak in Wuhan. The tactics, although unpleasant, were believed to have been effective. When copied also by Italy, the architects of lockdowns have admitted they realised that Western democracies too could do the same.

Few paused to question the reliability of the data and the credibility of official claims. China's leadership couldn't have imagined in their wildest wet dreams how successful they would be in wrecking Western economies, social cohesion and democratic institutions and practices. After worldwide publicity of our police brutality, lecturing China on human rights evokes mocking ridicule.

The key to successful lockdown politics hasn't been science but fear. Victoria proves conclusively to the world, albeit not yet to most Victorians, that lockdowns are indeed a dead end, exactly as predicted by the settled science before madness set in last year. They delay but don't eliminate Covid, while drawing out the overall health, mental health, social, political and economic damage from repeating lockdown cycles. Follow the money, not the science. As proven by the collusion between the scientific-publishing-technological complex on the lab leak theory, much of science has been seduced and corrupted by Mammon with Chinese characteristics.

John Tierney recalls how Anthony Fauci and Robert Redfield (the last CDC director) fed alarmism in the 1980s about a heterosexual AIDS epidemic that never happened but greatly boosted the careers of both and gained them fat research grants. Alarmists paid no professional or personal price. I read with headshaking disbelief that Neil Ferguson was back before a cross-party UK parliamentary committee on 5 October with more gloom and doom predictions but many sceptics were pilloried, hounded out of office and ruined professionally. Being proven right years later was little help or consolation. Talk of history rhyming as farce.

Like other respiratory diseases, Covid can be managed as an endemic illness by a mix of natural immunity, vaccination, and treatment. Both local elimination and global eradication are unrealistic.

The just-approved malaria vaccine was developed over more than three decades by GlaxoSmithKline and has only 30% efficacy. In the 1950s, around 50mn annual cases of smallpox killed millions. After an eleven-year effort that cost just $300mn, smallpox was eradicated by 1980. Dr Monica Gandhi, an infectious disease expert at the University of California San Francisco, explains why Covid-19 isn't comparable to smallpox. The latter virus lacked an animal reservoir available to coronavirus; it had sharply distinguishing symptoms whereas Covid overlaps with symptoms from other respiratory diseases; the two have a short versus a prolonged period of infectiousness; and those who survived smallpox had lifelong immunity against it.

On the vaccines side of the equation, mRNA vaccines use revolutionary new technology; the safety trials for Covid vaccines were fast-tracked; the subjects in the trial did not reflect the risk distribution of Covid by age and comorbidities; and no longitudinal studies have been done yet. Compared to smallpox, Covid vaccines also have much more limited efficacy in strength, reduced risks of infection and transmission, and duration.

University of Melbourne epidemiologist Prof. Tony Blakely now concedes "You can't deny that Covid just does what it wants. Basically." No sh*t, Sherlock. Welcome to the dark side of the Covid street where for 19 months we've said virus gonna virus. Or, in more formal language, the trajectory of the virus has proven to be remarkably policy-invariant everywhere. Government interventions shape human behaviour without controlling virus behaviour. The NY Times now admits the virus surges and retreats in roughly two-month cycles, with no discernible correlation to lockdowns and mask mandates, that epidemiologists don't understand.

Prof. Mary-Louise McLaws, a University of New South Wales epidemiologist, is concerned that only 23% of 16–39 year old Victorians are fully vaccinated. Yet Stanford University's Cathrine Axfors and John Ioannidis estimate the survivability of under-50s is 99.918-99.997%. The cult-like fixation on one-size-fits-all approach to framing Covid policy has worsened health outcomes, hardships and inconveniences for everyone. Experts who hold sway and leaders who implemented their advice have been plain mulish in rejecting the sound recommendations of the Great Barrington Declaration to design protection around the most vulnerable groups.

The stubborn hostility to the undeniable power of natural immunity by the establishment, led by the CDC and Fauci, says Marty Makary from the Johns Hopkins School of Medicine, has "damaged the credibility of public health officials." "Trust the science" requires trusting scientists and scientific institutions that have become demonstrably politicised and faddish. Public confidence has eroded with flip-flopping advice, cherry picked data and silencing of dissenting voices.

US Health and Human Services Secretary Xavier Becerra wants to mandate vaccines and denigrates the unvaccinated as "flat earthers." He's shown ignorance (he confessed to being unaware of the major Israeli study on the power of natural immunity), arrogance (I know better than 100mn Americans) and authoritarianism (do as I tell you, or else). As a concluding thought experiment, imagine the irony if the religious and political authorities when the flat earthers reigned supreme had had at their disposal the vast powers of persuasion, surveillance, censorship, thought control, and punishment for non-compliance available to today's government-pharmaceutical-social media complex. We'd all still be true flat earthers, the Enlightenment would have missed its date with history, plagues and pestilence would periodically kill up to a third of a population, and life would still be nasty, brutish and short for most of us.

Questioning Covid[47]

In lighting the way out of the nightmare of serial lockdowns, new NSW Premier Dominic Perrottet has said and done three interesting

[47] *Spectator Australia*, 23 October 2021, https://www.spectator.com.au/2021/10/questioning-covid/

things. Australians are born into freedoms, not granted them as a privilege or concession by governments. Health policy is a subset of the total responsibility of governments which also includes the social, economic and human impacts of public health measures. Following from this, the principal responsibility for health decisions lies with ministers; health experts should be on tap but not on top, to tender advice that ministers accept, modify or reject.

Chief Health Officer Dr Kerry Chant was notably absent from Perrottet's inaugural press briefing. Several journalists seemed shocked. Over 20 months of being spoon-fed official handouts on the pandemic and fuelling the global panic, reporters have lost professional curiosity, instinct to interrogate the official narrative and capacity for independent research. Sharri Markson has done world-beating investigative work to highlight the scientific establishment's collusion in suppressing questions on the origins of the virus. In *Unfolding Catastrophe*, John Stapleton tells the story of Australia's response through the eyes of a veteran reporter. This still leaves scope for broader inquiries into pandemic management strategies. Here's a list of hard-hitting questions for journalists to pursue.

Q1: Governments listened to scientists. What science did the latter base lockdown decisions on to overturn the settled science summarised in the WHO report *in September 2019? That argued against lockdowns and social distancing because they "can be highly disruptive, and the cost of these measures must be weighed against their potential impact."*

Starting with Professor Neil Ferguson of Imperial College London in March 2020, models have turned out to be spectacularly wrong. Many US experts predicted a worsening situation in August–September. "And what actually happened? Cases plunged" by 40%, hospitalisations by 30% and deaths by 13%, wrote David Leonhardt in *The New York Times* on the 8th. Locally, "Modelling gets Covid hospitalisations peak wrong," read a headline on NSW in *The Australian* on the 12th. How many, other than the modellers, were surprised?

Q2: How critical, accurate or flawed has Australian modelling been in developing Covid policy?

In an article on 4 October, Leonhardt noted "the Delta variant led to a surge in cases lasting somewhere from one and a half to two and a half months." This can be seen in most places around the world, with no discernible correlation with the timing or severity of lockdown restrictions and mask mandates (cue Sweden, Florida). Most recently, Norway's cases have continued to fall since lifting all restrictions.

Q3: Data from around the world are persuasive revalidation of the pre-Covid consensus on the futility of lockdowns. Can we definitively abandon lockdown as a policy tool?

Outlawing peaceful protest and the harsh enforcement of restrictive measures by police, riot police and the military has drawn unfavourable global attention to Australia.

Q4: Are Australians concerned about shifting the needle of governance settings to the CCP model of enforcing obedience to government diktats?

Dr Jenny Harries, CEO of the UK Health Security Agency, said on the 10th that Covid is no longer the most significant threat to health. The UK's top killer in May–June 2020 and January–July 2021, Covid has occupied the second spot after Alzheimer's/dementia since 25 July. Covid ranks a lowly 26 among Australia's leading causes of death.

Q5: Were we panicked into unprecedented health-driven restrictions on our daily lives and activities by dodgy data and claims from China totally disproportionate to the criticality of the virus threat to Australians' health? How can we avoid a repeat of such catastrophism in the future and retain balance and perspective?

The singular focus on the global pandemic prioritised Covid over other health threats. Many health and mental health outcomes worsened by diverting resources, putting regular screenings on hold and cancelling or deferring scheduled treatments. British experts fear that with reduced immunity, there could be 60,000 flu deaths over the coming winter, making it potentially the worst flu season in 50 years. The ABS reports 4,199 (6.2%) excess Australian deaths from 1 January to 30 June 2021, compared to the same period in the 2015–2019 average. Cancer, diabetes and Alzheimer's/dementia have been particularly hard hit.

Q6: Should we launch an urgent investigation into the reasons for and prevention of thousands of deaths above historical averages?

Vaccines are neither necessary nor sufficient to deal with Covid. This is evident from the shape and chronology of infection and mortality curves of India and Indonesia, their upward and downward slopes, and their respective vaccination rates.

Q7. Can health experts explain India's and Indonesia's striking success in driving down infections and mortality with very low vaccination coverage?

Q8. Doesn't this affect assessment of the necessity for and levels of vaccination in Australia and undermine the argument for domestic vaccination certificates?

Q9. Are there lessons to learn from India and Indonesia on Covid-19 prevention and treatment options, medicines and protocols?

On the other hand, evidence from Israel, UK, Japan and elsewhere confirm vaccines reduce severity of illness and deaths but not infections and transmission. In fact recent data from the UK Health Security Agency show that in the 40–79 age groups, the vaccinated have 78-109% *higher* infection rates than the unjabbed. Vaccines don't protect against future variants. Natural immunity from prior infection is at least as robust, lasts longer and probably has more protective efficacy against mutant variants.

Q10. Is it better to prioritise universal coverage among the over-60s while making vaccines available to all?

Q11. Could population-wide herd immunity be reached sooner and be sturdier through a mix of vaccination of high-risk and infection in the extremely low-risk age groups?

Q12. Does waning vaccine efficacy after six months raise concerns about possible long-term harms?

Q13. Does the negative efficacy of vaccines in relation to infections for over-40s suggest that mass testing and contact tracing should end and the focus should be on symptomatic cases only?

The empty moral posturing of attacks on vaccine hesitants[48]

Our so-called leaders are so blinded with the lockdown cult that they would stubbornly refuse to see reality even if it hit them hard on their faces and knocked them out.

Last Saturday, just before Melbourne became the city with the world's most number of days in lockdown, Victoria reported 1,488 new cases in the previous 24 hours. Canberra, in lockdown since 12 August with just one case, reported a record 52 new cases each on 1 and 2 October, with 27 of the combined total of 104 having been in quarantine for their entire infectious period.

Meanwhile, the public finger-wagging and hectoring of Gladys Berejiklian by Dan Andrews notwithstanding, NSW daily cases fell to 813. Yet by some perverse and twisted logic, those of us who have questioned the effectiveness and demanded evidence of benefits versus harms analysis of lockdown are the ones attacked for denying reality.

The same "logic" has been operating on vaccines. Riddle me this. On the one hand, the big multinational pharmaceutical companies

[48] *Spectator Australia*, 9 October 2021, https://www.spectator.com.au/2021/10/the-empty-moral-posturing-of-attacks-on-vaccine-hesitants/

making the Covid-19 vaccines insist they are highly effective and perfectly safe. On the other hand, they demanded and were granted indemnity against liability from harmful effects caused by the vaccines. If Big Pharma is so sure of their vaccines' safety why insist on an indemnity? It's a testament to the power of manipulation when Big Pharma, Big Tech and Big Government converge on a single point of "vaccine truth" that the masses have come to believe everyone must be vaccinated, by choice or coercion.

There are three issues in particular surrounding vaccine hesitancy that deserve dissecting: the anti-vaxxer smear, the fallacious free-rider argument, and the "selfishness" accusation.

All of us lie on occasion. Only those who do so habitually are "liars," although anyone who claims never to have lied may also be called a liar. Similarly, anti-vaxxers are those who object to vaccination in general and reject most vaccines in practice. Those who have no problem with most standard childhood and flu vaccines for the elderly in principle or practice, but remain doubtful of the risk-benefit equation of Covid vaccines, are mocked as anti-vaxxers only by those who are intellectually lazy, in which case they should be ignored, or those who are intentionally malicious and should be called out.

The curious thing is that from the beginning, lockdown sceptics have tried to reason with science and data while governments and their cult followers have deployed tactics of mass psychological nudging and emotional blackmail to vilify the conscientious objectors. For governments this has been helpful in deflecting attention from their own neglect of public health; for people it leads to fear and anger displacement from the government to the non-compliant.

A misleading claim would point to Technical Briefing 23 from Public Health England that of the 2,542 Covid-related deaths 1 February–12 September, 63% were fully vaccinated and 28% unvaccinated. This does not mean that the vaccinated are 2.2 times more likely to die if infected. The bald statistic must be doubly disaggregated. For one thing, 97% of the vaccinated deaths are in the over-fifties. For another, among under-fifties, the vaccinated are 23% of the dead and the unvaccinated 65%.

It's more accurate to look at fatalities among the infected by this age divide. There's no difference in mortality for the under-fifties but over-fifties are 3.2 times more likely to die if unvaccinated. As someone in my seventies, I conclude Covid is 4-5 times likelier to prove fatal without vaccination and, against the tiny risks of serious side-effects, the rational decision on the present state of knowledge is to get vaccinated. No one else—not my GP, not the government—has a greater interest in my health than me. The risk-benefit calculus is different again for the under-forties and becomes very heavily skewed lower down the age ladder.

As argued in several previous articles in this magazine, vaccines have failed to live up to their initial inflated claims on efficacy and risks. As the efficacy against transmission fell apart, the argument for compulsory vaccination shifted to the moral hazard of free-riding to "take advantage of the majority of people behaving appropriately to break the rules and thus attain a personal advantage." Free-riding arises when one actor benefits from the provision of a collective good without paying a fair share of the cost. The US has often accused NATO allies of unfair burden-sharing. The free-riding charge was also levelled by Australia and the US at anti-nuclear New Zealand in the 1980s. With vaccines, there's zero extra cost borne by the vaccinated. On the contrary, the taxes of the unvaccinated subsidise "free" vaccines for others and the extra risks of severe illness and death are also borne by the unvaccinated. In both respects all the health and financial advantage is gained solely by the vaccinated.

Calls to exclude the unjabbed from the vaccinated economy are rooted in spite. The scolds and sneers detest the deplorables but dress up their intolerance as virtue to feel good about it. This is best seen in demands by some that the unvaccinated who get seriously sick should be denied hospital care. Imagine there are four beds available in ICU. Seven ambulances arrive with a drug addict who has overdosed, a lifelong heavy smoker with breathing difficulty, a failed suicide attempt, an obese person with heart issues, an unvaccinated person with Covid, a vaccinated person with blood clotting and a badly burned firefighter. Which three, and by what vice-virtue calculation, should be denied hospitalisation? It's simpler, faster and morally better to treat those in urgent need of medical care based on triage.

Are not the vaccine-hesitant being selfish? No. Selfish is demanding everyone be put under house arrest because I don't feel safe. Selfish is the petulant provincialism of state border closures so Queensland hospitals can be reserved for Queenslanders.

Selfish is the rich outbidding poor countries for booster third jabs before the latter's first jabs. Selfish is the panic run on toilet paper rolls. Selfish is destroying the future of young who are least at risk for a few more months of existing without living by the elderly most at risk. Nature expects adults to protect the young. Covid mania has turned nature upside down. This is depraved and a sign that society has lost its moral moorings.

So don't come a-waltzing morality on me.

Hey scientists, it's OK to express dissent[49]

The public policy madness of the Covid years seems less and less believable with each passing week and month. Many policies were absurd, idiotic and farcical, including advice to "dodge and don't touch" if an errant football came your way. Others were inhumanely cruel and heartless, their pain made all the deeper with blatant breaches of many regulations by sports and entertainment celebrities, political leaders, and even top health bureaucrats. Most inexplicably, many of the central pillars of Covid management policies went off at a tangent from established scientific consensus and the empirical

[49] *Spectator Australia*, 16 March 2024, https://www.spectator.com.au/2024/03/hey-scientists-its-ok-to-express-dissent/

data base, spreading misinformation and disinformation and often gaslighting citizens in suppressing information on harms while overstating the benefits. Most alarmingly, the state expanded and often abused its power at the cost of citizens and private enterprise, especially small family-owned and operated businesses.

There's one recent study and three recent news items that together highlight the continuing confusion over the gravity of the Covid threat and the public health interventions to combat it. On 11 February, Frederik N.G. Andersson and Lars Jonung from Lund University in Sweden published a study in *Economic Affairs* examining the benefits and costs of lockdowns across 25 countries in Europe, with a particular focus on Sweden as the outstanding outlier on Covid policy. Their conclusions emphasise the importance of avoiding panic amidst a crisis and not letting short-term decisions harm long-term outcomes. Instead, measures introduced without a firm evidentiary basis as a temporary necessity lasted for two years and authoritarian China served as the model for curtailing civil liberties and citizens' rights. Europe's democracies instituted needlessly stringent lockdowns that produced negligible positive health effects but the decline in economic activity did correlate with the severity of lockdowns. This pathology was compounded by efforts to counter the downturn in economic activity with excessively expansionary fiscal and monetary policies that led to ballooning public debt. By contrast, Sweden's lockdown restrictions were modest and mostly voluntary and its fiscal response was also restrained. This gave Sweden remarkably low cumulative excess mortality, small losses in economic growth and continued strong public finances. Sweden's GDP today is around six per cent bigger than in 2019. The three news items are in relation to the mRNA injections for Covid. We now know that in reality, these are faux vaccines that neither prevent the vaccinated from being infected nor stop them from infecting others. This is why we seem to be into the ninth shot. By this logic, how long before the daily insulin injection is called a vaccine? Just weeks after reiterating the need for students registering for the fall semester to be vaccinated, Harvard University reversed that decision. In March, the university announced that incoming students will no longer be required to receive the Covid vaccine. Harvard's status in the world of higher education is such that some optimism is justified about the ripple effects of its decision on other universities still requiring vaccination.

Unfortunately, this was more than offset by the shocking example of Pfizer advertising to recruit children as Big Pharma lab rats. Playing on parents' fears, it noted that "getting vaccinated is one of the best ways to protect your child from serious illness." It then invited them to enrol their unvaccinated child in "one of our ongoing vaccine clinical trials." There are separate trial groups for 6-23 months, 2-4 years and 5-11 years-old children. This raises several troubling questions. Why would parents who have resisted the vaccination for their kids agree suddenly to let Pfizer experiment on their precious child? The latter cannot possibly give consent. But how "informed" will the parents" consent be if they are not provided with accurate statistics on the likelihood of a healthy baby, toddler or young child dying or suffering serious injury from Covid and a Covid vaccine, respectively? The available evidence suggests that the latter is up to 60 times more likely than the former. This explains why the Covid vaccine has not been authorised by the EU for children under five and permitted less than enthusiastically for young people under 18. Dr Clayton Baker, former clinical associate professor of Medical Humanities and Bioethics at Rochester University, is quoted by Thomas Buckley as saying that the heavily skewed harm-benefit ratio of Covid vaccines for children means, "There is no ethical reason whatsoever to continue clinical trials of these products in children, and all such trials should be stopped."

Third, and most importantly, has been an interesting set of poll data from the UK. A wide-ranging survey conducted by the *Telegraph* and Censuswide and published in the *Telegraph* on 2 March found that a third (33%) of scientists believe that officials had focused on only a minority of opinions, wrongly equating scientific scepticism with science denialism. Modelling was all too often mistaken for scientific research and modelled scenarios for hard data and scientific conclusions. This was the basis for claiming that lockdowns, mask and vaccine recommendations-cum-mandates were based on the science. A majority of scientists now profess to believing that more attention should have been paid from the start to the full and true cost of lockdowns. Yet, few were courageous enough to put their head above the parapet at the time. Science is always work in progress, never an encyclopaedia of immutable facts. The sceptics had considerable tacit support in the scientific community. "This was, however, muted by concerns about loss of patronage, access to research grants and difficulty in publication as the cost of speaking out," says Professor Robert Dingwall. It is always important to prevent any public abuse and persecution of scientists who are prepared to challenge the dominant consensus. But we should not hold our breath and expect an outbreak of common sense in the public health clerisy with the next pandemic scare.

Sarah Knapton, the *Telegraph*'s science editor, concluded on 2 March: "My advice to scientists? Be brave, stand up. There are more people on your side than you realise." While right to chastise the scientific community in their collective lack of courage, she was far too charitable to her own professional colleagues in ignoring the role of media, including the *Telegraph*. Adam Creighton's article from a year ago is still in the top 15 of the most popular articles published by the Brownstone Institute. He faulted "a too credulous, incurious mainstream media, naive to the political and financial forces that pushed governments to eschew the more sensible path of voluntary Covid-19 vaccination" and behavioural restriction measures. *The Spectator Australia* was a lonely standout against the contagion of cowardice and complicity that afflicted media across the Western democracies.

7: THE TRIALS, TRIBULATIONS AND TRIUMPHS OF "NOVAX" DJOKOVIC

I like watching tennis, especially the Australian Open owing to the most convenient hours of all the four majors for people in Australia. And of course I had been following the Covid debates on lockdowns, masks and vaccines very closely indeed, trying to make sense of it as public policy. Not surprisingly, I was incensed by the scientifically idiotic and politically authoritarian treatment of Djokovic by the Australian government.

Djokovic's rare victory against Australia's Covid-19 tyranny[50]

A federal court in Australia on Monday quashed the government's decision to cancel the visa of Serbian tennis star Novak Djokovic, who had been held in detention at Melbourne Airport since 6 January, and ordered his immediate release so he could begin preparing in earnest to defend his Australian Open title.

The government's lawyer, Christopher Tran, informed the court immediately after that the immigration minister reserves the right to exercise his personal power to cancel the visa again and deport Djokovic from Australia. This would bar him from entering Australia

[50] *The Japan Times*, 13 January 2022, https://www.japantimes.co.jp/opinion/2022/01/12/commentary/world-commentary/novak-djokovic/

for three years and he would also have to declare this henceforth on many countries' visa application forms.

In some ways the breathtaking arrogance of this is more frightening than the original blunder. It would be a deliberate two-finger gesture to the rule of law backed by an independent judiciary to arbitrate the exercise of state power over individuals. What it shows is that governments, bureaucrats and technocrats have become habituated to ruling by decrees without challenge and accountability, no matter how arbitrary, autocratic, capricious and cruel.

Clearly, people have a fight on their hands if they wish to roll back the vast expansion of state power in the shadow of the pandemic. "Rules are rules," Australian Prime Minister Scott Morrison said pompously as soon as news broke about Djokovic's detention.

Australia's international and state entry rules in the time of Covid-19 are frustratingly complex, hostage to subjective interpretation by airline and border staff, and have often been enforced with conscience-shocking brutality. The lack of clear rules means that people who plan a visit down under and are permitted to board flights enter a minefield on arrival at an Australian airport with no certainty of being let in.

The government's submission claimed Djokovic poses a "greater health risk" of spreading the virus than a vaccinated person, a risk that would "burden the health system." On the second claim, the facts are that on 9 Jauary, Australia's rate of 3,062 daily new cases per million people was one of the highest in the world, higher than the United Kingdom and United States rates of 2,607 and 2,132, respectively. Djokovic would be more at risk of catching than spreading the virus in Melbourne.

On the first claim, UK Health Security Agency data for the final four weeks of 2021 show that double vaxxed people in Djokovic's age group had a 2.4 times higher infection rate than the unvaccinated. Djokovic maintains a strict regime of diet and exercises to stay in peak physical condition. Vaccines do not stop people from catching and spreading the virus. Not every unvaccinated person is infected.

Also, a tennis spectator's risk of catching the virus does not depend on the vaccination but the infection status of the persons around them. They are safer with two unvaccinated but uninfected people on either side than two vaccinated but infected. There is no medical or ethical justification for requiring Djokovic to be vaccinated as a condition of playing in Melbourne. Governments have imposed that rule not because it's scientifically necessary but because they can.

Djokovic was trapped in a Kafkaesque nightmare of different jurisdictional requirements between federal and state governments and different departments dealing with him. Even Tennis Australia had tried to seek the cooperation of relevant authorities and cleared him for participation in good faith. The international embarrassment of a diplomatic farce could have been avoided with consistent and coherent policies and clear lines of communications between the different authorities. This has been conspicuously missing for two years. His lawyers argued that exemption had been granted to the player by two separate medical boards following a recent coronavirus infection; he had presented all the necessary medical evidence to officials and he had "engaged with everything that was required of him by Tennis Australia."

The court agreed. Judge Anthony Kelly concluded that Djokovic had obtained the necessary exemptions for travel before catching a flight; had been courteous and cooperative with border officials on arrival at Melbourne Airport; told airport officials he "had complied with all the rules about being permitted to enter into Australia" and wouldn't have flown into Australia otherwise; but had been treated unceremoniously and unreasonably and denied procedural fairness. At one point the judge asked: "The point I am somewhat agitated about is, what more could this man have done?"

Serbs were united in outrage, with President Aleksandar Vucic condemning Djokovic's treatment as a "political witch hunt."

Leading tennis players past and present were divided. Some took the pragmatic line that the whole mess could have been avoided by Djokovic just getting vaccinated. Few seemed to have the clarity of mind to recognise that the issue is a fundamental principle of freedom of choice and the right to medical privacy. Djokovic showed remarkable courage of conviction and has provided an example to all role models on how to stand up to collective hysteria, mob pressure and diktats from autocratic governments—without seeking to knowingly violate rules.

Many Australians are distressed by the verdict as yet another example of entitled celebrities being able to flout rules that are far too costly for ordinary people to challenge. This is back to front. Proportionately more of the poor and marginalised groups are unvaccinated and the target of efforts to stigmatise and exclude them from society. Governments get away with draconian powers secure in the knowledge that legal challenges are intimidatingly unaffordable for ordinary folks. Legal costs for the taxpayer of the Djokovic case could be more than 250,000 Australian dollars. His victory in the law court is a win for everyone against government overreach and arbitrary conduct of the administrative state. Victory on the tennis court would be the icing on the cake.

Omicron has utterly humiliated the "Fortress Australia" lockdown establishment and, arguably, just a few months away from an election, authorities decided to make an example of one of the greatest tennis players of all times by a very public humiliation to cover their own failures. Fortunately for Djokovic, their autocratic instincts were executed with a staggering degree of ineptness that unravelled spectacularly in court.

In the past two years, Australia has descended into a country I no longer recognise: authoritarian, bureaucratic, petty, meanspirited, and vindictive. It used to be said the interesting thing about the Australian accent is you can hear the sunshine in it. Now it would appear Australia might have been in the sun a bit too long.

Rules are rules[51]

Omicron has spread everywhere, smashing through the multiple layers of protection. It also completely demolishes the case for vaccine passports and reinforces doubts about mask mandates that symbolise compliance with the diktats of biofascist states but lack reliable scientific backing. Hospitals have come under pressure not from the virus but the crazy patchwork of rules to kill it that created unsustainable staff shortages because of overzealous contact-cum-isolation rules.

"Rules are rules," intoned Scott Morrison as his thoughtful response to the growing international embarrassment over Djokovic's wish to defend his Australian Open title. Set aside the intellectually shallow, conviction-free and political coward Morrison's politicised violation of this dictum when he shamelessly attacked Australia Post CEO Christine Holgate for acting within existing rules. More than a rebuke of Djokovic, Morrison's comment is an endorsement of the transformation of a vibrant democracy in which people have rights and governments have obligations, into a system of rule by, of and for the laptop class.

Just as truth that may not be questioned is dogma, not science, so rules beyond challenge are anti-democratic. They are not divine commandments but the products of bureaucrats and politicians. They've been autocratic, arbitrary, inconsistent, often anti-scientific and sometimes outright bizarre: punishing people for trying to exercise outdoors while socially distanced, despite obesity being a major Covid risk; watching a sunset; not wearing a mask while fishing and golfing alone and the like. They've been enforced with conscience-shocking brutality. Interpreted with inhumane rigidity for ordinary battlers, a conga line of chief health officers, politicians and celebrities were granted exemptions on whim.

---

[51] *Spectator Australia*, 15 January 2022, https://www.spectator.com.au/2022/01/rules-are-rules/

Ordinary mortals have problems understanding the complex rules hostage to subjective interpretation by airline and border staff. Having experienced it first-hand, *The Australian*'s Jacquelin Magnay wrote: "the process is stressful, long and, at times utterly, confusing." More than a war on the virus, lockdowns proved to be a war on the poor to protect the privileged followed by crackdowns on dissenters. It's a sign of just how far centre-left parties have abandoned the working class that they've been the most insistent advocates and authors of draconian restrictions.

Vaccine mandates are a violation of health privacy, bodily integrity and individual autonomy. In a short video clip published on 5 December, Euro MP Christine Anderson declared that Australia's "once free and liberal democracy has been transformed into a totalitarian regime" that "tramples on human rights" and civil liberties. Thanks to the global coverage of one of the greatest tennis players of all time and one of the greatest contemporary athletes, that message has been amplified around the world.

Given his age and supreme physical fitness; the extremely age-segregated and comorbidity-concentrated Covid risk; the waning efficacy of vaccines coupled with the small but real risks of side effects; and the failure of "vaccines" to prevent people being infected or infecting others, there is no medical, scientific, legal, or ethical justification for the shameful treatment of Djokovic like a disease-carrying rabid criminal. Because vaccines do not stop infections in either direction, your risk of catching the virus from someone depends not on their vaccination status but on their infection status. Because double vaxxed people in Djokovic's age group have a 2.4 times higher infection rate than the unvaccinated, the rational conclusion is that in a random group, you are more likely to be infected by the vaccinated. The paranoid delusion is that it's all the fault of the selfish and ignorant unjabbed.

Told to get vaccinated in order to return to normality, we discover the goalposts have been uprooted and transplanted in a different, distant playing field. There is an unresolvable contradiction at the heart of the "pandemic of the unvaccinated" lie. If true, the vaccinated wouldn't need protection from the unvaxxed. It's been an extraordinarily successful ploy by governments, experts and vaccine manufacturers, to shift the blame for previous neglect of health infrastructure and the failure of lockdowns and vaccines, to the refuseniks. Even now, governments would do better to strengthen the resilience of institutions rather than restricting everyday lives. Stigmatising and targeting the unvaxxed for punishment has also bolstered the self-righteous virtuousness of the masked and vaccinated "I've done the right thing" crowd.

Djokovic's case from the top end of the global village marks a useful bookend to another one last year from main street. Anthony and Natalie Reale are proud, warm-hearted second-generation Italian-Australians. They've never taken a government hand-out and worked hard to build Village Fix as the best coffee shop in Shellharbour. They were arrested in June, fined $1,000 each and charged with a criminal offence with strict bail conditions that left them vulnerable to imprisonment. In a reckless example of public humiliation of the non-compliant, the police gave prior notice to the Illawara Mercury which covered their arrest, plastered their names and faces on its front page and the couple received threats and their car tyres were slashed.

The locals responded by increasing their patronage. All this because of mask mandates that rely on suspect lab studies untethered to the real world in which cloth masks—routinely used multiple times with constant fidgeting, lowering and raising—are on balance vectors of transmission rather than a layer of protection. The empirical evidence is clear, compelling and pretty much universal that ordinary masks have shown no ability to halt the rising curve or accelerate the falling curve of infections. As Sir Desmond Swayne MP said: "I've decided I'm exempt from wearing a mask due to my genetic predisposition to liberty... Every time I ask [ministers] for the evidence, I'm told it's about sending a message. Well, I don't like the message."

At best, non-pharmaceutical interventions have only a modest effect on the life cycle of each viral outbreak. The various waves triggered by new variants rise and fall according to an inner logic irrespective of the severity of the restrictions imposed. They are self-limiting and eventually burn out of their own accord. The starkest illustrations of this are Sweden and Florida. Simple rules to live by? Stay home if sick, be careful around the vulnerable, wear a high-grade mask if infected and, above all, treat the person not a lab result.

GOAT becomes scapegoat[52]

Is God a djoker? First, we've had the historical irony that during the cowboy days of the wild west, banks feared masked robbers. Over the last two years they've called the cops on maskless customers. Then we had the sleight of hand by Big Pharma where for the first time in history, the failure of a pharmaceutical product was blame-shifted on those who never took them. This was followed by the insistence that people who feel well must be tested and if the result is positive, they must self-isolate and all close contacts be tested also.

Now we have the surreal inversion of the drugs in sports equation. The reigning champion, world No. 1, among the greatest tennis players of all time, one of the greatest contemporary athletes across all sporting codes and quite possibly the healthiest human being on the planet, is being prevented from defending his Australian Open crown because he refuses to take a drug with an unknown long-term safety profile. An astonishing 445 athletes, by definition the fittest people, have suffered cardiac arrest or serious injuries and 261 have died following Covid vaccination. EU regulators recently warned that frequent booster shots could adversely affect the immune system.

---

52 *Spectator Australia*, 22 January 2022, https://www.spectator.com.au/2022/01/goat-becomes-scapegoat/

The claim that Djokovic poses a threat to Australia's public health is false to the point of being risible. With Australia experiencing one of the highest infection rates in the world, the failures of its current Covid policy settings pose a threat to Djokovic's health, not the other way round.

A new study supported by the CDC in the US concluded: "clinicians and public health practitioners should consider vaccinated persons who become infected with SARS-CoV-2 to be no less infectious than unvaccinated persons." In remote Antarctica, two-thirds of 25 staff at a scientific research station caught the virus from one infected person. All were fully vaccinated, passed multiple PCR tests and were quarantined before entry to the station. Professor Ehud Qimron, a leading Israeli immunologist, wrote an excoriating letter on 6 January calling on the health ministry to admit failure: "a respiratory virus cannot be defeated."

The nine-time champion was invited by Tennis Australia to defend his title. He cooperated with them and the Victorian government to ensure his exemption was valid to get an entry visa. The Byzantine rules and jurisdictional confusion between regulators, state and federal governments, tennis authorities and airlines created an unseemly mess that reflects poorly on the government's competence. Denying Djokovic a visa would have been unfortunate but a clear-cut decision that would have averted this sorry fiasco. The government didn't want to own the opprobrium of that decision, so they allowed the situation to drift into an international PR disaster. Concerned more about the disaster at the voting booth in a few months' time, they have whipped up a hysteria and climbed so high up the moral high horse that they cannot dismount for fear of falling flat on their face.

Tennis players seem to believe they can comply their way out of tyranny. Shame on them for not speaking up in defence of a champion of champions of their sport. Pace Martin Niemöller, someone should ask them: When they come for you, will anyone be left to speak for you? Maybe they just fancy their improved chances of adding a major title with the defending champion absent. Problem is, victory *sans* Djokovic in these circumstances will see the halo displaced by an asterisk, the trophy tarnished and the tournament diminished.

Shame on the Professional Tennis Players Association and the International Tennis Federation for failing to stand up for Djokovic. Both should have made it clear that banning Djokovic would mean the end of the 2022 Open and call into question its future.

The foundational principle of a national healthcare system is compassion. The stubborn persecution of Djokovic and the wholesale stigmatisation of the unvaccinated, all in the name of protecting that system, shows just far we have moved from compassion. The true test of tolerance and inclusivity is looking out for people with opposing points of view. He is not trying to impose his values and choices on others. They are the ones either joining in the mob hysteria or failing to speak out. Sporting codes were at the forefront of boycotting apartheid South Africa. Tennis players are condoning and complicit in medically unjustified and morally abhorrent vaccine apartheid.

Shame most of all on the Morrison government hell-bent on making an example of Djokovic in a panicked ploy to deny the failure of their narrative and policy. As even a BBC analysis made clear, Immigration Minister Alex Hawke's decision is essentially political. They are terrified that a twice-infected but unvaccinated Djokovic, leaping and bouncing all over court to a record 21st majors triumph, will bring to a shuddering halt the constantly escalating Covid terror. To be fair, though, Morrison's foot-in-mouth prowess is the equal of Djokovic's athleticism and the two are evenly matched on the charm scale.

The visa was initially cancelled after Djokovic asked: "So you're giving me legally 20 minutes to try to provide additional information that I don't have ... where at 4 in the morning I can't call director of Tennis Australia, I can't engage with anyone from the Victorian state government through Tennis Australia." After the stinging defeat in court on the 10th, the government shifted the grounds of its second visa cancellation on the 14th as Djokovic's legal team pointed out in the emergency hearing that evening. With Djokovic scheduled to play on the opening day on Monday, even the delay in announcing the cancellation decision until Friday smacked of petty-minded vindictiveness. Accepting that Djokovic "poses a negligible individual risk of transmitting Covid-19" to others, Hawke nonetheless considered "his presence may be a risk to the health of the Australian community." Because Djokovic has a "well-known stance on vaccination," his very presence could whip up more anti-vaccination sentiment in Australia, therefore his participation is not in the public interest.

And there we have it. Djokovic must be kept from our shores not because he could infect others but because he is a visible reminder of the failure of lockdowns and vaccines. Team Morrison wants to ensure that, like the Ardern Government in NZ, there is only a single source of Covid truth in Australia.

If we get Covid, so be it[53]

On 7 August, after a series of round-robin matches in two groups followed by knockout matches in the semi-finals, Australia and India met in the final of the women's T20 cricket competition in the Commonwealth Games in Birmingham, UK. Before the final, Australia's most valuable player through the tournament had been Tahlia McGrath. Like all Australian athletes at the Games, she was likely required to be double-vaccinated and boosted.

On the day of the final, McGrath experienced mild Covid symptoms and a test duly confirmed the diagnosis: she had the dreaded disease that has been treated in Australia like the local coming of the Black Death.

Was she pulled out of the match? Was she put into one or two-week isolation?

Hell no. McGrath took the field but not without the rest of the performative protocols that we have been witness to for two and a

[53] Brownstone Institute, 10 August 2022, https://brownstone.org/articles/if-we-get-covid-so-be-it/

half years. She wore a mask during the singing of the national anthem and while on the playing field, to prevent cross-infecting her teammates and opponents. And she social distanced, waving away her teammates as they swarmed towards her in a congratulatory-cum-celebratory mob after she took a catch to dismiss an opponent. Her teammates experienced a brief moment of panic when she came too close during the coin toss.

What's more, it worked! No one else has tested positive. Such consideration. Such unselfish compassion for others. Not.

Instead what it lays bare is the idiocy of Australia's manic Covid protocols and the hypocrisy of its entire policy when a gold medal was at stake.

In January last year the visiting Indian men's cricket team expressed great resentment at the tough Covid protocols and restrictions and there was some muttering they might return home, or at least the venue shifted away from Brisbane, whose pandemic protocols were exceptionally restrictive.

Because India is the financial powerhouse in world cricket, this would have been a financial disaster for Australia. Even in Sydney, confined to their hotel rooms other than when training or playing, the Indians complained of being treated "like animals in the zoo."

The average Australian response was: Stop being a sook and suck it up. You are in our country, respect our laws while out here.

Last December Pat Cummins, the captain of the Australia men's cricket team who holds the status of a demi-god in Australia, had to withdraw from a match against the visiting English side because he'd been in proximity to someone in an Adelaide restaurant who later tested positive. Despite testing negative, Cummins was deemed a close contact and not allowed to play.

After the T20 final, Indian journalists—Saikiran Kannan of *India Today*, online commentators like Mantavya and many fans—pointed to the contradiction of unvaccinated but Covid-negative tennis superstar Novak Djokovic being prevented from playing in the Australian Open. So did the prominent British commentator Piers Morgan.

At the same Commonwealth Games a week earlier, Aneesh Pillai wasn't allowed to take part in the men's discus throw final after returning a positive case despite being asymptomatic.

Furthermore, if you are subjected to daily testing for Covid and one day you do test positive, but are allowed to compete in a team match anyway: what exactly is the point of all the testing?

Can you blame the many Indians who voiced suspicions of outright racism? Surely not. After all, this is the sport that mandated taking the knee to show solidarity against racism.

Yet, the situation is impossible to imagine in reverse. If an Indian player had tested positive and the team wanted to field her, Dame Edna Everage's "Possum" Australia would have refused point blank.

The Australians arrived in Birmingham deeply troubled by the English approach to "living with the virus." Maybe they will return home with the epiphany that in the final analysis, that is the only way to live.

And oh, the gold medal prize was duly won. India has to make do with silver.

On winning the match, McGrath jumped into the team huddle to hug her teammates. Australian bowler Megan Schutt was philosophical afterwards: "If we get Covid, so be it."

The verboten magic words that would have saved the world so much misery if countries had been as philosophical instead of collapsing into mass collective panic in March 2020.

If only…

Djokovic and the US Open: Let him play[54]

So "Novax" Djokovic has won Wimbledon, the second tennis major this year to be plagued by self-inflicted wounds following the Australian Open whose crown Djokovic was unceremoniously prevented from defending.

[54] Brownstone Institute, 18 July 2022, https://brownstone.org/articles/djokovic-and-us-open-let-him-play/

I concluded then that God must be a Djoker. How else to explain that banks that once feared masked robbers insisted on masked customers in 2020–21, Big Pharma blamed the failure of a product on those who refused to take it, and sporting bodies that banned drug-injecting competitors mandated a drug with no long-term safety data?

According to one site that tracks the adverse events associated with sportspeople, by mid-July 2022 1,174 athletes—by definition one of the fittest cohorts in society—had suffered cardiac arrests and other serious side effects, of whom 779 had died.

The claim that "No-vax" Djokovic poses a threat to others' health is risible. Yet now he faces the repeat prospect of the Biden administration barring him from entering to compete in the US Open, even though unvaccinated Americans can compete.

That would be unfortunate. The vaccination mandate for international arrivals made little sense back in January and is now demonstrably reliant on voodoo science. Until the southern spring of 2021, belief in the efficacy of vaccines as the exit ramp from Covid seemed to be validated by the data. Hence the phrase "pandemic of the unvaccinated," which made its inevitable way to Australia.

Australia's most populous state is New South Wales (NSW, where I live). For the period 16 June 16 to 27 October 2021, in which the Delta variant was dominant, 63.1% of infections were among the unvaccinated and just 6.1% among the double-vaccinated. Conversely, only 5.7%, 3%, and 11.4% of Covid patients in hospital, ICU and dead were double-vaccinated.

Yet by year's end it was abundantly clear that breakthrough infections of the highly contagious new Omicron variant were rampant around the world and had significantly breached the vaccination protective barrier. Omicron was first identified in November 2021 in South Africa. Bizarrely, having shown themselves to be model international citizens in promptly notifying the world of this, unlike, say, China at the start of the Covid outbreak in 2020, South Africa was stigmatised by conflating first detection with place of origin of the Omicron variant.

Putting that aside, the key fact is that at that time, international travel was restricted to the double-vaccinated and everyone had to be masked in flight. Yet Omicron spread rapidly right around the world within two months, was quickly seeded in every continent, even Antarctica, and became the dominant variant, thereby blowing up the narrative that vaccination stopped transmission of the virus dead in its tracks.

Meanwhile, for all its boastful claims about having tamed Covid into submission, Australia has experienced an explosion in cases, hospitalisations, ICU admissions, and deaths this year, despite having reached 91% double-vaccination coverage of people over age 16 by the start of the year and 95% by mid-year. There have been nearly four times as many Covid deaths in the first six months of 2022 as in the previous 24 months.

New Zealand's fall from Covid grace is even more dramatic. Both prove the truth of the early insistence by sceptics that "virus gonna virus," governments could defer but not avoid its deadly toll, and long societal shutdowns would create an immunity debt from lack of exposure to commonly circulating pathogens.

Figure 7.1: NSW Covid-19 weekly hospital admissions by vaccination dose status, for weeks ending 28 May–9 July 2022

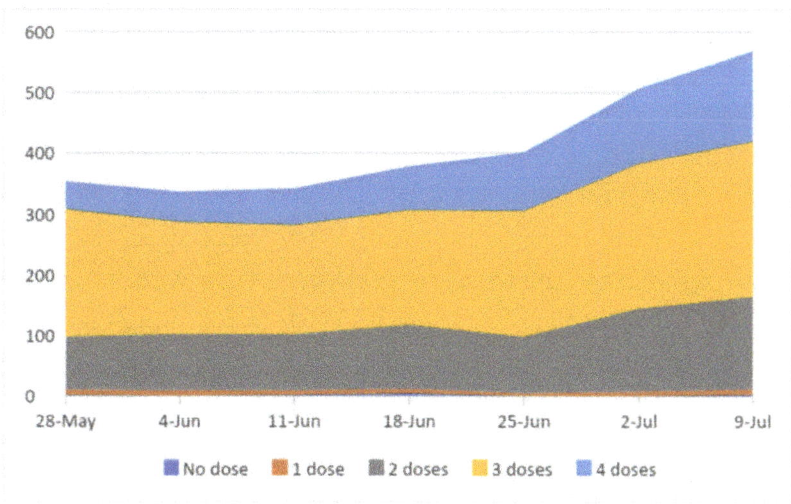

NSW has continued to provide detailed weekly reports on the status of Covid with helpful breakdowns by age group and vaccinations status (Figure 7.1). For the week ending 9 July, only 2 of the 1,325 Covid-19 deaths in the state over 15 weeks were aged below 20, while 1,268—96%—were aged 60 and above. This casts deep doubts on the "science" behind the drive to vaccinate the young, a point that Drs. Marty Makary and Tracy Beth Høeg make so powerfully in their recent article for Bari Weiss's Common Sense Substack site.

Claims that vaccinations help to reduce the strain on hospitals and significantly reduce mortality also seem to defy the data. In the seven-week period, of the 2,885 NSW residents admitted to hospital whose vaccination status was known, a grand total of 8—that's right, eight—were unvaccinated.

By contrast, a total of 2,820—a whopping 97.7%!—were double, triple and quadruple vaccinated. Remember, this is at a time when around 95% of people over 16 are at least double-vaccinated.

The Covid death toll is not quite so lopsided, but even there, vaccination provides limited protection. Clearly, if unfortunately, the real-world performance of Covid vaccines has not been as brilliant as the enthusiasts, including the manufacturers, had led us to believe.

Martin Kulldorff, an early supporter of Covid vaccines, recently argued on this site that new studies raise serious questions about the mRNA vaccines. The manufacturers and the FDA have failed in their responsibility to address legitimate safety concerns.

It's indisputable that vaccination does not provide protection against getting infected or infecting others. If health authorities were honest, then to be consistent with their 2021 messaging, they would now be using the language of the pandemic of the vaccinated.

The scale of the problem is such that suspicions arise that rapidly waning efficacy, especially after repeated boosters, might not be the only issue. In addition to the studiously ignored problem of adverse events, many serious and some fatal, could the vaccines themselves be sustaining and driving the pandemic?

Against this hard data that is now available, the decision in January to stop Djokovic from coming into Australia seems even more perverse. A court overturned the entry ban on procedural and substantive grounds. The government then made an end run around the legal system by relying on ministerial discretion that had deliberately been made nonjusticiable.

Djokovic's deportation was petty, vindictive and an example of medical tyranny. The international humiliation inflicted so publicly on him in pursuit of vaccine apartheid was morally corrupt. It lacked both scientific justification and hard data in support. It indulged a government's every illiberal instinct to control information and bully people into compliance.

More than authoritarian, it was totalitarian, in that it injected the state into the body of an individual in total repudiation of the principles of informed consent and "My body, my choice." To the extent that the policy was enforced in my name as a citizen, I remain regretful, embarrassed and ashamed.

This is why I would like to see Americans reject a repeat of the fiasco for the US Open but am not holding my breath. The capacity of authorities and governments to stubbornly—even cussedly—ignore facts, data and evidence throughout the pandemic has been awe-inspiring. It's an example of George Orwell's bon mot, in an article in *The Tribune* on 22 March 1946: "To see what is in front of one's nose needs a constant struggle."

Postscript

In January 2023, Djokovic reclaimed his Australian Open crown in Melbourne. On the night of Sunday 12 June 2023 in Paris, Djokovic won the French Open title for the third time. This increased his majors tally to 23, putting him in front of any other man in tennis history, making him the only man ever to have won all four majors at least three times, and returning the world number one ranking to him as well. Justice has been served.

8: REGULATORS: FROM PUBLIC HEALTH WATCHDOGS TO DRUG ENABLERS

The longer the health authorities pushed Covid-19 vaccines, exaggerating its benefits, downplaying its rapidly waning efficacy, and ignoring safety signals on its list of harms, the more attention turned to the role of drug regulators enabling pharmaceutical interventions more than acting as watchdogs on behalf of public health and safety. It contributed mightily to the growing loss of trust in public health institutions.

Health disgrace: bureaucrats in bid to silence our doctors[55]

Efforts to control the pandemic narrative began with a systematic suppression of any suggestion that it might have originated in a research lab of the Wuhan Institute of Virology, then moved on to denigrate, silence and smear critics of lockdowns, masks and vaccine efficacy and mandates.

A bill up for debate in the Queensland parliament on 11 October takes censorship to another level. The Australian Medical Network says under the new law "health bureaucrats will determine how doctors should approach treatment recommendations for their patients,"

[55] *The Weekend Australian*, 8–9 October 2022, https://www.theaustralian.com.au/inquirer/health-disgrace-bureaucrats-in-bid-to-silence-our-doctors/news-story/78f92a5c92bb900b5c497ba0f47ec3b3

and health regulators will be given "the power to sanction doctors for expressing their professional opinion based on their assessment of the best available science."

California's legislature has just passed a similar law empowering the state's medical board to revoke the licence of physicians who expresses opinions "contradicted by contemporary scientific consensus to the standard of care." So now it's official. They have outlawed opinions. We are on the cusp of revolutionising the everyday practice of medicine by subordinating the professional judgment of doctors on the best treatment options for their patients to the directives of bureaucrats and health regulators.

Let's look at the practical implications of this in relation to the vexed issue of vaccines for young people. Denmark and Norway have banned Covid vaccines for healthy under-50s/65s. On 30 September, Sweden announced an end to vaccine recommendations for 12 to 17-year-olds from 1 November. All three have excellent public health infrastructure and aggressively promote best-practice public health measures.

Yet our own Therapeutic Goods Administration (TGA) has approved vaccines for children aged six months to five years. The four countries cannot all be "following the science." New South Wales (NSW) Health data backs the Scandinavians' conclusion that the Covid risk to children is minuscule. In the past four months, just 0.1% of the 2,201 Covid deaths were aged 0 to 19. Almost all would have had serious underlying conditions. An article in *Vaccine* suggests that, for Moderna and Pfizer vaccines, added risks of serious adverse events are two and four times higher, respectively, than the reduced risk of hospitalisation. In a follow-up note, two of the authors note that the manufacturers' clinical trials showed 125 adverse events per 100,000 vaccinated people, while preventing between 22 to 63 hospitalisations.

Another study in preprint by US, Canadian and British scientists estimates that to prevent one Covid hospitalisation in 18 to 29-year-olds,

22,000 to 30,000 of them must be boosted. But for every one hospitalisation prevented, there are 18 to 98 serious adverse events: a net expected harm. Another new study of almost 900,000 children aged five to 11 in North Carolina, in the *New England Journal of Medicine*, adds to concerns that vaccines don't just rapidly lose effectiveness; they might also be destroying natural immunity against reinfection.

Among children who had been infected by the Delta variant and didn't get vaccinated, protection against reinfection fell from 95% in September last year to 53% at the end of May this year. In infected children who were also vaccinated, effectiveness had fallen to zero by May. The likely, albeit not definitive, explanation is that the vaccines themselves are damaging natural immunity. Ioannidis

He notes that Pfizer's own trial showed slightly more deaths in the treatment than in the placebo arm and no statistically significant reduction in all-cause mortality.

Some experts point to a worrying trend of rising excess mortality among under-14s in Europe. Aseem Malhotra is a British cardiologist who initially promoted the Covid vaccines on TV to help overcome public hesitancy. Using British data, he estimates the risk of a Covid death in 12 to 15-year-olds is one in 76,000, against the risk of myocarditis of one in 27,000: nearly three times more. The number needed to vaccinate (NNV) to prevent just one Covid death against the Delta variant reflects the steep age-segregated risk profiles, from 230 for over-80s, to 93,000 for 18 to 29-year-olds. Against this, the risk of myocarditis ranges in different studies from one in 6000 to one in 2700 for 12 to 27-year-old males, once again demonstrating net harm.

In the two–part peer reviewed article in the *Journal of Insulin Resistance* on 26 September, Malhotra concludes: "There is a strong scientific, ethical and moral case to be made that the current Covid vaccine administration must stop until all the raw data" has been released and "subjected to fully independent scrutiny." He calls on the medical and public-health professions to "recognise these failings and eschew the tainted dollar of the medical-industrial complex."

Malhotra argues that the rollout of vaccines under emergency-use authorisation without access to the raw data, the growing evidence of harms, and the resort to mandates whose major impact is to boost manufacturers' profits "have highlighted modern medicine's worst failings on an epic scale, with additional catastrophic harms to trust in public health." A poll by the Pew Research Centre in February mapped falling confidence in medical scientists since 2020.

To summarise, for children the risk of severe illness or death from Covid is very slight—while the risks of serious reactions to vaccines are higher. Protection against risk of reinfection is at least as robust and may last significantly longer for children who are infected but not vaccinated, compared to those who are vaccinated. The long-term effects of Covid vaccines are unknown. Every one of these statements is contestable and subject to revision as the databank grows and more studies are published. Not one is so implausible as to be summarily dismissed.

In these circumstances, for health bureaucrats and regulators to claim a monopoly on scientific truth is scandalous. I have more confidence in my consultant's professional advice based on training, qualifications, experience and knowledge of my medical history, free of pressures to conform to the zeitgeist from bureaucrats and regulators, the latter often with compromising links to industry.

Those of us without medical credentials arouse understandable scepticism towards our critiques. This makes it all the more imperative not to silence medical professionals, but instead to welcome and encourage contestable policy recommendations from them.

Agree with us or hold your tongue[56]

Every crisis, they say, is an opportunity. Governments, health bureaucrats and drug regulators all over the world have exploited the Covid-19

[56] Brownstone Institute, 19 October 2022, https://brownstone.org/articles/agree-with-us-or-hold-your-tongue/

crisis to grab power and gain control over our lives. Predictably, rather than to most people's surprise, many are proving singularly resistant to relinquishing their extraordinary powers, instead extending the emergency and broadening its scope to embrace other issues.

Efforts to control the pandemic narrative began with a systematic suppression of any suggestion that it might have originated in a research lab of the Wuhan Institute of Virology, then moved on to denigrate, silence and smear critics of lockdowns, masks and vaccine efficacy and mandates.

Australia's amended Health Practitioner Regulation National Law

The latest iteration in Australia occurred on 13 October when the Queensland Parliament amended the Health Practitioner Regulation National Law Act to fundamentally reshape the relationship between doctors, patients and health regulators.

On 22 February, Australian federal and state health ministers had approved the Health Practitioner Regulation National Law Amendment Bill. The updates to the guiding principles included "an increase in the regulatory responses available to protect public safety."

At best, this is vague and ambiguous. At worst, it shifts the balance decisively from the individual-centric in liberal democracies to the collective safetyism of technocrats and experts, justifying restrictions on individual rights and agency for the greater good as determined by government agencies. Everything done by health bureaucrats and regulators since March 2020, in the name of ensuring public safety and stopping disinformation, indicates we should fear the worst and would be naive to hope for the best. This includes psychological manipulation of emotions and feelings to nudge people into compliance with health directives.

Doctors will be prohibited from expressing their opinion and using their experience, training, education and knowledge of the patient, if this contradicts what the health bureaucrats say is in the interests of "public confidence in safety." The latter will remote-control how doctors should approach treatment recommendations for patients.

There were several submissions arguing against various elements of the amendment. The Australian Medical Association queried what a "main guiding principle" means "in practice" and argued that the "concept of public confidence is not always clear cut." The Royal Australian College of General Practitioners submitted that the amendments would imbalance the system even further away from the protection of patient safety and toward "the prosecution of practitioners," to the detriment of doctors' confidence in the National Law.

The most substantial submission came from the Australian Medical Professionals Society and the Nurses Professional Association of Australia representing more than 10,000 health professionals. They expressed concern that "the broad and discretionary nature of claims to 'public safety and confidence'" can be abused "as a mechanism to enforce compliance with government directives." On the one hand, these could be disconnected from science and evidence.

On the other, they could be used to control health practitioners in direct "conflict with their ethical duties and code of conduct obligations." They weren't confident that the provisions for public health and safety would in fact either "improve public protection from clinical misconduct" or "increase confidence in the public health system." Instead the proposed powers would "serve to conveniently silence voices of expertise that wish to correct health authorities" and prove counterproductive by preventing "necessary information and communication from entering the public sphere."

Long-standing principles that have guided Australian doctors and ensured its health system is second to none will be undermined: the Hippocratic Oath's duty of "Do no harm," informed consent of the patient based on a harm-benefit evaluation of different treatment options, the risks associated with them in the best professional judgment of the doctor, and the sanctity of the doctor-patient relationship.

People's faith in their GPs could collapse once they realise doctors are barred from questioning putative benefits or pointing to possible risks of recommended treatments. Instead, they must stay within the boundaries laid down by bureaucrats and regulators, the latter often subject to industry capture. A recently enacted similar law in California was described by the *New York Post* thus: "California makes it illegal for doctors to disagree with politicians."

The debate on the harm-benefit balance of Covid vaccines

The effort to shut down legitimate debates on pain of excommunication from the medical profession represents a clear and present danger to public health. We are intent on revolutionising the everyday practice of medicine by subordinating the professional judgment of doctors on the best treatment options for their patients, to the directives of bureaucrats and health regulators. With public esteem for politicians at all-time lows, this is not likely to inspire confidence in the health service.

Consider globally contested opinion on the benefit-harm balance of Covid vaccines for children. Their risk of severe illness or death from Covid is tiny, of serious adverse reactions is higher and the long-term effects are unknown. On 7 October, Florida issued a press release recommending against mRNA Covid vaccines for 18–39 year-old males. Their analysis had found an 84% higher risk of cardiac-related death within 28 days of vaccination in this group. Over-60s have a 10% increased risk.

This complements Florida's guidance on paediatric vaccine guidance issued in March which recommends against Covid vaccines for healthy under-18s. They note the limited risk to infants and children of severe illness due to Covid, the high prevalence of existing immunity among them, reduced vaccine efficacy and "higher than anticipated" severe adverse events, including myocarditis.

Florida thus joins Denmark, Norway and Sweden in ending vaccine recommendations for 12–17 year-olds and also, in two of these, for under 50s and 65s. Albeit contested, there is a substantial and growing body of scientific studies that support their scepticism toward the net benefits of Covid vaccines for infants, children and adolescents.

Florida's guidance includes three recommendations that are directly relevant to Australia's National Law:

- People are encouraged to discuss all potential vaccine benefits and risks with their health care provider.
- The risk associated with mRNA vaccination should be weighed against that with Covid infection.
- Doctors should inform patients of the possible cardiac complications that can arise after receiving an mRNA vaccine.

Yet, Australia's Therapeutic Goods Administration has approved vaccines for children aged 6 months-5 years. Meanwhile, many of the claims advanced in support of the vaccines—they stop infection and transmission and prevent severe illness and death—have had to be abandoned one after another but were never "fact-checked" by social media platforms, while the early critics of these claims were assessed by the self-styled fact-checkers to be spreading disinformation and promoting conspiracy theories—until they aren't any longer.

Moreover, people who die inside 14 days of a vaccine dose are wrongly classified as "unvaccinated." This distorts the statistics on the net harm-benefit balance to an indeterminate degree. In a particularly egregious example, an article in *Nature* on September 23 explained that the authors (1) had classified unvaccinated and single-dose vaccinated into the one catch-all category of unvaccinated, and (2) unvaccinated individuals with previous infection had been classified as "fully vaccinated" (Supplementary Table 2).

This in a study whose main objective was to assess the comparative susceptibility to infection by the Omicron variant of the vaccinated versus the unvaccinated within Danish households in December 2021. They concluded that the vaccinated are less susceptible. I can empathise with the reaction of Julian Conradson that after such analytical legerdemain in a leading peer-reviewed journal, "Academia Is Dead."

Examples of off-limits topics

Examples of studies that doctors could not discuss without fear of investigation and repercussions include:

- In a new study in preprint that looked at 31 pre-vaccination national seroprevalence studies to estimate the infection fatality rate (IFR) stratified by age, John Ioannidis and his team found that the average IFR was 0.0003% at 0-19 years, 0.003% at 20-29 years, 0.011% at 30-39 years, and 0.035% at 40-49 years. The median for 0-59 year-olds was just 0.035%. These are well within and often lower than the seasonal flu range for the under-60s. The last sentence would be ruled out as disinformation, or misleading, or at the very least missing context.
- In the weekly report for August 14–20, NSW Health said: "The minority of the overall population who have not been vaccinated are significantly overrepresented among patients in hospitals and ICUs with Covid-19" (p. 2). Two pages later, the same report gives us the data for hospital and ICU admissions by vaccination status. The number of unvaccinated is exactly zero for both. Now, this makes it mathematically impossible for the unvaccinated to be "overrepresented" among hospital and ICU Covid patients. There is an important conceptual distinction between the statement on page 2 and the statistics in Table 1 two pages later. The first is part of public messaging by

> the health department of Covid vaccines being "safe and effective." The second is actual data. The way I read the amended National Law, and therefore the way that some AHPRA official could read it at some time in the future against any doctor, the latter must conform to the public message and not mention the actual data.

Imagine a family of 45-year-old parents with three young children aged 5-12 who visit their family doctor to discuss vaccination for their kids and boosters for themselves, both to protect themselves and their parents in turn as they take the kids to spend quality time with grandparents. In the name of public safety, will Australian doctors have to promote the mRNA vaccines to children, boosters to grown-ups and be forbidden to mention advice to the contrary in Scandinavia and Florida? In New South Wales, of the 2,311 Covid-related deaths since May 22, only 3 have been under 20 and 34 under 50. Has any healthy under-20 died of Covid in Australia through the pandemic? If children are at virtually no risk and vaccines don't stop transmission, why expose children to the risk of serious adverse events?

What of the startling revelation that Pfizer had never tested its vaccines for transmissibility and therefore the entire vaccine passport requirement was built on a conspiracy of lies? In an NBC interview on 26 February 2021, Pfizer CEO Albert Bourla clearly says "there are a lot of indications right now that are telling us that there is a protection against transmission of the disease" provided by the vaccine. In a CBS interview on 26 May 2021, Anthony Fauci said: "when you get vaccinated, you not only protect your own health, that of the family, but also you contribute to the community health by preventing the spread of the virus throughout the community … you become a dead end to the virus." Australian data too confirm that while vaccines and boosters continue to provide protective benefits against severe disease and deaths, despite 95% adult vaccination they do not provide immunity against infection, hospitalisation, ICU admission or even death.

In an article on news.com.au, Frank Chung has done Australians a great service by compiling a list of statements from Australian ministers and health bureaucrats repeatedly stating their firm conviction that vaccines stop transmission. Michael Senger has done us all a service with a similar look back at the demonization of the unvaccinated by various public authorities, only too eagerly amplified by the media, and all predicated in the false belief that vaccines stop transmission.

For readers with an interest in Australia, Richard Kelly provides a review of many head-shaking edicts and enforcement actions—such as fining a delivery man for washing his van at an empty car wash at 1.15 am and a teenage learner driver for going for a lesson with her mum—that were issued by public health officials. Their ignorance about the disease was exceeded only by their arrogance and hubris about their ability to control the behaviour of a coronavirus. Would Australian doctors be at risk of deregistration for mentioning any of this?

Oliver May of *News UNCUT* wrote an open letter to 20 British news editors on 12 October, asking them to explain why they had failed to run a story either on the powerful documentary on vaccine injuries called *Safe and Effective: A Second Opinion*, or on Dr. Aseem Malhotra's painfully honest peer-reviewed study calling for a pause in Covid vaccination because of serious adverse events until all the raw data has been subjected to fully independent scrutiny. Both would be interesting to the public and both are very much in the public interest. We shouldn't hold our breath for an answer. Maryland School of Pharmacy's Peter Doshi, senior editor of the *British Medical Journal*, is right to call out the legacy media for their lack of balanced coverage of Covid vaccines.

Remarkably, the Pfizer admission has been studiously ignored by the Australian MSM. In case I had missed the coverage of the bombshell interview in the Australian media, I did a search on the website of ABC (Australia's version of the BBC), *Age*, *Australian* and *Sydney Morning Herald* papers. I got zero hits for Robert Roos, the Dutch

MEP who asked the question in the European Parliament of Pfizer director Janine Small, and for the latter who confessed to lack of testing for transmissibility. Fading trust in our principal institutions is contributing to the multipronged global crisis of democracy.

The lack of media interest and coverage means there is little pressure for public accountability. Absent that, there will not be any punishment meted out to ministers and bureaucrats for the extensive range of malfeasance in inflicting cruel and inhumane harms on millions of their citizens; no prospect of emotional closure for the people for the trauma they have suffered, including deaths of despair and desolation born of loneliness; delayed prospects of the masses shedding their sheer dread of a virus that for most healthy people under 70 or 65 is not really a severe illness; and a refusal to institute the most powerful deterrent of all for any repeats of public criminality on a grand scale.

Instead we can all look forward to endless cycles of rinse and repeat of surveillance, compulsion and coercion of the masses on the whims of their technocratic betters.

Hippocrates cancelled[57]

How can they sleep at night? Or face themselves in the mirror in the morning?

I ask the question "triggered" by a report in *The Indian Express.* There's been a sharp surge in child trafficking in India following lockdowns. Westerners have forgotten what "hand to mouth" existence means, when the sole breadwinner must earn daily wages to buy food for the family, including elderly parents. With lockdown for months without end, children are inevitably at risk of being trafficked into labour bondage, street begging or sexual slavery. An

[57] *Spectator Australia*, 24 October 2020, https://www.spectator.com.au/2020/10/hippocrates-cancelled/

analogous development has been the growth in sex predators in Australia as restrictions on movements mean more kids are online for longer periods.

We now know the fear-mongers were disastrously wrong, but persist with their heartless cruelty nonetheless. In April, the UN Economic Commission for Africa said "between 300,000 and 3.3 million African people could lose their lives as a direct result of Covid-19." In February, Bill Gates warned of 10 million Coronavirus deaths in Africa. On 15 October, the real number was 38,977. Gates is a genius as a tech entrepreneur but his grasp of epidemiology is near the other end of the scale. Mind you, the tech sector is one of the very few to have done well financially from the lockdown.

The unbearable cruelty imposed by health bureaucrats without a distinguished medical research record has sucked the very humanity out of society: delaying interstate visits until too late to see a dying father or save one of the twins in the womb in need of urgent attention. As British MP Charles Walker said in a BBC radio interview on 12 October, for many elderly people, "being told that you've got to spend the next six or 12 months without human contact, without seeing the people that you love, without embracing your grandchildren, is a price too high."

The US Centers for Disease Control (CDC) estimates 93,814 non-Covid excess American deaths. In the UK, "up to 150,000" could suffer non-Covid-19 premature deaths, the *Financial Times* reported. In Australia, there were 134 fewer deaths from all respiratory illnesses in the first half of the year compared to the five-yearly average annual deaths for 2015–19, but an additional 617 cancer deaths.

Of course, the biggest tragedy will be across the developing world over the next decade, with over 100 million more people pushed into extreme poverty, tens of millions of additional dead from increased infant and maternal mortality, hunger and starvation with more poverty and disrupted crop production and food distribution networks, sharp cutbacks in immunisation and schooling, and destruction of the informal sectors of the economy in which daily wage earners earn a pitiful living. Most countries will also need to prepare for potential spikes in mental health problems and suicides from the fear generated by exaggerated alarmism as well as the loneliness, isolation, financial ruin and despair caused by the lockdowns.

"Hundreds of thousands of cancer screenings were deferred after worries about Covid-19 shut down much of the U.S. health-care system this spring," *The* Wall Street Journal reported. "There's really almost no way that doesn't turn into increased mortality." UK Health Secretary Matt Hancock said on 6 October that cancer treatment would have to wait until coronavirus was "under control." Almost daily he has provided fresh evidence of being a thick politician without the intellectual nous to comprehend the sheer idiocy of his own statements. As London University oncologist Professor Angus Dalgliesh noted, Hancock "has had nine long months to educate himself out of his ignorance of the scientific implications of the Covid-19 pandemic. But this week he was still responding to reasoned argument with petulant contempt."

The top medical scientists cannot claim the defence of intellectual shallowness. Doctors who know better but have remained silent, are complicit in the crimes against humanity resulting from the brutal perverse consequences of the stringent measures. They might have pleaded ignorance of the extent of the consequences back in March, although some of us did warn of the possibility early on. The excuse of ignorance is no longer available. Nor is it good enough to go along with the mass cruelty in order to get along with professional colleagues. Kulldorff writes by email (15 October): "Among infectious disease epidemiologists that I know and interact with, the majority is in favour of an age/risk-targeted strategy of focused protection. For various reasons, some have been uncomfortable speaking out publicly."

I point them to Professor David Livermore, a microbiologist at the University of East Anglia. In an article for *The Telegraph*, he explains: "in conscience and surveying the wreckage, I can only quote Martin Luther: "Here I stand; I can do no other."" Pontius Pilate washed his hands of any responsibility for the death of Jesus. I didn't realise this is what the Australian and Victorian medical associations had in mind when they recommend frequent hand washing.

As Dr Matt Strauss of Queen's University in Canada (my alma mater) argues in *The Spectator*: "If lockdowns were a prescription drug for Covid-19 treatment, the FDA would never have approved it." Hence his conclusion as a medic with clinical practice: "mandatory government lockdowns amount to a medical recommendation of no proven benefit, of extraordinary potential harm, that do not take personal values and individual consent into account."

"First do no harm"—good counsel, that.

Drug regulators failed the public on Covid-19[58]

Rasmussen is among the most respected public opinion pollsters in America. In findings of a poll conducted between 27–29 March and published on 31 March, 11% of respondents said a member of their household had died with Covid, and 10% said someone had died from a vaccine side-effect. This is a remarkably even breakdown of deaths with Covid and from vaccine-related injuries.

Earlier, on 21 February, Norwegian scientists Jarle Aarstad and Olav Andreas Kvitastein published a preprint of their findings that vaccination rollouts across 31 countries in 2021 were associated with rising all-cause mortality in the first nine months of 2022. A one percentage point increase in vaccination uptake in 2021 was associated with a 0.105% increase in monthly mortality in 2022. The association remained robust even after controlling for alternative non-vaccine-related explanations for the increased mortality rate.

[58] Resistance Press, 12 April 2023, https://resistancepress.com/article/drug-regulators-failed-public-covid-19

This follows a March analysis from the Vaccine Damage Project which concluded that among 16–64 year old, employed Americans, 82% of people did not suffer any vaccine injuries. The next largest group of 18% suffered mild injuries, but 0.93% (1.36mn) suffered disabilities and there were 310,000 (0.05-0.1%) vaccine-related excess deaths in the two years of 2021–22.

If we were to add to the total those who have died from the enduring consequences of lockdowns (cancelled cancer and cardiovascular screenings, delays of scheduled operations, added difficulties in accessing healthcare, reduced beds and staff in hospitals from isolation and social distancing rules), it would be clear that the scale of non-Covid excess deaths was substantial.

Yet, unlike the breathless daily press briefings in 2020–21 on Covid cases and death counts as this disease was the only one that governments, health bureaucrats and the media seemed interested in, there are no urgent efforts to investigate just what is going on with these vaccine/lockdown-related deaths and how best to address the problem. The lack of curiosity from the press and parliamentarians adds to the institutionalised indifference to lockdown and vaccine harms that amounts to outright contempt of the public. And isn't it remarkable that we still don't have all the necessary details and raw data from the Pfizer and Moderna vaccine trials whose claimed efficacy results continue to be seriously disputed by reputable scientists? Not to mention allegations of fraud in Pfizer's clinical trials, as reported by Germany's Die Welt.

Disturbing data from Australia

On 8 February, the Australian Technical Advisory Group on Immunisation (ATAGI) quietly published updated advice on boosters. In this, ATAGI finally acknowledged that the harm-benefit equation for boosters doesn't compute for young people: "Adolescents and younger adults [especially males] have a lower age-related risk of severe Covid-19, and a comparatively higher risk of myocarditis following vaccination." It declined to recommend booster doses for under-18 year olds; recommended it for over-65 year olds and 18–64 year olds with comorbidities; and advised the bulk of the healthy 18–64 year olds to "consider a 2023 booster dose ... based on an individual risk benefit assessment with their immunization provider."

A January 2021 (sic) "Nonclinical Evaluation Report" from Australia's TGA was also published recently, following a Freedom of Inquiry request (which is a scandal in itself). The TGA states:

- The microscopic lung inflammation in monkeys after infection was "almost similar" in immunized and control groups;
- Long-term immunity after a second dose was questionable because the antibody and T cell responses "declined quickly over 5 weeks."
- Data was not available on:
- Distribution and degradation of "the S antigen-encoding mRNA," so the half-life and pattern of distribution was unknown;
- Medium- and long-term protection against serious illness, hospitalization, and death;
- Toxicity of the repeat dose;
- Potential for autoimmune diseases and other long-term effects.

Concentration of radioactive tracer (incorporated into the lipid nanoparticles) was detectable in tissue and blood as soon as 25 minutes after the initial dose and up to as long as 48 hours later in several parts of the body, including heart (peak total lipid concentration of 1.40 microgram of lipid equivalent/gram (or mL) after 2 hours), kidneys (2.05μg after 2 hours) and liver (26.54μg after 8 hours).

In other words, the TGA knew, back in January 2021, that we lacked full efficacy and safety data for both the short and the long term, there was evidence already of rapid waning of efficacy, and there was evidence of lack of effectiveness (the first bullet point above). And, if the TGA knew, then so must its counterparts across the Western world have known.

These are serious and egregious omissions. They suggest that the authorities should have been less emphatic and more guarded with the "safe and effective" messaging. They would not then have experienced the drip-drip erosion of public trust that has occurred.

This also raises another issue of medical ethics. Western medicine has been predicated on the norm that the doctor's primary responsibility in assessing benefits against the risk of harms of treatment options is the welfare of the individual patient, and only secondarily with community welfare. The messaging on "My mask/vaccine protects you and your mask/vaccine protects me" turned this long-standing principle of Western medicine on its head.

It is also a violation of Articles 3 ("The interests and welfare of the individual should have priority over the sole interest of science or society"), 5 (The autonomy of persons to make decisions, while taking responsibility for those decisions and respecting the autonomy of others, is to be respected), and 6 (Any preventive, diagnostic and therapeutic medical intervention is only to be carried out with the prior, free and informed consent of the person concerned, based on adequate information) of the Universal Declaration on Bioethics and Human Rights (2005).

This is centrally relevant, for example, to the benefit-harm equation of vaccines by age groups: it violates core medical ethics to recommend them to healthy children, adolescents and young people up to 50, and to pregnant women and women of child-bearing age, on the reasoning that doing so helps to protect the whole community. This is further reinforced by the Convention on the Rights of the Child (1989: "the most widely ratified human rights treaty in history," says Unicef), Article 3.1 of which affirms: "In all actions concerning children ... the best interests of the child shall be a primary consideration."

The primary consideration should always have been:

- The risk exposure to the Covid disease to the individual;
- The efficacy of the vaccine for them against infection, hospitalization, ICU admission, and death;
- The number within their age group that would need to be vaccinated (NNV) to prevent one hospitalization, ICU admission, and death; and
- The corresponding numbers of serious adverse events for that NNV.

The potential for protecting the wider community should not have entered the discussion unless the patient raised it with regard, for example, to a parent or grandparent.

The TGA report validates the early vaccine scepticism from the top British medical and scientific advisers. On 29 February 2020, responding to a report that Israeli scientists were weeks away from developing a Covid vaccine and the question of if this was credible, Chief Scientist Sir Patrick Vallance replied "Short answer is no." Chief Medical Officer Chris Whitty explained: "For a disease with a low ... mortality a vaccine has to be very safe so the safety studies can't be shortcut."

Raising questions in Parliament

On 17 March, a Member of Parliament in the UK, Andrew Bridgen, presented figures on the net benefit-harm equation of vaccines to show that for healthy people, the probability of being harmed by the vaccine is much higher than the risk of serious harm from Covid. Bridgen concluded: "in the light of the Government's own data, Covid vaccinations and boosters are not effective. From the evidence of the yellow card system, they are not safe, and for the UK taxpayer, they are not value for money."

Pericles declared that "Your empire is now like a tyranny: it may have been wrong to take it; it is certainly dangerous to let it go." That is certainly proving true of the empire of Covid tyranny. The MPs in the House appeared to stage a mass walkout as Bridgen began his speech, unwilling to contemplate the harms they had failed to check in the name of keeping the people safe.

Continuing their habit of questioning critics of official policy rather than their journalistic duty to investigate official claims with a genuinely open mind, the media have smeared Bridgen as a conspiracy theorist and criticized him for spreading dangerous misinformation. BBC Radio 4 broadcasted an hour-long program on his speech on 23 March, for which they declined his offer to join in the discussion.

Subsequently five experts mounted a robust defence of Bridgen in *The Daily Sceptic* and took apart the criticisms of his speech that was aired on Radio 4. There is a growing body of studies that support Bridgen's scepticism as, for the first time, there is genuinely open debate among experts. For example on 27 March *The Telegraph* reported that young women in England aged 12–29 faced a risk of death from heart issues that was 3.5 times higher after an AstraZeneca Covid vaccine.

The slippage between vaccine efficacy and effectiveness

There's a technical distinction between vaccine "efficacy" in controlled clinical trials and vaccine "effectiveness" in the real world. Non-sterilizing Covid vaccines could and should never have been expected to significantly reduce infection or transmission. The real world data show that with rapidly waning effectiveness and requirement for boosters every four months, they are closer to a treatment than a vaccine as traditionally understood. Tetanus and polio vaccines do not require multiple annual shots. For all the eye-watering amounts of money expended, Covid vaccines bear little causal relationship to mortality outcomes.

If we look at groups of countries by income levels, the difference in Covid mortality rates is shockingly stark, even accounting for their respective age differentials. And it correlates positively with vaccination rates. According to Our World in Data, the number of vaccine doses administered per 100 people as of 31 March went down from 224 in high, to 214 in upper middle, 142 in lower middle and 38 in low income countries. The number of Covid deaths per million people also went down, from 2,274 to 1,050, 390 and 65, respectively. Not exactly a stunning demonstration of vaccine success in reducing Covid mortality.

The vast majority of Covid deaths in many countries by now are among the vaccinated and boosted. On the harms side, a CDC report on 16 March showed US maternal mortality jumped by 40% from 861 in 2020 to 1,205 in 2021. The 2021 rate of 32.9 maternal deaths per 100,000 live births is the highest maternal mortality rate since 1965 and coincides with the year of the vaccine rollout. Similarly, lagged temporal correlations are clearly visible in several European countries between vaccine uptakes and falling births nine months later.

Dr. Ros Jones, a retired consultant paediatrician from the Health Advisory and Recovery Team (HART) guides us soberly through a discussion of how this could be explained by a combination of societal (choice, restricted opportunities due to lockdown effects) and medical causes (exacerbated problems with male/female fertility and conception, miscarriages, terminations, stillbirths). Her conclusion is the key message. As the public and the specialists have not been given access to the raw data, "when is the Government going to order a proper investigation to put an end to speculation over whether correlation does or does not reflect causation"?

According to the latest data from the Australian Bureau of Statistics (ABS) that was published on 31 March, there were 190,394 deaths from 1 January to 31 December 2022. This is 25,235 or 15.3% more than the five-year historical average (2015–19). Of these, the number of Covid-related deaths was 10,095 or 40% of the total excess deaths.

Thus 60% of the excess deaths could be the after-effects of the disastrous lockdowns and vaccine injuries. We don't know and, infuriatingly, the government refuses to order a proper investigation of what should be an urgent preoccupation for the public health clergy.

The tragic case of 24-year old Amy Sedgwick whose death came after painful side-effects following two doses of the Pfizer vaccine was featured in The Weekend Australian on 25 March. The Australian kept the story going with another feature article on 1 April about the manifold failings of the compensation scheme for the vaccine-injured. Adam Creighton pointed out that this story would have been disappeared from the Internet in 2021 owing to the censorship collusion between Big Pharma, Big Tech and public health authorities.

Even truth was no defence with accounts of vaccine injuries, if their effect was to promote narrative scepticism. The social media Big Tech censored, suppressed, shadow banned and slapped labels of "false," "misleading," "lacking context" etc. to content at variance with the single source ministries of truth. "Fact checking" was weaponized using fresh young graduates—with no training, skills or capacity to sift between authentic and junk science—to put such judgmental stamps on pronouncements from world-leading experts in their field.

Like Bridgen's figures on the net vaccine harms-benefits equation in the UK, we too urgently require the same age-stratified data for Australia on numbers needed to vaccinate to prevent one hospitalization, ICU admission and death. This should be accompanied by the corresponding numbers put at risk of hospitalization, ICU admission and death by the vaccine.

It is an outrageous and ongoing scandal that the public has not been given this information. How can anyone provide "informed consent" absent that vital data?

Journalists attending the ritual of daily press briefings by the health ministers and chief medical officers were "all graduates from the Uriah Heep school of obsequiousness," to borrow a phrase from

Angus Dalgleish. The professor of oncology at St George's Hospital Medical School in London adds that the boosters are against the Omicron variants. These "not only fail to protect from new variants but actively encourage them by Antibody Dependent Enhancement (ADE) which explains why boosted patients are 50% more likely to catch Covid after their vaccination than those who refuse." In addition, it "induces T-cell suppression and antibody class switching," causing cancer relapses.

India's contra example poses some difficult questions for Australia's drug regulators

Several Indian states deployed ivermectin repurposed as a preventative and early outpatient treatment for Covid. With around four billion pills sold around the world over several decades, its safety profile is well established. Large scale observational data from India and Africa offers some evidence for its effectiveness. As an off-patent drug, it is incredibly inexpensive. This might explain Big Pharma's hostility but does not excuse the TGA's failure to fund more reliable randomised control trials, particularly in light of some convictions and a long list of out of court settlements by Pfizer.

No one has as yet explained why, if the manufacturers were so convinced that their vaccines were safe and effective, they required legal indemnity against vaccine injuries. Did the ban by the TGA cost Australian lives, as asked by Kara Thomas and Andrew McIntyre in *Spectator Australia*, by preventing doctors from recommending it to patients based on their best professional judgment of each individual case?

Some of the fiercest vaccine promoters are starting to turn somewhat sceptical and hesitant, as reported in this article from Apoorva Mandavilli, herself an enthusiastic vaxmonger, in the *New York Times* on 24 March. It's when they go back to blaming President Donald Trump for the vaccines and its assorted failings and injuries, that we will know the circle has been closed.

One final question for regulators[59]

On 25 July 2021, Scott Morrison said the government will buy another 85 million Pfizer booster doses in 2022 and 2023. That's more than three boosters for every Australian or more than four for every adult, after their initial two-dose vaccination. Thus the government was already aware of the vaccine's waning effectiveness against the existing strain and its likely ineffectiveness against new variants. This of course is also the understanding about annual flu vaccines: they are reformulated every year because the pathogen is unstable and keeps mutating, which in turn rules out an eradication strategy. This is why we learnt long ago to live with the flu, focus public health efforts on protecting the most vulnerable through annual vaccines and leave the rest of society to carry on with the normal routine of life.

Meanwhile the safe and effective messaging on Covid vaccines looks increasingly suspect. Confidence has diminished in health authorities, parliaments, medical establishments and media for their manifold failures to interrogate the official claims and report on the rising toll of vaccine injuries. As from last month, the AstraZeneca vaccine is no longer available in Australia owing to the "rare but serious side effect" thrombosis. Despite the ABS reports of 15.3%) excess deaths in Australia in 2022, the government and opposition MPs rejected a motion from Senator Ralph Babet to hold an inquiry into this concerning phenomenon. Meanwhile from 1 April Switzerland has withdrawn all vaccine recommendations. Doctors can administer Covid vaccines only in individual cases under specified conditions and bear the risk of liability themselves.

Even if Covid had proven to be as deadly as the Spanish flu and the vaccines 90% effective, coercion and mandates would still have been unethical. Revelations that authorities knew this to be false in

[59] *Spectator Australia*, 22 April 2023, https://www.spectator.com.au/2023/04/one-final-question-for-regualtors/

early 2021, means there was little medical justification either. This makes the public policy scientifically perverse and ethically immoral. Social media Big Tech made it worse by actively censoring, shadow-banning, downgrading and slapping labels from self-identifying fact checkers better described as misinformers and disinformers. (India has gone one logical step better. The government will create a fact-check body for regulating online content. Opposition parties have denounced the move as censorship and accused the ruling party of being the biggest purveyor of fake news.)

On the one hand, Big Pharma and public regulators meant to oversee them colluded to hide and delay important information. On the other, they ferociously attacked independent researchers who tried various forensic techniques to "mine" the relevant data and offer a counter-narrative, with the goal of discrediting and demonising anyone with the temerity to question the official "truth." The Censorship-Industrial Complex was weaponised into a powerful tool of state power in an evolving system of governance that is a threat to the very survival of free society. I am not impugning doctors and researchers who put their faith in the underlying integrity of the regulatory agencies and medical establishments, even if that faith turns out to have been misplaced and abused. I too feel betrayed by the WHO and disillusioned with its patchy performance, to put it kindly.

On 5 April Maryanne Demasi published an article on Substack, republished by Children's Health Defense, that the triumphalist 95% efficacy narrative of the Pfizer vaccine, which would give us all an exit ramp from the coronavirus pandemic with universal vaccination, had already gone off script by June 2021. Some highly vaccinated countries like Israel were experiencing a fresh wave of infections that was fuelling vaccine hesitancy and slowing take-up. By July Israel was reporting effectiveness of 64% and in August only 39%. Regulatory filings show that Pfizer and the FDA had evidence already in April 2021 on waning effectiveness. This was not publicly disclosed until much later. The press release from Pfizer on 1 April 2021 announcing results of its six-month Phase 3 trial repeated claims of 91.3% efficacy against the Covid disease and up to 100% effectiveness against severe disease.

The top authorities continued to downplay the lack of evidence to demonstrate vaccine effectiveness against viral transmission and long term protection. While acknowledging the possibility of breakthrough infections, Fauci said on national TV on 16 May 2021: "when you get vaccinated, you not only protect your own health, that of the family, but also you contribute to the community health by preventing the spread of the virus throughout the community ... you become a dead end to the virus. And when there are a lot of dead ends around, the virus is not going to go anywhere." The official report from Public Health Ontario in March shows Covid hospitalisations and deaths in 2022 were 31 and 39% higher respectively than in 2021, despite 76% of Ontarians being double-vaccinated.

Neither the pharmaceutical industry nor public health agencies are releasing all the data nor undertaking the important safety studies and acting on safety signals in a timely fashion to restore trust in their good faith, competence and integrity. Independent researchers are still having to do medical detective work instead. With widely varying and contested definitions and measurements of Covid and vaccine-related deaths, they look instead for clues in all-cause excess deaths. Professor Norman Fenton calculates the number of deaths caused directly by vaccines until 23 March 2023 to be 120,000 in the US and 16,000 in the UK. Dr. Ros Jones examined the lagged temporal correlations in several European countries between vaccine uptakes and falling births nine months later.

On 28 March WHO experts published a revised roadmap which prioritises vaccines for the elderly and people with comorbidities, relegates healthy children and adolescents down to low priority because of their low disease burden and recognises natural immunity from prior infections. In a sign they might be awakening to the risk of cross-vaccine hesitancy because of disillusionment with Covid vaccines, the guidance acknowledges: "The public health impact of vaccinating healthy children and adolescents is comparatively much lower than the established benefits of traditional essential vaccines for children."

My final question is to the public health clerisy. If you become transparent on efficacy, investigate safety signals urgently and fully and publish the findings honestly: In the long run, will your credibility worsen or will you begin to regain public trust and confidence?

Reality check on the vaccine narrative[60]

On 23 October, an online poll on Covid controls and vaccines was published on news.com.au with some intriguing results. Conducted over one day, the survey attracted more than 42,000 votes for every question and more than 50,000 for some. Although the scale of the responses is impressive, the results show that the respondents were highly unrepresentative of the general population.

Official data from the health department show that nationwide, 95.2% of over-16s had received at least two doses of a Covid vaccine as of November 2, 72.2% were triple-vaccinated, and 41.7% had received four doses. But in the online survey, the percentages were 62, 26 and 16 for two, three and four shots, respectively. Clearly, therefore, the site's readership is not representative of the population and the survey attracted a disproportionate share of the Covid vaccine-hesitant.

Even with that caveat, some of the results are striking. "An overwhelming majority" are no longer concerned about Covid and do not wear masks in public. Half said they had caught Covid, with 6% getting it more than once. Around 37% said they were unvaccinated. Over two-thirds said the governments' pandemic response had been too heavy-handed, 25% said the leaders had done the best they could, and 8% thought Australia had handled the pandemic as well as any other country.

---

[60] Brownstone Institute, 10 November 2022, https://brownstone.org/articles/reality-check-on-the-vaccine-narrative/

Most strikingly of all, *only 35% of the 45,000 vaccinated respondents in the poll said they would make the same decision again, while not a single unvaccinated person expressed regret for the decision.*

Why do so many people feel this way? The latest weekly data from NSW Health covering the week of 23–29 October highlights four major disconnects between two critical claims in support of the official narrative and what their own data show.

Claims (p. 2)

"COVID-19 vaccines are very effective in preventing the severe impacts of infections with the virus."

"Over 95% of people aged 16 and over in NSW have received two doses of a COVID-19 vaccine."

Data (p. 4)

Table 8.1: NSW Covid-19 weekly data, 23–29 October 2022

NSW COVID-19 WEEKLY DATA OVERVIEW
Epidemiological week 43, ending 29 October 2022
www.health.nsw.gov.au/coronavirus

	Admitted to hospital	Admitted to ICU	Deaths
Age group (years)			
0-9	12	0	0
10-19	3	0	0
20-29	11	0	0
30-39	14	0	0
40-49	10	3	0
Vaccination status^			
Four or more doses	105	4	8
Three doses	53	6	3
Two doses	22	2	4
One dose	0	0	0
No doses	0	0	0
Unknown	47	6	2
Total	**227**	**18**	**17**

Source: NSW Health, *NSW Respiratory Surveillance Report – week ending 29 October 2022*, p. 4 https://www.health.nsw.gov.au/Infectious/covid-19/Documents/weekly-covid-overview-20221029.pdf

Not a single Covid-19 patient in NSW for the week—not one—who was admitted to hospital, or was admitted to ICU, or died, was unvaccinated: exactly 0% on all three metrics.

Every single one of the Covid-19 patients in NSW for the week, whose vaccination status was known, who was admitted to hospital, or was admitted to ICU, or died, was at least double-vaccinated: 100% on all three metrics.

Eight of the 15 Covid-related deaths—53.3%—had received four or more doses of the Covid vaccine. As of 2 November, the share of NSW residents eligible for four doses of the vaccine (30+ years old) to have received them was 43.3%. Thus, compared to their population, the four-dosed are over-represented by 23.1% in the Covid-related mortality in this reporting week. *However*, it's surely reasonable to say that it's almost certain that neither of the two who died with their vaccination status not known would have been four-dosed. If so, the share of the quadruple-vaccinated deaths drops halfway closer to their population share.

Not a single person whose death with Covid-19 in NSW was recorded in this week was under 50 years old.

Questions

Can you spot the gap/inconsistency/cognitive dissonance (pick your own preferred descriptor) between the claims that seek to bolster the highly effective vaccines slogan, and the data?

What do you think the chances are that if consulted, "fact-checkers" will judge this to be "misleading," "lacking context," and perhaps even "dangerous?" No doubt they could also find a couple of "useful idiots" to provide a helpful quote or two.

Of course, one weekly report cannot possibly have anything to say about trend lines. More than five months of NSW data can and do. They cast serious doubts on claims of vaccine effectiveness with regard to hospital admissions, ICU admissions and even deaths. The claims of trials-based efficacy were hugely exaggerated by using relative rather than the more honest absolute risk reduction, while ignoring the age-stratified number needed to be vaccinated in order to prevent one hospitalization or death.

Because of the long-term harms caused by the fear narrative and the severity of the coercion employed to encourage multiple rounds of vaccine and booster take-up, governments really do need to subject vaccine regulators and public health bureaucrats to serious scrutiny. Otherwise, they will continue to suffer from falling trust in public institutions.

At the individual level, vaccines may still offer some protection to the elderly, especially to people with serious underlying health conditions. But with the known and suspected risks of side-effects in the short and medium terms, the as yet unknown long-term safety profiles, and rising numbers with natural immunity from infection, the decision really is best left to individuals after full discussion with their doctors. The latter must not just be free, but must be encouraged to go over the balance of benefits and harms for their patients in order to get their informed consent.

Fearing the onset of relevance deprivation syndrome should the country conclude the pandemic is over and time to move on, or rather move back to pre-Covid normality, some experts are inevitably issuing grim warnings about newer, dangerously infectious variants that will come ashore over the Southern Hemisphere's autumn and winter.

What Is a safety signal and why does it matter?[61]

The pandemic has been an extended three-year "teachable moment" for many of us who previously had been content to go along with the public health messages from our nearly universally trusted medical experts, drug regulators and public health institutions.

Safety signals

In a peer-reviewed recent article, David Bell and colleagues concluded that "based on costs, disease burden and intervention effectiveness,"

[61] Brownstone Institute, 18 April 2023, https://brownstone.org/articles/what-is-safety-signal-why-does-it-matter/

mass Covid-19 vaccination campaigns did "not meet standard public health requirements for clear expected benefit." Several eminent experts warned about the likelihood of such a conclusion from the start and opinion has gradually been shifting towards this view, as I tried to summarise earlier.

Here I want to look specifically at the concept of "safety signals" because I don't believe the significance of this concept in medical science and public health interventions is widely understood in the general public.

I first became interested in this after watching Dr Peter McCullough in a TV interview with *France Soir* in June 2021. He pointed out that the CDC's Vaccine Adverse Events Reporting System (VAERS) normally records about 25 deaths per year from all vaccines. During the Covid pandemic, by 11 June 2021 it had verified 5,993 deaths, 20,737 hospitalizations, 47,837 urgent care visits, 1,538 anaphylaxis cases, and 1,868 cases of Bell's palsy.

Because VAERS is a passive-surveillance system, he said, the general consensus is that the numbers are vastly underreported. He warned that this is "a major safety signal … that has exceeded all boundaries of acceptability." Quizzed on the causal link to vaccines, he answered: "it's biologically plausible, temporally associated, internally consistent month by month" and also "externally consistent" with data from the US, Europe and England. "The vaccine is in the causal pathway to death … The majority of these 6,000 Americans, they were healthy enough to walk into a vaccine centre and within 2-4 days they're dead."

That was almost two years ago.

The European Medicines Agency defines "safety signal" as:

> *Information on a new or known adverse event that is potentially caused by a medicine and that warrants further investigation. Signals are generated from several sources such as spontaneous reports, clinical studies and the scientific literature.*

The WHO says:

> *a* ***safety signal*** *refers to information on a new or known side effect that may be caused by a medicine and is typically generated from more than a single report of a suspected side effect.*

A safety signal does not in and of itself establish a direct causal relationship between a medicine and any side effect. But it does generate "a hypothesis that, together with data and arguments, justifies the need" for an evaluation of "what is called causality assessment."

To complete the trilogy of authoritative pronouncements on the meaning, role and critical importance of safety signals, Australia's drugs regulator, the TGA directs medicine sponsors that:

You should establish and manage a pharmacovigilance system to help you meet your pharmacovigilance responsibilities…

In terms of monitoring and collecting safety information, your pharmacovigilance system should allow you to:

- *identify and collect all information related to the safety of your medicine from all possible sources, including*
- *spontaneous reports of adverse reactions (including consumer reports to you, or to people who work for you or have a contractual relationship with you)*
- *internet and social media reports*
- *reports from non-medical sources*
- *solicited reports, such as from post-registration studies or post-market initiatives*
- *reports in international and local literature*
- *individual adverse drug reaction reports in the TGA's Database of Adverse Event Notifications (DAEN)…*

*If you verify a signal that may change the benefit–risk balance of a medicine, you **MUST** report it to us as a significant safety issue together with any actions you propose to take, or justification for no further action.*

That seems pretty clear and comprehensive. If only it had been followed with respect to the Covid-19 mRNA vaccines.

The three wise monkeys

In recent times I have been ruminating over the intersection of the failure-cum-refusal of the public health officials to heed the safety signals in light of the cultural symbolism of the three monkeys. The origins of "The Three Wise Monkeys" are commonly attributed to Japan, although the proverb might have been brought there by Buddhist monks from India via China. Mizaru sees no evil by covering his eyes, Kikazaru hears no evil by covering his ears, and Iwazaru speaks no evil by covering his mouth.

The moral of the proverb is how to remain steadfast and morally upright even in the midst of evil. Instead, operating in the shadow perhaps of the militarized biosecurity state, the health authorities have seemed to have been operating under the injunction to "See No Harm, Hear No Harm, Speak No Harm," thereby inverting both their own professional obligation to "First, Do No Harm" (*Primum Non Nocere*) and the wisdom of the three monkeys.

"See No Harm"

Without reprising ground that has been extensively covered in the dissenting literature already and is now reaching a broader and more receptive audience, let us recall the following. The original trial data of the manufacturers has been extensively analysed to point to shortcomings, failures, refusal to publish the full raw data for independent cross-verification, allegations of fraudulent practices, and the deployment of the vaccine-sympathetic number of relative risk reduction while ignoring and downplaying the more vaccine-sceptical numbers of absolute risk reduction and the number needed to vaccinate in order to prevent one hospitalization, ICU admission and death.

The deliberate blind eye turned to the lagged temporal correlation between vaccine uptake and all-cause excess mortality is married to the focus on population-wide statistics instead of the age-segregated data for a disease whose burden shows a steep age gradient.

Regulators and authorities have proven to be just as determined to ignore the massive surge in the number of serious adverse events being reported as critics have been persistent in pointing to this as a critical safety signal that warrants further investigation and follow-up action. The phenomenon of fit and apparently healthy young athletes collapsing with alarming suddenness and frequency has provided visually powerful evidence of the possible harms from the vaccines.

The surge in miscarriages and fertility problems alongside the fall in birth rates nine months following vaccine rollouts is also being documented with increasing frequency and has the potential, Frijters, Foster and Baker argue, to rouse the slumbering public to righteous anger and calls for criminal accountability.

"Hear No Harm"

In the beginning, as vaccines began to be administered, some GPs and specialists, for example Dr Luke McLindon who has his own fertility clinic in Brisbane as well as Dr McCullough already referenced above, started speaking out about the alarming rate of serious adverse events and vaccine-related injuries they were noticing.

They quickly discovered that the drug regulators and their own medical licensing boards were deaf to all such reports. Their old fashioned fidelity to *Primum Non Nocere* was quaint but failed to charm the regulators.

"Speak No Harm"

Instead the regulators threatened them with professional disciplinary action and the threat was indeed carried out in a few instances. The modest numbers of doctors who lost their licenses does not invalidate the tactic. Authorities had adopted Sun Tzu's advice to "Kill one, terrify a thousand." We must appreciate how seriously worried these doctors of conscience must have been and the depth of courage they demonstrated in their duty of care to their patients that they risked their jobs and livelihoods in order to speak their truth to the powers that be. Bravo!

The understandings of the distribution of diseases in the population have a technical precision that they lack in general usage. We might think that in ordinary usage, 5% is rare. A disease is defined as "rare" if it affects about 1 in 2,000 people or about 0.05%, although it can range between 0.01–0.1%. "Very rare" is less than 0.01%; "uncommon," 0.1–1.0%; "common," 1–10%; and "very common," 10% upwards.

I have come to believe with the benefit of hindsight that the authorities intentionally conflated the common public understanding with the technical precision of the medical specialists in insisting that serious side effects have been very rare.

This was facilitated with the pandemic of media malfeasance. The Censorship-Industrial Complex was weaponized into a powerful tool of state power in an evolving system of governance that is a threat to the very survival of free society.

More questions for the public health clerisy

This raises some important questions. Was the mantra of "See No Harm, Hear No Harm, Speak No Harm" the result of:

- Regulatory capture by Big Pharma?
- Callous apathy, indifference and negligence by the regulators, public health institutions and medical establishments?
- Staggeringly gross incompetence?
- All of the above?

Most importantly, which ones of the above do not cross the threshold of criminality? What should be done about the reality that in refusing to be responsive to safety signals, the guardians and watchdogs of public health failed to discharge the solemn responsibility that had been entrusted to them?

N.B. This article grew out of a conversation on 15 April with Julie Sladden, Secretary of Australians for Science and Freedom, and Kara Thomas, Secretary of the Australian Medical Professionals Society.

Postscript

On 1 January 2021, the new chief of the The Medicines and Healthcare products Regulatory Agency (MHRA), Dr June Raine, said: "We are transforming the MHRA, making the regulator an enabler of innovation." Fast forward to January 2023 and a group of current and former advisers to the US Food and Drug Administration wrote to the FDA requesting that vaccine product labels be revised to more accurately reflect the known uncertainty on efficacy and harms in line with statements on the FDA's own site. The official "response was a sophisticated version of 'who cares'!"

How Covid broke our trust in the medical profession[62]

On 9 July, President Joe Biden's former Covid czar Ashish Jha conceded that vaccine mandates, which he had backed, "bred a lot of distrust" in the long run and did cause harms as well. Studies continue to be published to the effect that policy interventions to fight the pandemic—lockdowns, masks, vaccines—saved millions of lives. Thus a study by Watson *et al.* published in *Lancet Infectious Diseases* in

[62] *Spectator Australia*, 10 August 2024, https://www.spectator.com.au/2024/08/how-covid-broke-our-trust-in-the-medical-profession/

June 2022 estimated, using mathematical modelling of course, that just in its first year to 8 December 2021, vaccinations saved 14.4 million lives. Christopher Ruhm, in an article in *JAMA Health Forum* on 26 July, found that if all US states had followed the restrictions of the ten most restrictive states, there would have been 118,000-248,000 fewer US deaths in the two years to 8 December 2022. Perhaps.

Other studies claim that to the contrary, the number of deaths that policy interventions have caused and are likely to cause in the long term from the combined downstream effects, including severely disrupted healthcare and pharmaceutical supply chains, missed childhood immunisations, learning disruptions, hunger and poverty, will greatly exceed the sum of lives saved. On 19 July a 521-page paper by three Canadian researchers, based on data from 125 countries for 2021 and 2022, calculated the number of all-cause excess deaths "associated with Covid vaccines" to be 16.9 million—four times the number of Covid deaths until February 2024 as per the World Health Organisation (WHO). An article published online on 21 June in *Forensic Science International* , based on a systematic review of autopsy data, found that 73.9% of all Covid-related deaths were either caused or significantly impacted by Covid vaccines.

In September 2021, the UK government, acting on the advice of Chief Medical Officer Chris Whitty who overrode the more cautious Joint Committee on Vaccines and Immunisation (JCVI), authorised the vaccination of 5–11 year-old children. This was done despite a warning from a group of 26 Tory MPs that overruling expert advice from the JCVI risked "dissolving the bond of trust" between the public and the government. A new preprint on 20 May from a team at Oxford University reports on a study of a total of 415,884 vaccinated and unvaccinated children. They came to three important findings: there was not a single Covid-related death in either group among otherwise healthy children; the vaccinated had marginally better health outcomes on hospitalisation (1 additional child per 10,000) and A&E attendance (1 per 20,000); but these were mostly offset by the incidence of myocarditis and pericarditis which put 1 in 25,000 vaccinated kids into hospital. The economic cost worked out at £1.3/0.6 million per each hospital visit/A&E attendance (not death) that was averted. The moral of the story: trust neither the science nor the scientists.

Record-level data for ten million people in the Czech Republic were analysed by Steve Kirsch to show that all-cause deaths among 45–69 year olds given Moderna vaccines were more than 50% above those from Pfizer vaccines. Treating the latter as the placebo group allowed him to control for other potentially confounding variables and limit causality to vaccines. An Israeli study published on 26 June in the high-impact journal *Nature* explained how the Pfizer vaccine causes menstrual irregularities. For one compilation of scientific studies documenting vaccine injuries, with hyperlinks, see: https://ladycasey.substack.com/p/scientific-studies-on-vaccine-injuries.

Yet, articles and reviews critical of the official narrative on masks and vaccines, authored by well-credentialled experts and published in leading scientific outlets after rigorous peer review processes, were sometimes retracted or had cautionary notes added by nervous editors, only to be vindicated months or a year later, greatly diminishing their impact during the critical period. The eminent British oncologist Angus Dalgliesh wrote on 11 July that there's been a systematic suppression of the truth about the link between Covid vaccines and cancer and death.

In an interview with the *Brisbane Times* on 30 April 2020, Queensland's then-Chief Health Officer (and now Governor) Jeannette Young made it clear that her logic on school closures was primarily political. She accepted the evidence that schools are not a high-risk environment for the spread of the virus but argued that closing them helped to convince people how grave the situation was. "So sometimes it's more than just the science and the health, it's about the messaging." There's additional evidence of the creeping politicisation of the medical profession. The British Medical Association has rejected the Cass review into gender-identity services in England. Last week it called on the government to lift the ban on puberty blockers for adolescents disoriented about their sexuality. In another sign of the creeping ideological takeover of medical science, an article published in *JAMA Pediatrics* on 1 July substituted "pregnant people" and "pregnant persons" for pregnant women.

On 1 August, the Australian Medical Association warned that the nation's overstretched health system is at a tipping point with a real risk of life expectancy falling over the next ten years. Yet the AMA went along with all the questionable Covid eradication policies that wasted billions of dollars that could otherwise have been used to strengthen the public health infrastructure and also with un- and even some anti-scientific interventions and mandates that damaged trust in the medical profession. A 24-wave survey of 443,455 US adults across the 50 states, published recently in the *Journal of the American Medical Association*, found that overall, trust in physicians and hospitals had plummeted from 71.5 to 40.1% between April 2020 and January 2024. Trust had fallen in every sociodemographic group in the survey by age, gender, race and income. Unsurprisingly, lower levels of trust correlated with lower rates of vaccination. There's little reason to believe the situation in Australia is much different.

The media could have helped to contain the deepening loss of public trust in the medical profession and the public health clerisy by adopting its customary role of interrogating official claims and reporting fearlessly and neutrally on the significant minority of medical and scientific opinion that expressed disquiet at the abandonment of established public health consensus on managing pandemics. Instead, as Adam Creighton argued in a powerful essay in *The Australian* on 3 April 2023, "a too credulous, incurious mainstream media," with too many journalists acting as "cheerleaders for the health bureaucracy and politicians," must wear much of the blame for the "Covid vaccines" wall of infallibility" that has caused so much lasting harm.

9: APPROACHING ENDEMICITY

At which point do authorities conclude either that a pandemic disease has been eradicated, or else that it has become endemic? Whichever of the two is the conclusion, the result should mean an end to the emergency measures proclaimed to deal with the pandemic. Yet, many of the interventions to deal with Covid-19 seemed to have been kept in place long after their shelf life had expired.

A Covid stocktake[63]

In an article in the *Epoch Times* on 9 September, Julie Ponesse tells Canada's students that Covid control measures by university administrations "will stop as soon as you say 'no'." Moments we should all have said no was when put under house arrest, banned from the bedside of dying family members and the healing rituals of funerals (remember a masked Queen sitting all alone at her husband's service?), stopped health-sustaining access to beaches and parks and mandated facemasks, QR codes and digital vaccine certificates, etc: self-harms for the greater good.

The lockdown and vaccine narratives are falling apart at the seams. Canada's new opposition leader Pierre Poilievre is staunchly libertarian, anti-lockdown and anti-vaccination mandates who supported the truckers' Freedom Convoy. My jaw is still on the floor after

[63] *Spectator Australia*, 24 September 2022, https://www.spectator.com.au/2022/09/a-covid-stocktake/

hearing Jacinda Ardern say "we all just need to respect people's individual decisions." In the UK, former Chancellor Rishi Sunak's break from official policy led Liz Truss to rule out future lockdowns. On 11 August , the US Centers for Disease Control and Prevention (CDC) issued revised guidance to return much of the responsibility for risk reduction from institutions to individuals and shifted from sweeping population-wide precautions to targeted advice for vulnerable groups. "The effects of lockdown may now be killing more people than are dying of Covid," says the UK *Telegraph*, including a rise in the rate of prostate cancer deaths from 7% to 26%.

In Australia the push to end all special Covid measures is led by New South Wales (NSW) Premier Dominic Perrotet against stiff resistance from some states and experts who insist there's "no scientific basis" to end them. What scientific basis was there to introduce them, pray tell? Last year, UK "experts" warned Prime Minister (PM) Boris Johnson of catastrophe unless he cancelled his planned ending of restrictions and Anthony Fauci warned of disasters in states that rejected his recommended restrictions. Both were proven dead wrong.

In a press briefing on 6 September, White House Covid response coordinator Dr. Ashish Jha explained people can get their flu and Covid booster vaccines in one visit: "I really believe this is why God gave us two arms—one for the flu shot and the other one for the Covid shot." Was this a Freudian slip revealing the religious dogma that lies behind Covid policy? Used in ancient and medieval times, mass closures were discredited in Western epidemiology in the last century and replaced by the concept of herd immunity built through naturally-acquired and vaccine-induced infections. An analysis by Michael Senger concludes that, based on bioterrorism fears in the national security community after 9/11, the CDC had insinuated China's lockdown measures during the SARS epidemic as US federal policy by January 2004. They called it "social distancing" to disguise its origins.

Debbie Lerman has distilled a lockdown blueprint centred on a relentless fear campaign reinforced by stressing uniqueness, worst-case scenarios, not knowing what to expect and "we're all equally at risk," on the one hand; and the abandonment of all previous policies in favour of universal mandates to isolate, test, trace, mask up, vaccinate etc. Based mostly in junk science, they terrified the people into demanding draconian "health" measures whose primary, intended purpose was to cynically exploit emotional distress to ensure compliance with unprecedented, untested, ineffective and destructive policy interventions. They succeeded.

Covid poses such miniscule risk to children that vaccinating them is "all risk, no benefit." An article in the *British Medical Journal* shows 12-15 year old healthy boys are four times more at risk of myocarditis after a second Pfizer vaccine than of hospital admission for Covid.

The global drug industry has a particularly scandal-ridden history. In a class action case against Merck in Australia in 2009, court documents revealed that the US drug giant had prepared a "hit list" of doctors who criticised Vioxx, a Merck product, for its deadly cardiovascular side-effects. On 4 February 2021, Merck—which makes patent-free low profit Ivermectin and has been selling it for years—publicly questioned its safety. How often does a drug company badmouth its own product? The *British Medical Journal* documented a compromising 96% of the TGA's 2020–21 budget came from industry sources, raising serious questions about regulatory capture. Last year the TGA banned the use of ivermectin for Covid treatment.

A month later Merck announced the development of a new antiviral drug for which it sought emergency use authorisation from the Federal Drug Administration (FDA). This cannot be granted if an existing treatment is available. Banning ivermectin and hydroxychloroquine was essential to grant emergency use authorisation for high-profit Covid vaccines and drugs. Yet a major large-scale study from Brazil published on 31 August found that, compared to regular users, non-use of ivermectin increased the risk of Covid-related mortality by 12.5 times and dying from Covid by seven times.

The Therapeutic Goods Regulation (1990) restricts provisional approvals to medicines for "the treatment, prevention or diagnosis of a life-threatening or seriously debilitating condition." This would appear to rule out provisional vaccine approval for children below five. On this basis, a group of lawyers is aiming to file a crowd-funded case in the High Court against the TGA's decision. On past form, don't hold your breath for the courts to uphold citizens' autonomy over the health bureaucracy's infinite if inscrutable wisdom.

Look back in anger[64]

Remember this joke: a teenager kills his parents and appeals to the courts for mercy as an orphan? The Australian Medical Association backed lockdown restrictions back in the day but is now complaining about the growing backlog in elective surgery. Here's a question. Had the vast sums thrown at Covid been redirected to the leading killer diseases, using the standard quality adjusted life years (QALY) metric, how many million deaths would have been averted around the world over the next decade? The lockdown harms are showing up in excess death counts, job losses, supply chains chaos, rising cost of living and have locked in generational poverty and inequality in and across nations.

Historical illiteracy is now a job requirement for "experts." Germany has burnt 17.25 million masks past their expiry date, while stockpiling more for future emergencies. Recalling Margaret Thatcher's comment on the trouble with socialism, politicians don't learn from mistakes made with other people's money. The media too lived down to their description as stenographers with amnesia. The state dictated every aspect of peoples' lives, down to the most ridiculous,

[64] *Spectator Australia*, 28 January 2023, https://www.spectator.com.au/2023/01/look-back-in-anger-5/

absurd and intimate details. With no known cure for blind faith in governments, people embraced compliance with draconian directives from politicians proffering iron fists as a magic bullet.

Lockdowns were a euphemism for a wholesale shutting down of social and economic activities and putting entire populations under house arrest. Neither based in science and best-practice medicine, nor commensurate with the age-stratified threat from the virus, they lasted on and off for two years with constantly shifting goalposts. Early data told us in February–March 2020 already that the most vulnerable were elderly people with comorbidities. In a modern day version of sacrificing virgins to appease the viral gods, the young have lost many more years of their life to buy a few more lonely, miserable months for the infirm old. A study in the *Proceedings of the National Academy of Sciences* showed that lack of household exposure to kids increased Covid hospitalisation of grown-ups by 27% and ICU admission by 49%. They should have said: "Don't be a Granny killer. Leave that to us."

The UK Influenza Preparedness Strategy 2011 encapsulated the prevailing consensus on masks: "there is very little evidence of widespread benefit from their use in [the community and household] setting." The lack of observed differences can be seen in a series of comparative charts in Ian Miller's Unmasked: The Global Failure of Covid Mask Mandates (2022). Governments "nudged" the public to exert peer pressure as a tool of social coercion, backed by sometimes brutal police action against pockets of resistance and protest. Mask mandates reflected and perpetuated the reign of fear and demonstrated broad compliance with the effort of governments to exercise population-wide social control. A highly visible symbol of collectivist compliance, masks became Mao suits for the face.

Japan has extraordinarily high levels of public compliance with government directives and mask wearing is all pervasive. Using Our World in Data figures, in Japan 2.5 times as many people died with Covid in the 13.5 months after than in the 21.3 months before 80% full vaccination. Yet they still refuse to entertain the notion that vaccines might be the problem, not the solution. The continued hold of the "safe and effective" vaccine mantra and facemasks efficacy for controlling the coronavirus is cause for despair in official cussedness and public gullibility. The transient effectiveness of vaccines has necessitated boosters every few months. Often vaccine rollouts coincided with upsurge in infections and deaths, suggesting negative efficacy. Newer studies show successor doses are less effective and repeated doses may be driving infections by damaging the immune function. When vaccines began to be administered at the end of 2020, 1.9mn people had died with Covid globally. Another 4.8mn have died since then. Added to the growing toll of vaccine injuries, this has discredited officials and experts who claimed the vaccines would prevent infection, transmission, severe illness, and death. All that matters to zealots is how many arms are jabbed how often.

With help from the media, social media (thank you Elon Musk for the Twitter Files) and police, people were frightened, shamed and brutalised into submission to arbitrary and authoritarian diktats. Governments deployed state propaganda to instil fear of the disease and shame all effort to question edicts. Turning the debate from a scientific discourse into a moral imperative facilitated the demonisation and denigration of critical voices on the lethality of the virus, the effectiveness and ethics of lockdowns, masks and vaccine mandates, and the harms inflicted by these interventions.

Calls have grown for an immediate suspension of vaccinations until the unusually strong correlations with excess deaths, heart problems and female reproduction are properly investigated. Instead, suspicions become only stronger that regulators have become vaccine enablers first, more committed to defend vaccines from criticism than protect people from harmful vaccines. The media switched from exposing official lies to amplifying them instead. One dispiriting lesson from the last three years is people will "live happily ever after" as long as the media ignores how governments trample our freedoms and liberties while claiming to keep us safe.

.On every major point of contention in managing the pandemic, the Great Barrington Declaration was right. Fearmongers-in-Chief like Neil Ferguson, Anthony Fauci (whose omniscience deserted him during deposition) and their local "useful idiots" were wrong. The common sense distilled into the few words of the Declaration was an uncommon virtue. The three scientist-authors—from Harvard, Oxford and Stanford!—were taken down savagely and belittled as "fringe epidemiologists."

The malfeasance was compounded by the cowardice of political leaders hiding behind "Follow the Science" that mistook a slogan for policy and let loose upon democratic societies previously unimaginable acts and scenes of censorship, coercion and brutality that has gradually eroded trust in authorities and institutions. Recovery and healing will be difficult without accountability, punishment and robust and resilient institutional guardrails against repeating episodes of the abuses.

Conspiracy theories become conspiracy facts[65]

At first slowly but in recent weeks with seemingly gathering pace, two trends have emerged. On the one hand, many of the core claims behind lockdowns, masks, and vaccines are unravelling and the prevailing narrative has been in retreat on all three fronts. But there is still a long way to go, as indicated by the refusal of the Biden administration to let Novak Djokovic play at Indian Wells.

On the other hand, the explosive lockdown files in the UK have blown apart the official narrative. We the sceptics were right in our dark suspicions of the motives, scientific basis, and evidence behind government decisions, but even we did not fully grasp just how venal, evil, and utterly contemptuous of their citizens some of the bastards

[65] Brownstone Institute, 9 March 2023, https://brownstone.org/articles/conspiracy-theories-become-conspiracy-facts/

in charge of our health, lives, livelihoods, and children's future were. "Hell is empty, And all the devils are here" (Shakespeare, *The Tempest*) indeed. They will have to build a new circle of hell to accommodate all the perpetrators of evil let loose upon the world since 2020.

A mistake is when you spill coffee or take the wrong exit ramp off the highway. Lockdown was a policy pushed hard by politicians and health chiefs even against scientific dissent and substantial public opposition, using tools from every tyrants' playbook of disinformation and lies whilst attacking and censoring truth. The depth of public opposition went unrecognised because the fear-peddling media colluded in not reporting on protests.

Genuine mistakes were few and are forgivable. Most were deliberate distortions of reality, outright falsehoods, and a systematic campaign to terrorise people into compliance with arbitrary diktats interspersed with efforts to vilify, silence, and cancel all critics by using the full powers of the state to co-opt, bribe, and bully. All in pursuit of the most maddening public policy insanity of modern times because it ignored existing canons of pandemic planning in blind panic just when calm was most needed. To call lockdown a mistake is to trivialise the shock to society.

Before coming to that, a few preliminary observations to summarise where we are at.

What is now known and generally but not universally admitted

Covid is now endemic. It will circulate throughout the world and keep returning with mutating variants. People who have been infected and/or vaccinated can contract and transmit it. Consequently we have little choice but to learn to live with it. What is important is to make sure the right policy lessons are learnt so that never again, neither for a novel coronavirus nor for any other infectious disease, do we go down the path of public policy insanity to lock up an entire city or country with the discovery of 1-10 cases and bring all social, cultural and economic activity to a shuddering halt—or give total power and control to sociopaths and psychopaths.

Meanwhile what is particularly striking is just how many suspicions voiced by sceptics from early 2020 onwards and mocked as conspiracy theories have turned into plausible claims and accepted facts:

- The virus may have originated in the laboratory of the Wuhan Institute of Virology;
- Covid modelling was dodgy and dressed up outliers as reasonable case scenarios;
- Lockdowns don't work;
- Lockdowns kill through perverse consequences and inflict other damaging harms, including interruptions to critical life-saving children's immunization campaigns in developing countries;
- School closures are particularly bad policy. They did not curb transmission but they did cause long-term harm to children's education, development and emotional well-being;
- Masks are ineffective. They stop neither infection nor transmission;
- Infection confers natural immunity at least as effective as vaccination;
- Covid vaccines do not stop infection, hospitalisation, or even death;
- Covid vaccines do not stop transmission;
- The safety of vaccines using new technology had not been definitively established, neither for the short term nor for the long term;
- Vaccine harms are real and substantial but safety signals have been summarily dismissed and ignored;
- mRNA vaccines are not confined to the arm but spread rapidly to other parts, including reproductive organs, with potentially adverse consequences for fertility and births;

- The harm-benefit equation of vaccines is, like the disease burden itself, steeply age-differentiated. Healthy young people did not need either initial or booster doses;
- Vaccination mandates don't increase vaccine take-up;
- Vaccine mandates can fuel cross-vaccine hesitancy;
- Suppression of sceptical and dissenting voices will lessen trust in public health officials, experts and institutions, and possibly also in scientists more generally;
- Estimates of "Long Covid" were inflated (CDC estimate of 20% of Covid infections against UK study's estimate of 3%) by using generalised, non-specific symptoms like mild fatigue and weakness;
- Health policy interventions involve policy trade-offs just like all other policy choices. Cost-benefit analysis is therefore an essential prerequisite, not an optional add-on.

The Lockdown Files

The last three years have seen lives lost in the millions with tens of millions more yet to be accounted for in the coming years, civilised lifestyles destroyed, previously inviolate freedoms shredded, civil liberties turned into privileges to be granted on the whim of bureaucrats, law enforcement officers corrupted into street thugs brutalising the very people they are sworn to serve and protect, businesses destroyed, economies wrecked, bodily integrity violated.

The Lockdown Files, a treasure trove of over 100,000 WhatsApp messages in real time between all the principal policymakers on Covid in England while Matt Hancock was the Secretary of Health (2020–26 June 2021), offer an unparalleled and gripping window into the amoral and cynical arrogance circulating in the corridors of power. The daily drip-feed of revelations in the *Telegraph* is akin to watching with fascinated horror a slow-motion train wreck. Schadenfreude doesn't come any more delicious.

The files are littered with flippant remarks, mocking comments and contempt for citizens. Among the revelations about the Johnson government:

The government knew there was no "robust rationale" for including children in the "rule of six" (the maximum number of people who could meet at any given time), but backed the controversial policy anyway.

Facemasks were introduced in secondary schools in England after PM Johnson was told it was "not worth an argument" with Scotland's Nicola Sturgeon over the issue, despite England's Chief Medical Officer (CMO) Chris Whitty saying there were "no very strong reasons" to do so. In other words, political calculations were knowingly prioritized over schoolchildren's needs.

A plan to lift restrictions were dropped after Johnson was told it would be "too far ahead of public opinion."

Consultants were paid over £1 million a day for more than a year on the totally ineffectual test and trace program, turning the scheme into the embezzlement of public funds to line private pockets.

We now know just how punch drunk on tyranny the political, bureaucratic, scientific, and journalist class was during the pandemic. The ruling elites, when liberated from democratic accountability and media scrutiny, morphed seamlessly into morally cavalier and inhumane petty tyrants. Averse to alternative ways of thinking outside the echo chamber, they developed neuralgia to any idea that might challenge lockdown fanaticism.

Lockdown sceptics like the authors of the Great Barrington Declaration (GBD) who argued for the elderly and frail to be protected were demonised as dangerous "Covid deniers" who wanted to "let it rip" in a callous and cruel strategy of herd immunity. But government officials whose policies had a direct, catastrophic impact on the health of the elderly and frail were treated as heroes and unimpeachable voices of moral authority.

Sociopath, psychopath, or both?

Among the revelations about Hancock:

- More than 40,000 residents of care homes in England died with Covid. Hancock was advised by Whitty in April 2020 to test everyone entering the care homes. He rejected the advice because testing capacity was limited and, for political (PR) reasons, he prioritised reaching his grandiose, self-imposed target of 100,000 daily tests in the lower risk general community over protecting the care home residents, despite repeated claims of having thrown a "protective ring" around the homes. Patients discharged into care homes from hospitals were tested but not those coming in from the community. That is, "focused protection" of the GBD was the right way to go. Instead Hancock rubbished the GBD and belittled its three eminent epidemiologist authors.
- Social care minister Helen Whateley told Hancock that stopping visits to care homes by spouses was "inhumane" and risked the elderly residents "just giving up" after prolonged isolation, but he refused to budge.
- He rejected advice in November 2020 to shift from 14-day Covid quarantine for people who had been in close contact with anyone infected, to five days of testing because it would "imply we've been getting it wrong." Talk of a sunk cost fallacy. Over 20mn people in total were told to self-isolate even if they had no symptoms. God I feel vindicated for refusing flatly to join Australia's clunky test and trace program.
- In a discussion on how to ensure the public complied with ever-changing lockdown restrictions, Hancock suggested "We frighten the pants off everyone" and Project Fear was born. Simon Case, Britain's most senior civil servant, said the "fear/guilt factor" was "vital" in "ramping up the messaging" during the third lockdown in January 2021.

- Informed of the emergence of the alpha/Kent variant in December 2020, Hancock and his aides canvassed the ideal time to "deploy" the new variant in order to sustain public fear of the virus to ensure continued compliance with directives.
- A member of his team asked if they could "lock up" Nigel Farage after he tweeted a video of himself at a pub in Kent, because the troublesome politician was such a thorn in the government's side.
- Hancock and Case mocked people forced to isolate in quarantine hotels, joking about returning travellers being "locked up" in "shoe box" rooms. Case wished he could "see some of the faces of people coming out of first class and into a premier inn shoe box." Informed by Hancock that 149 people had entered "Quarantine Hotels due to their own free will," Case replied: "Hilarious."
- Hancock fought furious internal battles to hog the vaccine media limelight. He preened about his pictures in the media and boasted how the pandemic could propel his career "into the next league."
- He told other ministers to "get heavy with the police" to enforce lockdown restrictions and then boasted that "The plod got their marching orders." This raises questions about the legality of interfering with the operational instructions of police.
- Intoxicated by his own brilliance and infallibility, Hancock attacked vaccine czar Dame Kate Bingham, the chief of the National Health Service (NHS) Lord Stevens, and CEO of the Wellcome Trust (and now top scientist at the WHO) Sir Jeremy Farrar.
- He schemed with his aides, with the help of a secret spreadsheet, to deny rebellious party MPs funding for pet projects in their constituencies if they did not fall in line, including a new centre for disabled children and adults.

I can relate therefore to this online comment on one of these stories in the *Telegraph*: "Hancock was intellectually stunted pondlife before the pandemic and still is now, but with more slime and a bit of a stink to him." Or, to put it in more technical language: Hancock comes across as an ego-driven total f…wit.

The state criminalised quotidian activities like sitting on a bench in the park, walking on the beach and meeting with extended family. Public health messaging was weaponised to normalize and sacralise spirit-sapping levels of social isolation. Even East Germany's Stasi did not stop the elderly from hugging their grandchildren. Elderly patients were forced to die alone and surviving family members were banned from saying final farewells and denied the solace of a full funeral.

Hancock was able to get away with exercising his lust for power because his prime minister proved to be lazy, weak, and vacillating. The vivid description of Johnson by fired top aide Dominic Cummings—an out of control "shopping trolley" lurching from side to side in a supermarket aisle, depending on who he last talked to—has been amply validated by the leaked files. The instinctual libertarian rapidly morphed from a lockdown sceptic into a zealot.

Lessons

The Lockdown Files confirm that politics informed the policymakers in most of the key decisions on how to manage the pandemic. Accordingly, while medical specialists can debate the technical details of different medical approaches, policy specialists should be among the lead assessors in evaluating the justifications for and results and effectiveness of the policy interventions.

The existing frameworks, processes and institutional safeguards under which liberal democracies operated until 2020 had ensured expanding freedoms, growing prosperity, an enviable lifestyle, quality of life, and educational and health outcomes without precedent in human history. Abandoning them in favour of a tightly centralised small group of decision-makers liberated from any external scrutiny, contestability, and accountability produced both a dysfunctional process and suboptimal outcomes: very modest gains for much long-lasting pain.

The sooner we return to the conviction that good process ensures better long-term outcomes and acts as a check against suboptimal outcomes alongside curbs on abuses of power and wastage of public funds, the better.

Interventions rooted in panic, driven by political machinations, and using all the levers of state power to terrify citizens and muzzle critics in the end needlessly killed massive numbers of the most vulnerable, while putting the vast low-risk majority under house arrest. The benefits are questionable but the harms are increasingly obvious. The Johnson government in general and Hancock in particular revalidate Lord Acton's astute observation that power corrupts and absolute power corrupts absolutely.

They weren't following the science but Hancock's ego and career ambitions. He exploited Johnson's "stonking" laziness and shallowness. The Lockdown Files reveal a government gone rogue that viewed and treated the people as enemies. The UK, US, and Australia don't need an inquiry strung out over years, focussed on small details to the neglect of the big picture, with the tame conclusion that lessons will be learnt but blame cannot be apportioned. Instead we need criminal charges, and the sooner the better.

Britain's top civil servant acted more like a partisan political hack than an apolitical, neutral and loyal-to-the-elected-government of the day civil servant. Case's bias, immaturity, poor judgment, and unwillingness to support the PM with accurate, balanced, and impartial information were such as to warrant instant sacking. His hubris is such that he is yet to submit his resignation despite the publication of these appalling exchanges with Hancock who had effectively taken over the government.

The fact that as the "absolutely cringe-worthy" revelations came tumbling out, PM Rishi Sunak insisted Case has his confidence reflects poorly on Sunak's judgment.

In a modern-day version of sacrificing virgins to appease the viral gods, the young have lost many more years of their life to buy a few more lonely, miserable months for the infirm old.

If the vast sums thrown at Covid had been redirected to the leading killer diseases and upgrades to public health infrastructure, using the standard quality-adjusted life years (QALY) metric, many million deaths would have been averted around the world over the coming decades.

If we fail to heed the lessons of the last three years, we will indeed be condemned to repeat them, not just for new pandemics of infectious diseases but also for other crises like the "climate emergency."

The narrative in retreat[66]

The Lockdown Files have dished up a curious exchange among Britain's top policy advisers in early 2020. On 29 February, responding to a WhatsApp message from PM Johnson's chief adviser Dominic Cummings that Israeli scientists were just weeks away from developing a Covid vaccine and if this was credible, Chief Scientist Sir Patrick Vallance replied "Short answer is no."

CMO Whitty explained: "For a disease with a low (for the sake of argument 1%) mortality a vaccine has to be very safe so the safety studies can't be shortcut. So important for the long run." England's highest mortality rate was in April 2020 at 0.6%, falling to 0.55% in January 2021 and 0.04% by January 2023.

Based on the original Phase 3 trial data, Bart Classen showed as early as August 2021: "Results prove that none of the vaccines provide a health benefit and all pivotal trials show a statically significant increase in "all cause severe morbidity" in the vaccinated group compared to the placebo group."

This is nicely book-ended by a recent (16 March) CDC report showing US maternal mortality jumped to 1,205 in 2021 compared with 861

[66] Brownstone Institute, 22 March 2023, https://brownstone.org/articles/the-narrative-in-retreat/

in 2020 and 754 in 2019. The 2021 rate of 32.9 maternal deaths per 100,000 live births is the highest maternal mortality rate since 1965. Hmmm, let's see. What was the newly introduced pharmaceutical intervention in 2021 that begins with "v," that must not be named in connection with unexplained deaths, that also exacerbated the damage to healthcare access caused by the nonpharmaceutical interventions?

As Sonia Elijah comments, drug regulators withdrew 20 common cough and cold remedies earlier this month "because of concerns about a 'very rare' risk of anaphylaxis." The European Medicines Agency identified anaphylaxis as an important risk from Pfizer's Covid-19 vaccine way back when in December 2020 and flagged it again in August 2021.

So the vaccine was withdrawn immediately, you ask? I like your sense of humour. And please do try to remember that anyone dying within 14 days of a Covid injection was in reality "unvaccinated."

Thomas Buckley summarises it succinctly:

> *Tetanus boosters are not scheduled every four months … and polio is an awful memory of the past.*
>
> *Covid is still around and, most likely, will be forever, as will the growing list of health problems associated with the shot itself….*
>
> *From two weeks to stop the spread to get a not-vaccine shot every four months, the pandemic response has been full of lies and suffering for the general public and money and power for the autocrats and oligarchs and their clerisy.*

Setbacks to the narrative

Panic saw 100 years of evidence-based pandemic response programs junked. The accumulated wisdom was to quarantine the sick, not those feeling well; to prioritise the most vulnerable, not coerce the least vulnerable. I've gone back to read the CDC's 2017 "Community Mitigation Guidelines to Prevent Pandemic Influenza." Among its conclusions:

The CDC "might recommend the use of facemasks by ill persons as a source control measure during severe, very severe, or extreme influenza pandemics when crowded community settings cannot be avoided." However, "little evidence supports the use of facemasks by well persons in community settings."

"Persons in community settings who show symptoms consistent with influenza and who might be infected with (probable) pandemic influenza should be separated from well persons as soon as practical, be sent home, and practice voluntary home isolation."

While Sweden was a lonely outlier in sticking with existing science and plans, almost all others chose experimentation over decades of experience. Bizarrely, with lockdown normalised as the default response, Sweden was the one called on to explain staying with its existing plan.

This happened because superstition-driven diktat took over in the wish to be seen to be doing something. Fear was instrumentalised to terrify citizens. A Yale study in November 2021 concluded that public health messaging was effective in shaming and embarrassing people into getting vaccinated to protect themselves, in the belief that this would also expedite the date on which the entire community could be released from the restrictions.

Focusing on only one of three metrics

Yet, vaccines were tested for reducing the likelihood of infection leading to serious illness and death, not for protecting against infection and transmission. Robert Blumen has noted how manufacturers and health authorities ignored the more troublesome numbers of absolute risk reduction and numbers needed to vaccinate. Instead, they concentrated in weaponising the relative risk reduction of 95% so that people were misled into believing it meant 95% protection against infection, rather than a 95% reduction in the risk of those infected to progress to severe disease: "Covid injections were a treatment, not a vaccine."

There would never have been the widespread public backing for vaxports if people had not been misled into exaggerating the threat from Covid by several factorfold and mistaking relative for absolute risk reduction. This led them into the false belief that mass vaccination would end the pandemic and the unvaccinated were selfishly prolonging that day of release.

The brainwashing was so effective that to this day many insist that the high rate of vaccination protected Novak Djokovic from Covid.

The virus and the disease are two different things that became conflated in the public discourse. "Coronavirus" is a generic term that includes a large family of viruses with spiky projections on their surface that look like crowns. SARS-CoV-2 is a specific virus. Covid is the respiratory illness caused by the virus (just as measles is the disease caused by the virus rubeola).

Anyone could catch the virus, but the health risks from the disease were steeply age-dependent. So yes, the virus doesn't discriminate, but no, we were not in it together. The conflation of the virus and the disease led directly to the policy confusion that dismissed targeted protection in favour of universal prescriptions.

A Covid vaccination helps the body to build immunity against the disease. A person with enhanced immunity to developing the disease owing to being vaccinated can still carry and transmit the virus that causes the disease.

The three key and distinct numbers for assessing vaccine efficacy are absolute risk reduction, relative risk reduction, and number needed to vaccinate (NNV). The vaccine manufacturers and promoters engaged in a misleading campaign.

A *Lancet* article gave the relative risk reduction of five vaccines from 67% to 95%, but their absolute risk reduction ranged from 0.84% for Pfizer to 1.3% for AstraZeneca: not so impressive but far more realistic. A 95% efficacy within a 1% subgroup will barely register as a blip on the mortality curves.

On the number needed to vaccinate, CDC Director Rochelle Walensky tweeted on 25 June 2021 that among 12-17 year olds, one million vaccinated protect one death. To estimate the benefit-harm ratio, therefore, we would need to know the injurious side-effects for that age group.

This is where Aseem Malhotra's calculations are pertinent. In summary, Pfizer's original trial data suggested that there is "a greater risk of serious adverse events from the vaccine than from hospitalisation because of Covid-19."

The puzzle of why there was a worldwide cascading abandonment of a hundred years of accumulated knowledge by scientific and policy advisers will occupy researchers for many years. The result is that old lessons are having to be relearned. Judging by the rush of studies now coming through to contradict key tenets of the 2020–22 narrative, there's hope that the wall of silence rooted in groupthink and fear of consequences to career and reputation might have been irreparably breached.

Recent studies

At the community level, neither isolation nor vaccination but socialisation confers the best immunization. A study in the *Proceedings of the National Academy of Sciences* last July showed that lack of household exposure to kids increased Covid hospitalisation of grown-ups by 27% and ICU admission by 49%.

The state turned out to be the most efficient Granny killer along with the biggest purveyor of mis- and disinformation. A study of almost 300,00 people in California found that adults have sharply elevated risks of being diagnosed with heart, skin and psychiatric conditions in the three months following Covid injections. In February, three years later, the *Lancet* published a meta-analysis of 65 studies confirming that immunity conferred by prior infection is real, robust and long-lasting, at least as protective as two doses of the mRNA vaccines.

A study from George Mason University in February found that vaccine mandates in nine US cities did not increase vaccine take-up, undermining one of their key justifications. Data released in

February by the Office of National Statistics showed that in England, deaths among the vaccinated was disproportionately higher for all age groups for most of 2021 and 2022. Another study by a Slovenian team, published in preprint, found the mortality of vaccinated-infected groups to be 14.5% higher on average than that of non-vaccinated groups.

An earlier study in 2022 found that across 19 European countries, birth rates fell nine months after vaccine rollouts gathered speed. Pfizer began a clinical trial in February 2021 to examine the safety and efficacy of its mRNA vaccine in pregnant women and their newborns but the release of data from the trial is still awaited.

Perhaps the biggest surprise is an article in *Cell Host & Microbe* published on 11 January 2023, with Anthony Fauci as one of the co-authors. Contrary to the good doctor's many absolutist claims while still in office, this article concedes that "it is not surprising that none of the predominantly mucosal respiratory viruses have ever been effectively controlled by vaccines." Non-sterilizing Covid vaccines could and should never have been expected to significantly reduce infection or transmission. Here is a five minute compilation of Anthony Fauci's many inconsistencies, contradictions, and denialism.

Dr. Guy Hatchard has drawn attention to two studies by authors from the New Zealand Ministry of Health that show (1) a statistically significant association between Pfizer Covid vaccines and myocarditis and acute kidney injury, (2) correlation between vaccination status and mortality in 2021–23 inclusive, and (3) compared to the 73% of those eligible who had received Pfizer booster shots, the boosted account for a disproportionate 80% of all Covid deaths.

Other studies show successor doses are less effective and repeated doses may be driving infections. A study in December in *Science Immunology* by German scientists indicated that the third and subsequent doses of mRNA vaccines could be weakening the immune system, increasing the risk of infection and of prolonging and making the illness more serious.

A study published in February found that mRNA vaccines contain billions of particles of self-replicating DNA that can turn human cells into permanent factories for Covid-19 spike protein. This could explain the persistence of spike protein and mRNA in the body for months after injection.

An analysis of the situation in Western Australia is especially interesting, because although 4mn vaccine doses were administered in 2021, border closures to interstate and international travel were zealously enforced to protect the state as an infection-free-zone. Subsequent adverse events therefore cannot be attributed to Covid.

In an analysis posted on 14 March, Rebekah Barnett notes that the rate of adverse events for Covid vaccines (264.1/100,000 doses) was almost 24 times higher than all others (11.1). The number of adverse events in 2021—remember, there was almost no Covid in WA that year—was 10,726, 39 times higher than the average of 276 per year in the 2017–20 period. She quotes the annual WA Vaccine Surveillance Report: "The number of adverse events following immunisation ... was significantly higher in 2021 than in previous years ... due to the introduction of the Covid-19 vaccination program."

Figure 9.1: WA adverse events following immunisation by month, 2021, excluding active surveillance reports for routine vaccination reports

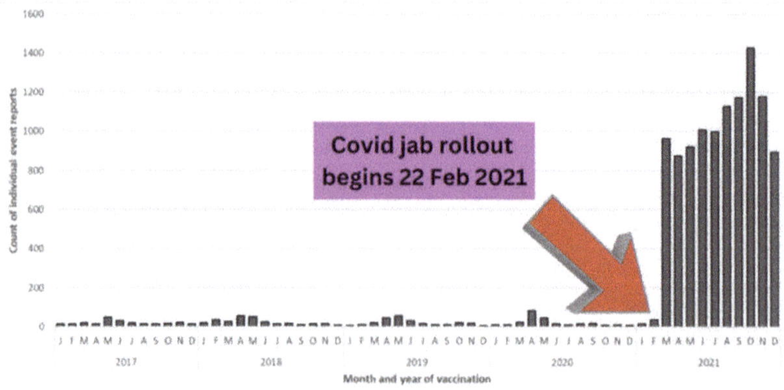

The impact of the Covid vaccination campaign in 2021 on reported adverse events is visually quite dramatic in her first chart (Figure 9.1). Some of the key takeaways are:

- Women were disproportionately affected (64%);
- Contrary to claims from the national drug regulator, 57% of those adversely affected required treatment in the emergency department of hospitals;
- The hardest hit age bracket was the 30–49 year olds;
- Background rates of myocarditis and pericarditis increased by 35 and 25%, respectively.

Figure 9.2: OECD excess deaths

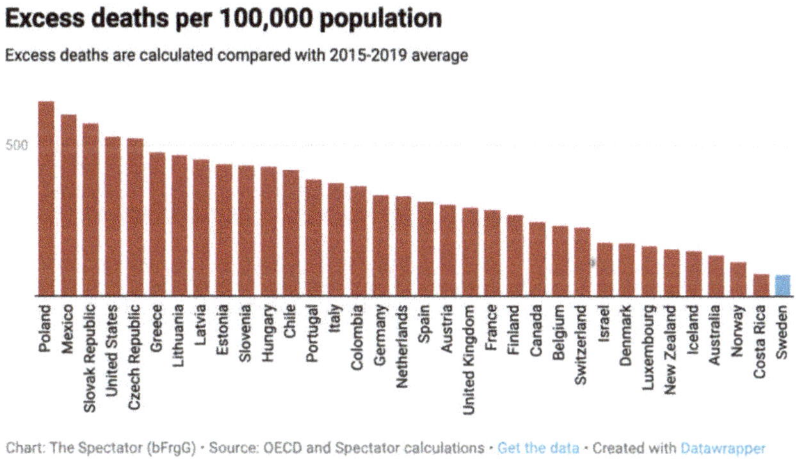

Source: Michael Simmons (*Spectator UK*'s Data Editor), 10 March 2023

The lockdown harms are showing up in excess death counts, job losses, supply chains chaos and rising costs of living. This may get worse in the next 2-5 years before it begins to normalize. Sweden is an absolute standout in bucking this trend (Figure 9.2).

I wonder why? Could it be that if we hadn't shut down the economy and healthcare, cancelled cancer and coronary work, induced mass fear in the general populace, stopped people exercising in the open air and not intensified social isolation by preventing people talking to one another, we might, just possibly might, have had lower excess deaths?

The Lockdown Files show UK Health Secretary Matt Hancock getting increasingly riled by the Swedish counterexample. I am sick of the "fucking Sweden argument," he said, and demanded "three or four bullet [points] of why Sweden is wrong." He didn't inquire if Sweden was wrong. Assuming that, he wanted to be able to show why it was wrong: a perfect example of policy-based evidence.

That said, Sweden's exceptionally low excess death count is also a strong cautionary note against popular arguments conflating vaccine-excess deaths correlation with causation. Will Jones, editor of *The Daily Sceptic*, explores several alternative hypotheses on the link between excess deaths, the virus, lockdowns and vaccines.

Conclusion

The vast majority of Covid deaths in many countries by now are among the vaccinated and boosted. This proves conclusively the ineffectiveness of vaccines at the community level, totally discredits the premise of vaccine mandates, but leaves open the possibility of net protective benefits for target groups like the elderly and people with comorbidities.

The policy conclusion is to lift mandates in public settings and prohibit companies from imposing them in most business settings, leaving it instead for people to make informed decisions in consultation with their doctors, without pressure on the latter from drug regulators.

For all the eye-watering amounts of money transferred from taxpayers to Big Pharma, the Covid vaccines would seem mostly to bear little causal relationship to mortality outcomes:

- Not every death listed as a Covid death was caused by Covid;

- Not every vaccinated person who died was killed by the vaccine;
- Not everyone who was vaccinated, infected by the virus and got sick with Covid but didn't die, lives because of the vaccines;
- Among the unvaccinated also, conversely, not everyone who died from Covid, did so because they avoided the jabfest;
- Not every unvaccinated person who was infected by the virus and got sick with Covid but didn't die, lives because of avoiding the vaccine.

The important point is the imperative need to investigate the phenomenon. The refusal of governments to do so is exasperating but perhaps also very telling: Never ask a question to which you don't know the answer.

With no known cure for blind faith in governments, people embraced compliance with draconian directives from politicians proffering iron fists as a magic bullet.

From Twitter Files #18 and #19 released by Matt Taibbi, we now know that government agencies, NGOs, academia, Big Tech, media, and the intelligence community colluded in the Virality Project led by Stanford University to censor as mis/disinformation even true stories if their effect was to promote vaccine hesitancy. This included true accounts of vaccine injuries.

As Andrew Lowenthal puts it, rather than highlight safety signals to protect the public, the censorship-industrial complex "ran cover to protect Big Pharma, smearing and censoring critics. The moral depravity is astounding and quite possibly criminal.

This misuse of government power is a genuine threat to democracy, not a confected one.

10: THE WHO IS NO LONGER FIT FOR PURPOSE

Figure 10.1: Historical timeline of pandemics

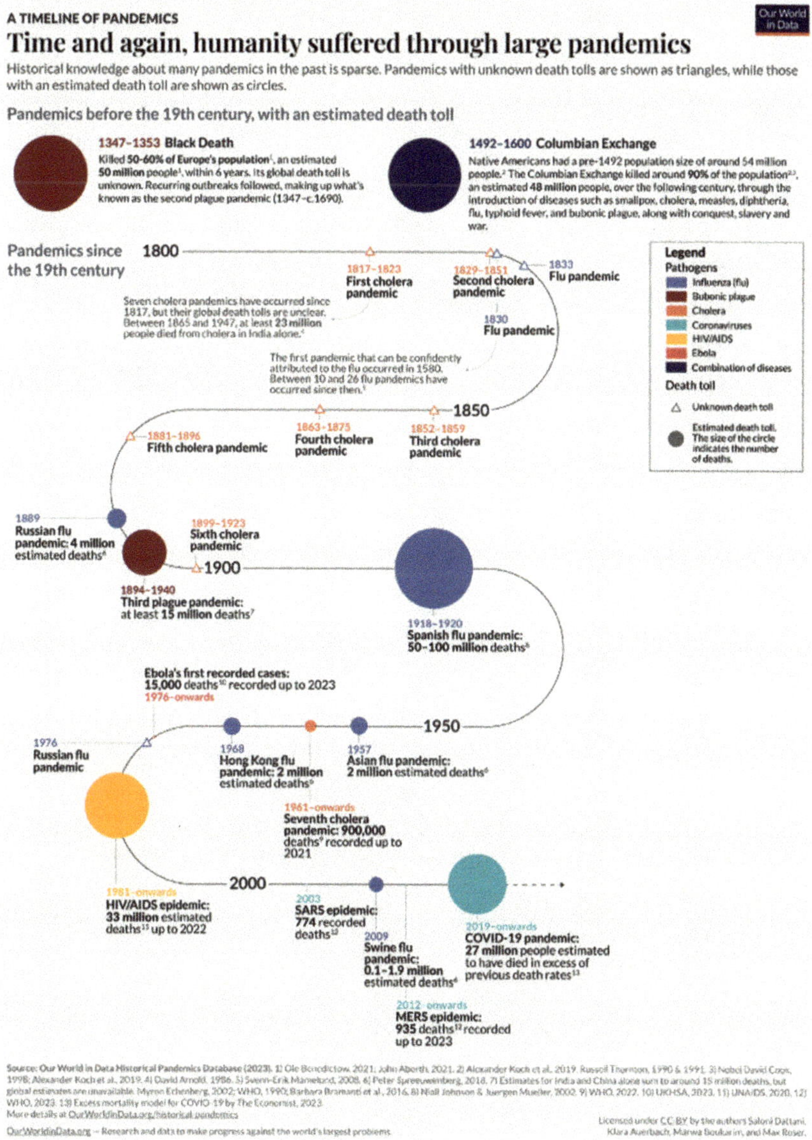

Pandemics are rare events. In the history of pandemics and pestilence (Figure10.1), Covid-19 was a relatively insignificant blip. The five years from early 2020 to mid-late 2024 were tumultuous not because of the scale of the mortality inflicted by the novel coronavirus, but because of the massive over-reaction by a succession of panicked governments around the world. The Australian-origin Dr David Bell argues that the pandemic industry's business model relies on persuading governments to prioritise made-up diseases over real ones by stoking fear and urgency. The dramatic drop in the pandemic-related morbidity and mortality toll since the Spanish flu (1918–20) is attributable mostly to improvements in sanitation, hygiene, potable water, antibiotics and other forms of expanding access to good healthcare. The top global agency, part of the United Nations system, for promoting preparedness in advance for health emergencies and crises and coordinating national responses, is the World Health Organisation. Unfortunately, its performance in helping the world to manage Covid-19 proved, to be kind, very patchy. Instead of acting as a check against panic-driven state excesses, the WHO functioned as an integral element of the global pandemic industry, helping to turn modelling-confected alarm into lucrative returns on investment. The concerted effort to expand its authority and boost its resources proved successful but provoked a backlash from the second Trump administration and the formal withdrawal of the US, the WHO's biggest state funder, from the organisation in January 2026.

WHO wants a new pandemic treaty?[67]

The Covid-19 crisis illustrates how the source and scope of many critical problems are global and require multilateral solutions, but the policy authority and requisite resources for tackling them are vested

---

[67] *Spectator Australia*, 18 June 2022, https://www.spectator.com.au/2022/06/who-wants-a-new-pandemic-treaty/

in states. An efficient architecture of global health governance would have detected the emerging epidemiological threat early, sounded the alarm and coordinated the delivery of essential equipment and medicines to population clusters in the most need.

The World Health Organisation (WHO) is at the centre of the existing architecture. It works worldwide to promote universal health care, monitor public health risks, prepare for emerging epidemiological emergencies, and coordinate responses. It sets international health standards and guidelines and provides technical assistance to countries in need. It's credited with eradicating smallpox and coordinating the response to SARS.

Its Covid performance, however, was somewhere between underwhelming and disgraceful. Its credibility was badly damaged by tardiness in raising the alarm; by shabby treatment of Taiwan at China's behest despite the potential lessons to be learnt from its prompt and effective measures to check Covid; by the initial investigation that whitewashed the origins of the virus; and by flip-flops on masks and lockdowns. For problems without passports, in Kofi Annan's evocative phrase, we need solutions without passports. Instead, international and domestic border closures, wholesale quarantine of healthy populations and mandatory vaccine requirements insinuated passport requirements into quotidian activities.

Health includes mental health and wellbeing and is highly dependent on a robust economy, yet the WHO-backed package of measures to fight Covid have been damaging to health, children's immunisation programs in developing countries, mental health, food security, economies, poverty reduction, educational and social wellbeing of peoples. Their worst effect was grievous assaults on human rights, civil liberties, individual autonomy and bodily integrity.

To make it worse, in promoting these policies the WHO violated, without providing any justification beyond China's example, (1) the guidance from its own report in 2019 that summarised a century's worth of worldwide experience and science; and (2) its own constitution which defines health as "a state of complete physical, mental and social well-being and not merely the absence of disease or infirmity." The vaccine push has similarly ignored accumulating safety signals about the scale of adverse reactions, on the one hand, and rapidly dwindling efficacy after successive doses, on the other.

Euro-US efforts, backed by Australia, to amend legally binding international health regulations and adopt a new pandemic convention would confer extraordinary powers on the WHO to declare public health emergencies of international/regional concern and command governments to implement their recommendations. WHO inspectors would have the right to enter countries without consent and check compliance with their directives. They would lock in the lockdowns-vaccines narrative and preempt rigorous independent retrospective reviews of their costs and efficacy.

The "reforms" amount to a WHO power grab at the behest of Big Pharma and Big Donors. Whether approved as two separate instruments or folded into one overarching new treaty, the changed architecture will greatly strengthen the WHO's core capabilities on public health surveillance, monitoring, reporting, notification, verification and response. The rush to amend the existing International Health Regulations (IHR) encountered significant pushback from developing countries, China and Russia last month but will come up again for discussion and approval. The new treaty under negotiation will be presented to the World Health Assembly, the WHO's 196 member governing body, in 2024.

Remarkably, there's been virtually no public debate on the ramifications of such far-reaching encroachments on national autonomy, state sovereignty and human rights. The Spectator has been an honourable exception. Well capacitated, technically proficient and democratically legitimate states should be wary of ceding control of the policy agenda, decision making authority, and enforcement powers to inefficient, cumbersome, and unaccountable international bureaucracies. Many governments argue that other issues like climate change, gun violence and racism also constitute public health emergencies which would expand the WHO's remit even more.

The two new instruments would give pride of place to pandemics above all else. Yet pandemics are rare events. The WHO listed only four in the 120 years before Covid-19: the Spanish flu 1918–19, Asian flu 1957–58, Hong Kong flu 1968–69 and swine flu 2009–10. They impose a low disease burden compared to the endemic infectious and chronic diseases. According to the World Life Expectancy, from 1 March 2020 to 9 June 2022, heart diseases, cancers, strokes, lung diseases and influenza and pneumonia killed more people around the word than Covid-19. Moreover, as is well known and unlike the earlier pandemics, about three-quarters of the 6.3mn Covid-related deaths were in people with comorbidities at or above average life expectancy.

Florida and Sweden resisted the lockdown groupthink and have come out markedly better on the balance of benefits versus harms. Yet the new regulatory framework would strip away their right to chart their own independent paths, just like lockdowns removed responsibility and agency from individuals to the public health clerisy.

Why empower a bigger and richer WHO to enforce wrongthink on the whole world? On 24 January, Director-General Tedros Adhanom Ghebreyesus said an urgent priority was to "strengthen WHO as the leading and directing authority on global health," for: "We are one world, we have one health, we are one WHO." On 12 April, he said the Covid crisis had "exposed serious gaps in the global health security architecture"; the new treaty would be "a generational agreement" and "a gamechanger" for global health security.

If adopted, they will consolidate the gains of those who have benefitted from Covid-19, concentrating private wealth, increasing national debts and decelerating poverty reduction; expand the international health bureaucracy under the WHO; shift the centre of gravity from common endemic diseases to relatively rare pandemic outbreaks; create a self-perpetuating global biopharmaceutical complex; shift the locus of health policy authority, decision-making and resources from the state to an enlarged corps of international technocrats, creating and empowering an international analogue of the administrative state that has already thinned national democracies. It will create a perverse incentive: the rise of an international bureaucracy whose defining purpose, existence, powers and budgets will depend on outbreaks of pandemics, the more the better.

The Woke Health Organisation?[68]

On 8 May, Senator Malcolm Roberts discussed the latest abortive effort by the UN system to promote "sexuality education" from birth. Yes, really. The origins of this go back to the document Standards for Sexuality Education in Europe funded by Germany's health ministry and published jointly with the WHO Collaborating Centre in Europe in 2010. In 2023 the effort to universalise these Euro-origin standards faltered in the UN Commission on Population and Development. The EU and "progressive" Western countries" (Sweden, Denmark, Norway, Canada) push to foist the woke agenda on the rest of the world failed due to resistance from non-Western countries like Iran, Pakistan, Nigeria and the Holy See.

Dr David Bell explains how last year WHO's abortion care guidance called for babies to "be killed up until the moment they emerge from the birth canal, without delay, whenever a pregnant woman requests it." It recommends abortions be available on request and advises against "gestational age limits." This is both a bureaucratic and a moral overreach. Only the governments concerned have the right and responsibility to make decisions on policy parameters between pro-choice and pro-life advocates.

The WHO has also determined that alcohol is dangerous for your health, regardless of how little or rarely you imbibe. If you believe

[68] *Spectator Australia*, 20 May 2023, https://www.spectator.com.au/2023/05/the-woke-health-organisation/

you drink responsibly, you are just the alcohol industry's useful idiot. The WHO says alcohol accounts for 5.1% of the world's disease burden and "contributes to 3 million deaths each year globally." A WHO news release in January insisted that "no level of alcohol consumption is safe for health." Over the last three years we have been conditioned to accept that public health safety trumps all other values and considerations, including such quaint old-fashioned notions as liberty, free choice, and individual responsibility for one's health and lifestyle choices.

On 15 April, in the latest iteration of its role as the world's nanny, the WHO published Reporting about Alcohol: A Guide for Journalists attacking the notion of "responsible drinking" as "a marketing tool and a tactic to influence public beliefs about the alcohol industry" that neither tells us when to stop nor acknowledges the option of abstinence. It also allegedly "ignores the inherent risks in consuming alcohol, mischaracterising its harms as the result of a small minority of individual drinkers who cannot control their intake." It stigmatises those who cannot hold their drink by putting "the entirety of the blame for alcohol problems on individual drinkers rather than more prominent ... factors such as advertising, pricing or availability."

Thus three key elements of the successful weaponisation of Covid for ensuring compliance with Science™ diktats from the WHO—scaremongering, shaming, and controlling the media narrative around it—are being replicated to socially engineer human behaviour on drinking, behaviour that is as old as human civilisation.

The *bureaucratic nature* of the WHO shows in the Preamble to the draft pandemic treaty: 49 articles over 4.5 pages. The current draft of the treaty uses language beloved of technocrats: "synergies between multisectoral collaboration—through whole-of-government and whole-of-society approaches at the country and community level—and international, regional and cross-regional collaboration, coordination and global solidarity, and their importance to achieving sustainable improvements."

The *progressive elements* of the treaty include ritualistic obeisance to inclusiveness, solidarity, transparency, accountability, "the importance of diverse, gender-balanced and equitable representation and expertise," "the determination to achieve health equity through resolute action on social, environmental, cultural, political and economic determinants of health, such as eradicating hunger and poverty, ensuring access to health and proper food, safe drinking water and sanitation, employment and decent work and social protection in a comprehensive intersectoral approach."

The treaty also makes several references to environmental and cultural factors. A research brief from the Australian Academy of Science in August 2020 concluded: "males with Covid-19 are more likely to be hospitalised, more likely to be admitted to an ICU and more likely to die." According to data from the Australian Bureau of Statistics (28 April), of the 13,456 people whose underlying cause of death was Covid-19, 7,439 were men and 6,017 women. According to Worldometers, in China the Covid case fatality rates for males was 2.8% compared to 1.7% for females. According to the CDC, 55% of US Covid deaths were males. Yet, the WHO says Covid has a worse impact on women.

WHO to govern the health of the world?[69]

The WHO has been captured by the woke activists, as can be seen in the following sentence from the executive summary:

> *In this guideline, we recognize that most of the available evidence on abortion can be assumed to be derived from research among study populations of cisgender women, and we also recognize that cisgender women, transgender men, nonbinary, gender-fluid and intersex individuals with a female reproductive system and capable of becoming pregnant may require abortion care (p. 4).*

[69] Resistance Press, 8 May 2023, https://resistancepress.com/article/who-govern-health-world

How can any organisation that spouts such anti-empirical rubbish as "women, girls or other pregnant persons" be accepted as an authority on science, biology, medicine, or public health? A search of the document reveals that the phrase "pregnant person" occurs 65 times, including Recommendation 2(LP) mentioned above. The WHO has become just another vehicle for global cultural imperialism of the US woke agenda.

Unicef published *The State of the World's Children 2023* report last month with the alarming conclusion that in the last three years, lockdown-induced disruptions to healthcare had resulted in a total of 67mn fewer childhood immunisations. This means that "in just three years, the world has lost more than a decade of progress."

Whisper it softly for fear of being cancelled, but does the WHO understand the difference between enjoying life and existing on life-support? Going by its woeful record on Covid, the answer is: No, it does not.

Yet, this is the body that wants to expand and entrench its powers to dictate our lives. What's more and contrary to what most Westerners believe with respect to the UN system, the push for the WHO as a nanny suprastate legally empowered to override national decisions on health measures is being led by Western governments and philanthropic foundations that have captured the organisation, including one Bill Gates. In fact, had it not been for a revolt led by African governments, the push would already have succeeded last year.

Euro–US efforts to amend legally binding international health regulations and adopt a new pandemic accord (that is, treaty) on "pandemic prevention, preparedness and response" would confer extraordinary powers on the WHO, acting through the director-general and the six regional directors (for Africa, the Americas, Europe, Eastern Mediterranean, Southeast Asia, and the Western Pacific), to declare public health emergencies of international/regional concern and instruct governments to implement their recommendations.

A new treaty would require approval by two-thirds of the WHA member states (that is, 131 countries) and be subject to their national ratification process. But the international health regulations can be amended by just 50% of member states (98 countries).

An open letter to the two houses of the UK Parliament from the Health Advisory and Recovery Team (HART) on 9 December was a welcome effort to educate parliamentarians. Rather surprisingly for such a radical recalibration of the relationship between sovereign governments and an international bureaucracy, parliamentarians and ministers have so far shown a singular lack of interest in learning just what their governments are signing up for.

To take just one example, the amendments propose that the present reference to "full respect for the dignity, human rights and fundamental freedoms of persons" in Article 3 of the IHR should be replaced by "equity, coherence, inclusivity." This would throw out the standard vocabulary of the international human rights movement as embedded in the Universal Declaration of Human Rights with the faddish catchphrase of the current woke agenda.

Many governments argue that other issues like climate change, gun violence, and racism also constitute public health emergencies which would expand the WHO's remit even more. Sure enough, on 2 May the *Guardian* reported that the next UN climate summit in November in Dubai will, for the first time ever, discuss health issues in depth.

The terminological change in the IHR (the draft new treaty sticks to "pandemics") from a pandemic to a "public health emergency of international concern" would make it easier for the WHO to assume extraordinary powers for health crises short of pandemics. The new regulatory framework would chip away at the right of sovereign states to chart their own independent paths, just like lockdowns shifted responsibility and agency from individuals to the public health clerisy.

Because pandemics are rare events, the requirement for every country to dedicate a minimum of 5% of its health budget to pandemic preparedness (Article 19.1c of the draft new treaty) doesn't make much sense. Why empower a bigger and richer WHO to enforce wrong groupthink on the whole world?

This is the stuff of bureaucrats' dreams: the legal authority to declare an emergency and the power thereafter to commandeer resources for oneself from sovereign states and to redirect resources funded by the taxpayers of one country to other states. The Covid years saw a successful bureaucratic coup that displaced elected governments with cabals of unelected experts and technocrats who lorded it over citizens and intruded into the most intimate personal behaviour and business decisions.

Deeply held differences—over whether it should be legally binding or voluntary, limited to actual emergencies or extended to cover potential outbreaks, whether the WHO should be the single source of authority on pandemic information with the power to advise governments on what constitutes unreliable information, misinformation and disinformation (proposed new IHR Article 44.2e); on equitable vaccine access vs. vaccine nationalism where rich countries can price out the poor; robust regulation of wet markets, strengthened information sharing requirements etc.—will likely make the negotiations protracted and contentious and may yet scupper the initiative.

We can but live in hope.

The WHO is engaged in a silent coup against the governments of the world. If it succeeds, an organisation set up to serve governments will boss it over them instead and compel their taxpayers to pay for the privilege. It is a basic axiom of politics that power that can be abused, will be abused—some day, somewhere, by someone. The corollary holds that power once seized is seldom surrendered back voluntarily to the people.

WHO accords warrant sovereignty concern[70]

On 11 March, my article criticising what appeared to be a slow motion coup d'état by the World Health Organisation (WHO) to seize health

[70] Brownstone Institute, 20 May 2024, https://brownstone.org/articles/who-accords-warrant-sovereignty-concern/

powers from states in the name of preparing for, conducting early warning surveillance of, and responding to "public health emergencies of international [and regional] concern" was published in *The Australian.* The coup was in the form of a new pandemic treaty and an extensive package of more than 300 amendments to the existing International Health Regulations (IHR) that was signed in 2005 and came into force in 2007, together referred to as the WHO pandemic accords.

The two sets of changes to the architecture of global health governance, I argued, will effectively change the WHO from a technical advisory organisation offering recommendations, into a supranational public health authority telling governments what to do.

On 3 May, *The Australian* published a reply by Dr. Ashley Bloomfield, co-chair of the WHO working group on the IHR amendments. Bloomfield was New Zealand's Director-General of Health from 2018–22 and received a knighthood for his services in the 2024 New Year's Honours list. His engagement with the public debate is very welcome.

Rejecting the charge that the WHO is engaged in a power grab over states, Bloomfield wrote that as a one-time senior UN official, I "would know that no single member state is going to concede sovereignty, let alone the entire 194 members."

I bow to the good doctor's superior medical knowledge in comparison to my non-existent medical qualifications.

Unfortunately, I cannot say the same with respect to reforms across the UN system, or sovereignty, or the relationship between "We the peoples" (the first three words of the UN Charter), on the one hand, and UN entities as agents in the service of the peoples, on the other. On medical and not health policy issues, I would quickly find myself out of my depth. I respectfully submit that on sovereignty concerns, Dr. Ashely may be the one out of his depth.

On the first point, I was seconded to the UN Secretariat as the senior adviser to Annan on UN reforms and wrote his second reform report that covered the entire UN system: Strengthening the

United Nations: *An Agenda for Further Change* (2002). The topic of UN reforms, both the case for it and the institutional and political obstacles frustrating the achievement of the most critical reforms, forms a core chapter of my book *The United Nations, Peace and Security* (Cambridge University Press, 2006, with a substantially revised second edition published in 2017).

I was also involved in a small Canada-based group that advocated successfully for the elevation of the G20 finance ministers' group into a leaders' level group that could serve as an informal grouping for brokering agreements on global challenges, including pandemics, nuclear threats, terrorism, and financial crises. I co-wrote the book The Group of Twenty (G20) (Routledge, 2012) with Andrew F. Cooper, a colleague in that project.

On the second point, I played a central role in the UN's reconceptualisation of sovereignty as state responsibility and citizens as rights holders. This was unanimously endorsed by world leaders at the UN summit in 2005.

On the third point, in *Utopia Lost: The United Nations and World Order* (1995), Rosemary Righter (the former chief leader writer at *The Times* of London) quoted Alexander Solzhenitsyn's description of the United Nations as "a place where the peoples of the world were delivered up to the designs of governments" (p. 85).

So yes, I do indeed know something about UN system reforms and the importance of sovereignty concerns in relation to powers given to UN bodies to prescribe what states may and may not do.

In agreeing to undertake to implement the WHO advisories, states will creating a new system of pandemic management under the WHO authority and binding under international law. It will create an open-ended international law obligation to cooperate with the WHO and to fund it. This is the same WHO that has a track record of incompetence, poor decision-making, and politicised conduct. The insistence that sovereignty is not being surrendered is formulaic and legalistic, not substantive and meaningful in practice.

It relies on a familiar technique of gaslighting that permits plausible deniability on both sides. The WHO will say it only issued advisories. States will say they are only implementing WHO recommendations as otherwise, they will become rogue international outlaws. The resulting structure of decision-making effectively confers powers without responsibility on the WHO while shredding accountability of governments to their electorates. The losers are the peoples of the world.

A "Litany of Lies" and misconceptions? Not so fast

Bloomfield's engagement with the public debate on the WHO-centric architecture of global health governance is very welcome. I have lauded the WHO's past impressive achievements in earlier writings, for example in the co-written book *Global Governance and the UN: An Unfinished Journey* (Indiana University Press, 2010). I also agree wholeheartedly that it continues to do a lot of good work, 24/7. In early 2020 I fought with a US editor to reject a reference to the possible virus escape from the Wuhan lab because of WHO's emphatic statements to the contrary. I later apologised to him for my naivete.

Once betrayed, twice shy of the message: "Trust us. We are from the WHO, here to keep you safe."

Sir Ashley was merely echoing the WHO chief. Addressing the World Governments Summit in Dubai on 12 February, Director-General (DG) Tedros Adhanom Ghebreyesus attacked "the litany of lies and conspiracy theories" about the agreement that "are utterly, completely, categorically false. The pandemic agreement will not give WHO any power over any state or any individual."

DG Tedros and Sir Ashley do protest too much. If Australia chooses as a sovereign nation to sign them, that does not mean there is no loss of effective sovereignty (that is, the power to make its health decisions) from that point on.

This is why all 49 Republican senators have "strongly" urged President Joe Biden to reject the proposed changes. The expansion of

"WHO's authority over member states during" pandemic emergencies, they warn, would "constitute intolerable infringements upon US sovereignty." In addition, 22 Attorneys-General have informed Biden that the WHO writ under the new accords will not run in their states.

On 8 May, the UK said it would not sign the new treaty unless clauses requiring transfer of pandemic products were deleted. Under Article 12.6.b of the then-draft, the WHO could sign "legally binding" contracts with manufacturers to get pandemic-related "diagnostics, therapeutics or vaccines." Ten percent of this is to be free of charge and another ten percent at profit-free prices. In the latest, 22 April draft, this last requirement comes in Article 12.3.b.i in slightly softer language.

The UK wants to retain the right to use British-made products first to address domestic requirements as judged by the government, and only then to make them available for global distribution. The draft, the government fears, will undermine British sovereignty.

On 14 May, five senators and nine representatives from the Australian parliament wrote a formal letter to PM Anthony Albanese expressing deep concern over the likely prospect of Australia signing the accords that "will transform the WHO from an advisory organisation to a supranational health authority dictating how governments must respond to emergencies which the WHO itself declares." If adopted and implemented into Australian law, they wrote, these would give the WHO "an unacceptable level of authority, power and influence over Australia's affairs under the guise of declaring "emergencies.""

"Legally Binding" vs "Loss of Sovereignty" is a distinction without a difference

They can't all be part of a global conspiracy to peddle a litany of lies. WHO is offering up a highly specious argument. Sir Ashley didn't really engage with the substance of my arguments either. He dismissed criticism of the proposed changes as "an attempt by the

WHO to gain the power to dictate to countries what they must do in the event of a pandemic" as a "misconception."

The G20 Leader's Bali Declaration (November 2022, paragraph 19) supported the goal of a "legally binding instrument that should contain both legally binding and non-legally binding elements to strengthen pandemic planning, preparedness and response (PPR) and amendments to the IHR." In September 2023, the G20 Delhi Leaders' Declaration (28:vi) envisioned "an ambitious, legally binding WHO" accord "as well as amendments to better implement" the IHR.

Lawrence Gostin, actively involved in the negotiations, was co-author of a report last December that said containing transnational outbreaks under WHO leadership "may require all states to forgo some level of sovereignty." A joint Reuters-World Economic Forum article on 26 May 2023 stated: "For the new more wide-reaching pandemic accord, member states have agreed that it should be legally binding."

The WHO itself describes the IHR as "an instrument of international law that is legally-binding on 196 countries." Last year it published a document which includes section 4.6 on "legally binding international instruments" such as a new pandemic accord.

I get the argument that sovereign states are voluntarily agreeing to this. In terms of legal technicality, it might well be more accurate, as Libby Klein suggests in her draft letter to Australian MPs, to use words and phrases like "ceding autonomy," "yielding "effective control over public health decisions," "outsourcing public health decision-making to the WHO," or "offshoring our public health decision-making." This is the legalistic distinction that Bloomfield is effectively making.

However, simply because states must voluntarily sign the new WHO accords doesn't mean they will not be ceding sovereignty once the accords are adopted. With all due respect to Dr. Tedros and Sir Ashley, this is a distinction without a difference. Every single "legally binding" requirement will mean a transfer of effective decision-making power on health issues to the WHO. That is a curtailment of state sovereignty and it is disingenuous to deny it.

Since the creation of the United Nations in 1945, states have been required to conduct themselves increasingly in conformity with international standards. And it is the UN system that sets most of the relevant international standards and benchmarks of state behaviour.

For example, for centuries countries had the absolute right to wage wars of aggression and defence as an acknowledged and accepted attribute of sovereignty. By adopting the United Nations Charter in 1945, they gave up the right to wage aggressive wars. I am very glad they did so. Just because the surrender of this aspect of sovereignty was voluntary, it doesn't mean there was no surrender of sovereignty.

Similarly, by signing the Nuclear Non-proliferation Treaty (NPT), Australia and around 185 states surrendered their sovereign right to make or get the nuclear bomb. Again, I am very glad they did so.

Article 10 of the treaty does permit withdrawal after a three-month notice to other states parties and the UN Security Council:

> *Each Party shall in exercising its national sovereignty have the right to withdraw from the Treaty if it decides that extraordinary events … have jeopardised the supreme interests of its country.*

Australia could still act as a sovereign state and pull out of the NPT but, absent exculpatory events, only at the reputational cost of acting illegally under international law.

North Korea first announced withdrawal from the NPT in 1993, suspended the withdrawal, withdrew in 2003, has conducted six nuclear tests since 2006, and acquired up to 50 bombs. Yet, the UN has refused to accept the withdrawal and it is still listed on the UN website as an NPT member, with the explanatory note that: "States parties to the Treaty continue to express divergent views regarding the status of the DPRK under the NPT."

Like these two important examples, states will lose key parts of the right to exercise their sovereignty over national policy settings and decisions on health if the WHO accords are adopted. It is their sovereign right to reject the treaties now. They should exercise it before it is too late. The complications entangling the post-Brexit referendum in the UK demonstrate only too vividly how challenging it can be for a state to extricate itself from a supranational authority despite the sovereign right to do so.

The best way to allay these fears and concerns would be to return responsibility to where accountability lies: with the national government and parliament. States should learn to cooperate better in global pandemic management, not hand effective decision-making powers and authority to unelected and unaccountable international technocrats.

The effort should be put on indefinite hold

It is an iron law of politics that any power that can be abused, will be abused by someone, somewhere, some time in the future. For current examples of overreach by a technocrat, look no further than Australia's eSafety Commissioner. The truly frightening thing about her example is the realisation of just how much her efforts have been deliberately embedded in a global campaign to "bureaucratise" and control the internet.

A softer conclusion is that powers once granted over citizens to authorities are far more difficult to claw back than not giving them the powers in the first place. Thus far from retreating, the censorship-industrial complex is simultaneously being broadened to embrace additional sectors of governance and public policy and globalised.

A report from Leeds University documented that pandemics are rare events. They are not becoming more frequent. For poor countries, their global disease burden is much lower than that of the big killer diseases like TB, malaria and HIV/AIDS. For industrialised countries like Australia, the disease burden has been greatly reduced since the Spanish flu with improved surveillance, response mechanism and other public health interventions.

There is no emergency justifying the rushed process. An immediate pause and a slow and deliberative process would lead to better policy development and deliver better national and global health policy outcomes.

"Pause for thought, argue for a wider delay, think it through properly. And don't sign till it's right." David Frost, who led the UK Brexit negotiations.

Just so.

We need an International Health Organisation that's fit for purpose—unlike the WHO[71]

As humans we commonly consider ourselves, our beliefs and our work of particular importance. It is not surprising, then, that when we form institutions, those within them seek to promote the institution's relevance, expand their work and centralise decision-making within their own "particularly important" group. Few want to divest power and resources, let alone put themselves and their colleagues out of a job. This fatal flaw infects all bureaucracies, from local through national and regional to international.

It is unsurprising then that the World Health Organisation (WHO), an international health bureaucracy of over 9,000 staff, a quarter of them in Geneva, should suffer the same problems. The WHO was originally intended primarily to transfer capacity to struggling states emerging from colonialism and address their higher burdens of disease but lower administrative and financial capabilities. This prioritised fundamentals like sanitation, good nutrition and competent health services that had brought long life to people of wealthier countries. Its focus now is more on stocking shelves with manufactured commodities. Its budget, staffing and remit expand as actual country need and infectious disease mortality decline.

---

[71] David Bell and Ramesh Thakur, *Daily Sceptic*, 18 May 2025, https://dailysceptic.org/2025/05/18/an-international-health-organisation-fit-for-purpose-for-todays-world/

While major gaps in underlying health equality remain, and were recently exacerbated by the WHO's COVID-19 policies, the world is a very different place from 1948 when WHO was formed. Rather than acknowledging progress, however, we are told we are simply in an "inter-pandemic period," and WHO and its partners should be given ever more responsibility and resources to save us from the next hypothetical outbreak (like "Disease X"). Increasingly dependent on " from national and private interests heavily invested in profitable biotech fixes rather than the underlying drivers of good health, WHO looks more and more like other public-private partnerships that channel taxpayer money to the priorities of private industry.

Pandemics happen, but a proven natural one of major impact on life expectancy has not happened since pre-antibiotic era Spanish flu over a hundred years ago. We all understand that better nutrition, sewers, potable water, living conditions, antibiotics and modern medicines protect us, yet are told to be ever more fearful of the next outbreak. Covid happened, but overwhelmingly affected the elderly in Europe and the Americas. Moreover, it looks to be, as the US Government now makes clear, almost certainly a laboratory mistake by the very pandemic industry that is promoting WHO's new approach.

Collaborating on health internationally remains popular, as it should be in a heavily interdependent world. It also makes sense to prepare for severe rare events—most of us buy insurance. But we don't exaggerate flood risk in order to expand the flood insurance industry, as anything we spend is money taken from our other needs.

Public health is no different. If we were designing a new WHO now, no sane model would base its funding and direction primarily on the interests and advice of those who profit from illness. Rather, these would be based on accurate estimates of localised risks of the big killer diseases. The WHO was once independent of private interests, mostly core-funded, and able to set rational priorities. That WHO is gone.

Over the past 80 years the world has also changed. It makes no sense now to base thousands of health staff in one of the world's most expensive (and healthiest!) cities, and it makes no sense in a technologically-advancing world to keep centralising control there. The WHO was structured in a time when most mail still went by steamship. It stands increasingly as an anomaly to its mission and to the world in which it works. Would a network of regional bodies tied to their local context not be more responsive and effective than a distant, disconnected and centralised bureaucracy of thousands?

Amidst the broader turmoil roiling the post-1945 international liberal order, the recent US notice of withdrawal from the WHO presents a unique opportunity to re-think the type of international health institution the world needs, how that should operate, where, for what purpose and for how long.

What should be the use-by date of an international institution? In the WHO's case, either health is getting better as countries build capacity and it should be downsizing. Or health is getting worse, in which case the model has failed and we need something more fit for purpose.

The Trump administration's actions are an opportunity to re-base international health cooperation on widely recognised standards of ethics and human rights. Countries and populations should be back in control, and those seeking profit from illness should have no role in decision-making. The WHO, at nearly 80 years old, comes from a bygone era, and is increasingly estranged from its world. We can do better. Fundamental change in the way we manage international health cooperation will be painful, but ultimately healthy.

Rewarding the WHO for Covid failures[72]

Using figures from Our World in Data, in the 105 years since the Spanish flu, a grand total of 10-14 million people have died around the world in pandemics including Covid-19: Asian and Hong Kong

[72] *The Daily Sceptic*, 1 June 2025, https://dailysceptic.org/2025/06/01/rewarding-the-who-for-covid-failures/

flu (1957–58, 1968–69), around two million each; swine flu (2009–10), 0.1-1.9 million; seventh cholera pandemic since 1961, 0.9 million; COVID-19 (2020–24), 7.1 million.

To put this in perspective, in 2019 alone, 7.7 million people died from infectious diseases: pneumonia and other lower respiratory diseases, 2.5 million; diarrhoeal diseases, 1.5 million; tuberculosis, 1.1 million; HIV/AIDS, 800,000; malaria, 600,000; and other infectious diseases, 1.2 million. Another 40.7 million deaths were caused by non-communicable diseases. The three leading causes of deaths in the year before Covid were heart diseases (18.5 million), cancers (10 million) and chronic respiratory diseases (3.8 million).

Based on these historical data, what percentage of the world's total health budget should be spent on pandemic preparedness, prevention and response? Would a higher percentage benefit the world's peoples or the international health organisation that acts as the world's "directing and coordinating authority on... pandemic prevention, preparedness and response"? Do we really need yet more national and international bureaucracy and meetings: national committees for implementing International Health Regulations (IHR) (Article 54 *bis*), five yearly conferences by States Parties of the World Health Assembly (Article 19.2 of the Pandemic Treaty) and engagement between the two structures?

These are the questions and considerations worth bearing in mind when discussing the newly adopted pandemic accords. Indeed, do the three years already devoted to meetings and negotiations on the pandemic accords not amount to a diversion of time, effort and resources from more urgent health priorities?

Speaking at a media briefing in Geneva on March 3rd 2020, Director-General (DG) Tedros Adhanom Ghebreyesus of the World Health Organization (WHO) said Covid's case fatality rate (CFR) was 3.4%, against under 1% for seasonal flu. Addressing an internal meeting on April 7th 2025, he said: "Officially 7 million people were killed [by Covid], but we estimate the true toll to be 20 million".

The two statements, delivered five years apart as bookends to the pandemic, amount to self-serving catastrophisation and fear-mongering. They underpin efforts to commandeer even more powers and resources for future pandemics to be declared on the sole judgment of the DG. Like New Zealand's Jacinda Ardern, the WHO must be revered as the single source of pandemic truth for the whole world. The WHA met in Geneva (19–27th May) and adopted the new treaty that, although diluted from its original iteration, will still reward the WHO for its gross mismanagement of Covid by strengthening the framework for global health cooperation under its auspices.

Whoever thought it was a good idea to give any bureaucracy and its head the power to declare a pandemic emergency that will expand its reach, authority, budget and personnel and shift the balance of decision making away from states to an unelected globalist bureaucrat? Or to adopt a One Health approach when the empirical reality is of sharply differentiated health vulnerabilities and disease burdens between regions?

According to statistics reported by Our World in Data, on life years lost by people in low income countries because of premature death, disease or disability, 56% was from infectious and 35% from noncommunicable diseases. For high income countries the figures were 10% and 81%, respectively. To better capture this empirical reality of sharply differentiated health vulnerabilities, we need devolution, not more centralisation, with the principle of subsidiarity determining the distribution of authority and resources at the different levels.

WHO's sins of commission and omission during Covid

As per the WHO's constitution, "Health is a state of complete physical, mental and social well-being and not merely the absence of disease or infirmity." In responding to a pandemic, there is a trade-off between public health, individual well-being and economic stability. It is the responsibility of health experts to focus solely on the first. Governments have the duty to balance all the competing demands and expectations and intuit the social fulcrum: the sweet spot at the intersection of dangerous complacency, alarmist panic and reasonable precautions.

In the case of Covid-19, almost all the mistakes and damage can be traced back to two extreme but mutually contradictory assumptions, neither of which was ever revised back to the mean. First, assume the absolute worst about the pandemic on infectivity, speed of progression in the infected and in rate of cross-infection, lethality and lack of treatment options. Second, assume the very best about the effectiveness of all policy interventions, regardless of existing science and data (not GIGO computer modelling) and the need for careful analyses of risk profiles by demographic cohorts and the harms-benefits equation of interventions.

The WHO should have stepped in immediately as the international institutional firewall against this. It did not. Instead its top leadership joined national health bureaucrats to insist they knew best and colluded in the takedown of dissenting voices. The consequences were catastrophic and have caused lasting damage to public health. In a recent *Politico* interview, Dr Jay Bhattacharya, the new director of the US National Institutes of Health (NIH), lists the NIH and WHO as among the leading examples of the dual institutional pathology.

The WHO failed the peoples of the world in becoming a cheerleader for panicked responses instead of holding the line on existing science, knowledge and experience as summarised in its own report of September 2019. It proved too credulous of early Chinese data on risk of human-human transmission, no Wuhan lab origin, lethality and effectiveness of brutal containment measures. The first WHO panel to investigate the origins of Covid was riddled with conflicts of interest of key panel members and gave China a free pass. A follow-up investigation was stymied by China's refusal to cooperate, for which it hasn't been held to account.

Other WHO sins of commission included exaggerations of Covid lethality by presenting highly inflated CFR; obfuscation on the age-stratified risk profile of Covid mortality; unscientific recommendations on mask mandates and vaccine passports; and complicity in the human rights abuses committed in pursuit of the fool's gold of Covid eradication. Sins of omission included downplaying warnings of short and long-term health, mental health, educational, economic, social and human rights harms of the drastic interventions. School closures, for example, have created a generation of pandemic children in the hundreds of millions.

Avoidable non-Covid deaths have escalated through disrupted food production and distribution globally; interrupted childhood immunisation programmes; deferred and cancelled early detection programmes and treatment of cancers; and deaths of despair among elderly people cut off from the emotional support crutches of loved family. The inflationary spirals are yet to subside from government support schemes to compensate for loss of incomes owing to economic shutdowns. The dramatic erosion of trust in public health institutions has lowered Australia's childhood vaccination rates to alarming levels, the ABC reported on 16th May.

The WHO's advice on Covid management also seemed to prioritise the high disease burden of industrialised over developing countries and the interests of the major global pharmaceutical companies over patients. Yet, there have been no admissions of culpability, no apologies for the extensive and lasting damage inflicted and no accountability for those responsible for unleashing and cheerleading the public policy insanity.

The pandemic accords: a solution in search of a problem[73]

The WHO has accomplished important work in its relatively long lifespan for an international organisation, including the eradication

[73] 'Flat White," *The Spectator Australia*, 7 June 2025, https://www.spectator.com.au/2025/06/the-pandemic-accords-a-solution-in-search-of-a-problem/

of smallpox. More recently, however, its "priorities have increasingly reflected the biases and interests of corporate medicine." The pandemic treaty adopted last month will reward the WHO for its gross Covid mismanagement by strengthening the framework for global health cooperation under WHO auspices. The treaty sets out the principles, approaches and tools for the international coordination of the global health architecture for pandemic prevention, preparedness and response. It will open for signature and ratification next year, if and when the Pathogen Access and Benefit Sharing (PABS) system is negotiated, drafted and adopted.

What follows is a five-part analysis of (a) the low salience of pandemics as a health risk, (b) WHO's Covid failures, (c) the reality of major disease burdens disaggregated by income levels of countries, (d) the dilution of sovereignty by the globalisation of health, and (e) the need to rebalance health sovereignty through subsidiarity as the organising principle of the distribution of responsibility, authority and resources for health decisions. The article concludes with an assessment of the impact of the US exit from the WHO.

1. The threat salience of pandemics

The pandemic accords focus on building a global surveillance system to detect emerging pathogens and respond swiftly with coordinated measures, including the development and equitable distribution of medical countermeasures. Yet, the premise of the accords is an inflated account of pandemic risk that is simply not supported, neither by historical evidence nor indeed by the experience of the last five years. As a result, its effect will be to badly distort health priorities away from the real health needs and other social and economic goals of many countries.

Using figures from Our World in Data, in the 105 years since the Spanish flu, a grand total of 10-14 million people have died around the world in pandemics: Asian and Hong Kong flu (1957–58,

1968–69), around two million each; swine flu (2009–10), 0.1-1.9 million; seventh cholera pandemic since 1961, 0.9 million; Covid-19 (2020–24), 7.1 million.

Nor did Covid pose an overwhelming threat even during the last five years. Of the 55 million total global death toll from all causes in 2019 (the last year before Covid) alone, 7.7 million people died from non-Covid infectious diseases. Another 40.7 million deaths were caused by non-communicable diseases. The three leading causes of deaths were heart diseases (18.5 million), cancers (10 million) and chronic respiratory diseases (3.8 million).

Table 10.1: Covid-19 and leading causes of death, Jan 2020–Jan 2025 (millions)

Covid-19	Noncommunicable diseases				Infectious diseases			
	Heart	*Cancer*	*Chronic respiratory*	*Total*	*Lower respiratory*	*Diarrhoeal*	*TB*	*Total*
7.08	92.9	50.4	19.2	203.5	12.4	7.7	5.5	38.5

Source: Extrapolation of 2019 statistics from Our World in Data

If we do a simple linear extrapolation, that means that in the same five-year period since January 2020 in which 7.1 million people died with Covid, about 203.5 million people would have died from non-communicable, and another 38.5 million from non-Covid infectious diseases. It's worth emphasising that the Covid death toll refers to deaths with Covid. Deaths from Covid would have been considerably fewer.

Based on these historical data and wider perspective, was it prudent health policy or medical malpractice to repurpose national health services into de facto Covid health services? What percentage of the world's total health budget should be spent on pandemic preparedness, prevention and response? Would a higher percentage benefit the world's peoples or the WHO? Do we really need yet more national and international bureaucracy and meetings: national committees for implementing International Health Regulations (IHR) plus periodic Conferences of States Parties?

These are the questions and considerations worth bearing in mind when discussing the newly adopted pandemic accords. Indeed, do the three years already devoted to meetings and negotiations on the pandemic accords not amount to a diversion of time, effort and resources from more urgent health priorities—opportunity costs?

2. WHO Covid failures

Speaking at a media briefing in Geneva on March 3, 2020, WHO Director General (DG) Tedros Adhanom Ghebreyesus said that Covid's case fatality rate (CFR) was 3.4%, against under 1% for seasonal flu. Addressing an internal meeting on April 7, 2025, he said: "Officially 7 million people were killed [by Covid], but we estimate the true toll to be 20 million."

The two statements, delivered five years apart as bookends to the pandemic, amount to self-serving catastrophisation and fear-mongering. They underpin efforts to commandeer even more powers and resources for future pandemics to be declared on the sole judgment of the DG. Like New Zealand's Jacinda Ardern, the WHO must be revered as the single source of pandemic truth for the whole world.

Yet, DG Tedros's judgment on such matters is demonstrably flawed. He unilaterally declared a global emergency in July 2022 over monkeypox after just five deaths. This was lifted in May 2023 after a worldwide total of 140 deaths. To grasp just how farcical this was, consider: an average of 501 Australians died daily in 2023, 140 Australians (the worldwide total of monkeypox deaths by the time the global emergency was lifted) died by suicide in 16 days, from accidental falls in three weeks and in road accidents in six weeks.

As per the WHO's own constitution, "Health is a state of complete physical, mental and social well-being and not merely the absence of disease or infirmity." In responding to a pandemic, there is a trade-off between public health, individual wellbeing and economic stability. It is the responsibility of health experts to focus solely on the first. Governments have the duty to balance all the competing demands and expectations and intuit the social fulcrum: the sweet spot at the intersection of dangerous complacency, alarmist panic, and reasonable precautions.

Almost all the Covid mistakes and damage can be traced back to two extreme but mutually contradictory assumptions, neither of which was ever revised back to the mean. First, assume the absolute worst about the pandemic on infectivity, speed of progression in the infected and in rate of cross-infection, lethality and lack of treatment options. Second, assume the very best about the effectiveness of all policy interventions, regardless of existing science and data (not GIGO computer modelling), careful analyses of risk profiles by demographic cohorts, and harms-benefits equation of interventions.

The WHO should have stepped in immediately as the international institutional firewall against this. It did not. Instead, its top leadership joined national health bureaucrats to insist they knew best and colluded in the takedown of dissenting voices by entering into partnerships with media houses and social media platforms. The consequences were catastrophic and have caused lasting damage to public health.

The WHO failed the peoples of the world in becoming a cheerleader for panicked responses instead of holding the line on existing science, knowledge, and experience, as summarised in its own report of September 2019. It proved too credulous of early Chinese data on no risk of human-human transmission, no Wuhan lab origin, lethality, and effectiveness of brutal containment measures. The first WHO panel to investigate the origins of Covid was riddled with conflicts of interest of key panel members and gave China a free pass. A follow-up investigation was stymied by China's refusal to cooperate, for which it hasn't been held to account.

Other WHO sins of commission included exaggerations of Covid lethality by presenting highly inflated estimates of fatality rates; obfuscation on the age-stratified risk profile of Covid mortality; unscientific and evidence-free recommendations on mask mandates and vaccine passports; and complicity in the human rights abuses committed in pursuit of the fool's gold of Covid eradication.

Sins of omission included downplaying warnings of short and long-term health, mental health, educational, economic, social and human rights harms of the drastic interventions. School closures, for example, have created a generation of pandemic children in the hundreds of millions.

Avoidable non-Covid deaths escalated through disrupted food production and distribution globally; interrupted childhood immunisation programs; deferred and cancelled early detection programs and treatment of cancers; and deaths of despair of elderly people cut off from the emotional support crutches of loved family. The inflationary spirals are yet to subside from government support schemes to compensate for loss of incomes owing to economic shutdowns. The dramatic erosion of trust in public health institutions has lowered Australia's childhood vaccinations to alarming levels, the ABC reported on May 16.

3. The distribution of disease burdens by income levels

According to statistics reported by Our World in Data, on life years lost by people in low-income countries because of premature death, disease or disability, 56% was from infectious and 35% from non-communicable diseases. For high-income countries the figures were 10% and 81%, respectively. To better capture this empirical reality of sharply differentiated health vulnerabilities, we need devolution, not more centralisation, with the principle of subsidiarity determining the distribution of authority and resources at the different levels.

4. Sovereignty v globalist One Health

Whoever thought it was a good idea to give any bureaucracy and its head the power to declare a pandemic emergency that will expand their reach, authority, budget, and personnel and shift the balance of decision-making away from states to an unelected global bureaucrat?

Or to adopt a One Health approach when the empirical reality is of sharply differentiated health vulnerabilities, nutritional deficiencies and disease burdens between regions?

In combination with the amended IHR that come into force this September and which must and will be read in parallel, the political reality is that member states will be enmeshed into the international pandemic management framework led by international technocrats who lack the legitimacy of democratically elected political leaders, are not in practice accountable, and who have been given this enhanced directive role without meaningful parliamentary scrutiny or public debate by citizens.

Nothing in the Covid experience inspires confidence about the willingness and capacity of political leaders to resist WHO recommendations in this global institutional milieu. Rather, a de facto realignment of chairs at the decision-making table will see the experts take up positions at the head of the table instead of merely being present at the table to aid and advise on but not set health policy. This is why the pandemic accords are the latest waystations on the journey to an international administrative state that consolidates the globe-spanning "new pandemic industry."

We need to do a better job in locating the sweet spot between inward-looking nationalism and sovereignty-destroying globalism.

5. Health sovereignty and the principle of subsidiarity

Health policy and healthcare that use subsidiarity as the organising principle would begin with individual agency and autonomy, informed consent and prioritisation of patients' individual health outcomes over collective public health benefits. The doctor-patient relationship in the clinic has to be sacrosanct and inviolate. If medical regulators violate that sanctity to invade the clinic, for example by prohibiting the doctor from discussing risk of collateral harms because this could increase vaccine hesitancy, they destroy patient faith in the doctor's professional integrity, increase public distrust of health experts and promote cross-vaccine hesitancy. All this has already happened and been documented in multiple polls in several countries.

Medical and drug regulators should prioritise patient safety over every other consideration. On this criterion, there was the unacceptable dereliction of the duty of care during Covid. To enable emergency use authorisation of vaccines, regulators hugely exaggerated health risks and threats, refused to draw accurate risk profiles by age and regions, dismissed legitimate concerns and questions about side effects and harms, condemned efforts to identify promising possible repurposed drugs as dangerous, and short-circuited the normal multi-year stringent safety and efficacy trials. Remarkably, all this was done based in pseudoscience and voodoo science.

Governments abdicated responsibility for pandemic policy to their health bureaucrats. The latter deferred to the international technocrats in and around the WHO. Thus they acted on the basis of the very opposite of the principle of subsidiarity, from the individual and the state to the regional and the global.

The US exit is a wake-up call

Before empowering the WHO to cause even more harm, we should first investigate its Covid failings and decide if major reform can overcome the accumulated vested interests or if we need a new international health organisation. Any organisation that has been around for nearly eight decades has either succeeded in its core mission, in which case it should be wound down out of existence. Or else it has failed, in which case it should be abolished and replaced by a new one that is more fit for purpose for today's world.

The WHO confronts a $2.5 billion shortfall between 2025 and 2027. Its financial situation is not helped by President Donald Trump's decision to pull the US out. Explaining why, Health Secretary Robert F Kennedy Jr says that the WHO has been corrupted by political and corporate interests and "is mired in bureaucratic bloat." "Too often it has allowed political agendas, like pushing harmful gender ideology, to hijack its core mission." The pandemic agreement "will lock in all of the dysfunctions of the WHO pandemic response." "We want to free international health cooperation from the straitjacket of political interference by corrupting influences of the pharmaceutical companies, of adversarial nations, and their NGO proxies.'

That is a clear and compelling rationale put forward by Kennedy for the US withdrawal from the WHO. As in most areas in the current era, the United States has the heaviest normative weight and strongest gravitational pull of any country in the world. For better or worse, the presence of the likes of Robert F Kennedy Jr, Jay Bhattacharya, Marty Makary, and Vinay Prasad in the top echelons of public health decision-making in Washington DC is bound to have ripple effects in other countries in recalibrating the normative settling point of national and global public health policy.

Moreover, the US exit from the WHO does not necessarily signify a retreat from the commitment to international cooperation in shared health goals. In a joint statement on May 27, Secretary Kennedy and Argentina's Health Minister Mario Lugones announced an initiative to launch a new alternative to WHO. They explained that the two countries' withdrawal from the WHO was due to the organisation's "increasing politicisation" and the "absence of meaningful reforms': "increasingly reliant on voluntary contributions and vulnerable to the influence of non-scientific agendas," the WHO "has shifted away from its founding mission." That said, withdrawal marks the beginning of a new path—towards building a modern global health cooperation model grounded in scientific integrity, transparency, sovereignty, and accountability. Our shared commitment is to cost-effective, evidence-based public health interventions that prioritize prevention, especially in children, by addressing root causes such as environmental toxins, nutritional deficiencies, and food safety standards.

The international managerial-technocratic elite (the "lanyard class" of officious, rules- and process-obsessed professional cadre that runs the national public sector and international secretariats) will circle the wagons to defend the expansion of the international administrative state. The political leaders in thrall to the expert class will genuflect to their advice. Those seduced by the idealism of international solidarity and others corrupted by the lucre of pharmaceutical lobbyists will not be persuaded by the Kennedy-Lugones diagnosis of what ails the WHO and their vision of a replacement international health organisation.

Competent leaders of self-confident countries, however, should take up the offer to nest the ethic of global health cooperation in a new specialised international organisation that better respects the health sovereignty of member states and the health needs of people. Other countries too should join the US to shift the focus to chronic diseases that sicken peoples and bankrupt health systems. This will better serve the needs of people instead of aiding and abetting the pharmaceutical industry's goal of profit maximisation.

WHO pandemic accords are badly flawed[74]

The decades-old International Health Regulations, as amended last year, came into effect on 19 September. A new Pandemic Agreement, adopted in May, will be opened for signature after a pathogens access and benefits sharing deal that is expected to be reached next year. The WHO Pandemic Accords, as the two documents are known, are a good example of the type of global governance initiatives on which there is a consensus among technocratic elites, but against which there is a rising populist revolt. Two other examples that were mentioned by President Donald Trump in his UN address on 23 September are immigration and climate change. The speech was a wide-ranging defence of national sovereignty against globalism.

[74] *Brownstone Journal*, 2 October 2025, https://brownstone.org/articles/who-pandemic-accords-are-badly-flawed/

Flawed assumptions

Yet, pandemics are rare events that, compared to endemic infectious and chronic diseases, impose a low disease burden. The rationale for the accords rests on the false understanding that the risk of pandemics is rapidly growing, predominantly from increasing zoonotic spillover events in which pathogens move from animals to humans. Well-founded suspicion that Covid arose from gain of function research and a lab leak negates the second part of this justification.

The assumption of increasing pandemic risk is also undermined by work from the University of Leeds. They show that the reports of the WHO, World Bank and G20 that back the pandemic agenda don't support the agencies' claims. Data show reducing mortality and outbreaks in the decade prior to 2020. Much of the recorded "increase" in episodes reflects improved diagnostic technologies, not more frequent and more serious outbreaks.

Previous major epidemic diseases like yellow fever, influenza, and cholera continue to decline overall. The historical timeline of pandemics shows that improvements in sanitation, hygiene, potable water, antibiotics, and other forms of expanding access to good healthcare have massively reduced the morbidity and mortality of pandemics since the Spanish flu (1918–20) in which fifty million people are believed to have died.

According to Our World in Data, in the 105 years since the Spanish flu, a grand total of 10-14 million people have died in pandemics including Covid-19. To put this in perspective, in 2019 alone, nearly eight million people died from non-Covid infectious diseases. Another 41 million deaths were caused by non-communicable diseases. In the five years 2020–2024 inclusive, 7.1 million Covid-related deaths were recorded. Projecting the trendlines from 2000–2019, in the 2020–24 five years, we could have expected a total of around 35 million deaths from non-Covid infectious diseases and another 220 million from non-communicable, that is, chronic diseases.

Calculations by Leeds university's REPPARE project also show how key claims of massive costs from pandemics are inflated whilst the costs of endemic infections are downplayed. Establishing a dedicated, treaty-based, and resource-intensive international machinery to prepare for a low-burden disease of infrequent outbreaks will distort public health priorities and divert scarce resources and finite attention from more urgent health and other goals. This is bad public policy that fails the basic test of cost-benefit analysis.

Expanded powers and increased resources for the WHO

Covid saw a successful bureaucratic coup that displaced elected governments with unelected experts and technocrats as de facto policymakers. The pandemic accords provide the WHO legal authority to declare an actual or apprehended emergency and the power thereafter to commandeer resources for itself from sovereign states and redirect resources funded by the taxpayers of one country to other states, on the basis of what the WHO chief alone considers simply a risk of potential harm.

Many governments argue that other issues like climate change, gun violence, and racism also constitute public health emergencies. These would expand the WHO's remit even more. In addition, the pandemic treaty commits to a One Health Approach that includes animal health.

At a time of growing public disquiet about the expansion of the administrative state and its export to the world stage, the accords put in place requirements to add still more planks to the scaffolding of international health governance. These include a committee of states parties, and a technical subcommittee, to meet biennially to oversee implementation; entities to serve as a national "Authority" and a "Focal Point" for the implementation and coordination of health measures within countries; consultations with Indigenous populations; and yet another conference of parties (COP) that will meet every five years to review and strengthen treaty implementation.

Countries are further required to submit periodic reports on implementation measures, maintain or increase pandemic funding, and mobilise additional resources for developing countries. To this end, a coordinating financial mechanism will be established. The treaty also requires states to put in place expedited regulatory review and authorisation of pandemic-related health products, the controversies attending emergency-use authorisation of the mRNA Covid vaccines notwithstanding.

Furthermore, clauses on misinformation and disinformation will lead to censorship, once again despite the harmful and enduring legacy of this during Covid. The reality of dissent, diverse opinions, and robust scientific debate was kept hidden from the people who no longer trust governments and experts, like they largely did before Covid, to level with them.

Jay Bhattacharya, delivering the keynote address at the National Conservatism Conference in Washington DC on 3 September as the director of the National Institutes of Health, recalled that in 2020–21, among his scientist friends, there

> *'were a lot of diverse opinions. But the problem was that the scientific debate you deserved to hear in 2020 and 2021—you were denied, because the free speech guarantees that this country normally has were taken away… The First Amendment was effectively a dead letter during the pandemic."*

The WHO believes in "the science of managing infodemics" (my emphasis). Its role as a lead participant in the worldwide censorship industrial complex comprising governments, academia, legacy media, social media, and tech platforms has imposed a high cost on the WHO in eroded public trust. The core problem is mistrust, not misinformation. Managed information is not the solution. On the contrary, it will worsen the pathology.

Judgement of history

It is impossible to know how the Covid experience will be assessed by historians in the fullness of time on the criterion of informed consent, a bedrock principle of medical ethics. In a very real sense, selective and manipulated release of data ensured that informed consent was corrupted into misinformed and disinformed compliance. The steep age gradient of the mortality risk profile from the disease was known, or should have been known, by any diligent public health authority and expert. Deliberately ignoring that and the attendant strategy of policies targeted towards the high risk groups, universal fear was ramped up to off the chart on the Richter scale of panic with breathless daily press briefings on new cases, hospitalisation, deaths, and containment measures.

Absolute risk reduction was conflated with and collapsed into relative risk reduction in highlighting the "95% efficacy" of vaccines. The same with regard to the great variability across continents. Heroic assumptions were made on the benefits of pharmaceutical and non-pharmaceutical interventions as against the absolute worst-case doomsday scenarios of not going soon, hard, and long in responding to the grossly inflated threat. Those responsible for the irresponsible fear-mongering have not been held to account. Instead, chief health officers in charge of the pandemic response received public veneration, promotions to governorships, and high national honours, while their critics, even those whose dissenting voices have been vindicated by now, were vilified as immoral and dangerous, dismissed from service and the public square, and remain mostly sidelined.

The WHO pandemic accords were negotiated by national and international public health officials and experts who shut down societies and imposed mask and vaccine mandates. The Covid years gave them a taste of high profile visibility and unprecedented powers to dominate the public policy and media attention and issue commands that must be obeyed for entire populations, including putting everyone under house arrest under the euphemism of "lockdowns." They were deferred to with great respect by prime ministers and health ministers, courted and feted by the media, and lionised and venerated by the public. The personal and career interests of the public health clerisy were best served by convincing governments and people that the frequency and severity of pandemic risks are accelerating and intensifying. Building resilience into health systems against future pandemic shocks requires more resources and powers for health bureaucrats, technocrats, and experts.

Or did we seriously expect them to say that pandemic risks are modest and can be adequately contained by existing budgets and institutional arrangements, and then to fade softly back into the shadows of pre-Covid obscurity? To ask is to answer.

Should Argentina leave the WHO?[75]

Argentina's government has become increasingly sceptical of the World Health Organization, reflecting a wider reconsideration of international health institutions in the aftermath of Covid-19. Although Argentina has not formally withdrawn, it has expressed dissatisfaction with the WHO's performance, its growing reliance on donor-funded agendas, and its push for expanded treaty authority.

This reassessment coincides with the even more consequential reality that the United States has initiated its withdrawal from the WHO. It is the first time since the Soviet Union rejoined the WHO in the 1950s that a major funder, in this case its most influential member, has stepped away.

[75] Roger Bate, David Bell, Ramesh Thakur, *Brownstone Journal*, 24 December 2025, https://brownstone.org/articles/should-argentina-leave-the-who/

The US departure changes the strategic environment in which Argentina must act. Washington's decision was driven by concerns that the WHO mishandled the pandemic, promoted extreme and damaging restrictions, tolerated poor scientific practice, and allowed private philanthropies and advocacy networks to shape policy. The United States may seek re-entry if future negotiations produce meaningful reform, and it may rejoin under a future administration, but for the foreseeable future the WHO will operate without its principal sponsor. This shift presents Argentina with new risks and new opportunities.

Argentina could leave immediately, but doing so now would limit its influence. Remaining as a conditional participant offers a more effective path. Conditional engagement means Argentina stays within the WHO while making clear that its membership depends on substantial changes in governance, transparency, and scientific integrity. This approach preserves access to certain technical networks, avoids needless diplomatic friction, and allows Argentina to align its stance with that of the United States during a period of global institutional realignment. Just as importantly, it leaves withdrawal as an option if the WHO remains unresponsive.

The case for this strategy rests on well-documented failures. During Covid-19, the WHO endorsed restrictive measures that imposed severe economic and health and social costs, particularly in low- and middle-income countries (LMICs). It resisted acknowledging successful alternative strategies, notably in Sweden and Tanzania, and later revised its historical guidance in ways that shielded institutional authority rather than enabling honest evaluation. In tobacco control and other areas, the WHO has become increasingly shaped by donor priorities that do not reflect the interests of sovereign nations.

The well-intentioned initiatives to limit the harms from smoking have led to unintended and perverse consequences that the organization has been reticent in acknowledging. The proposed expansion of the International Health Regulations and the Pandemic

Agreement—negotiated with limited transparency—would grant the organization unprecedented influence over national emergency responses. These dynamics undermine trust and justify Argentina's insistence on reform.

Conditional engagement allows Argentina to use its membership to demand these reforms. It can press for transparency in donor funding, scientific pluralism in decision-making, strict limits on the WHO's authority during emergencies, and priority attention and resources to the most lethal infectious diseases in the LMICs. It can refuse to implement WHO recommendations unless they pass independent national review. With the United States now outside the WHO, Argentina becomes one of the few reform-minded voices still at the table, giving it a degree of influence it would not have from the outside. Should meaningful reforms fail to materialize, Argentina can still withdraw later—and that withdrawal would carry more weight because it followed a period of principled engagement.

At the same time, Argentina should deepen bilateral and regional cooperation, especially with the United States, which is building alternative health partnerships to replace WHO mechanisms. These can provide stronger technical support than the WHO currently offers, including in surveillance, laboratory capacity, drug-quality monitoring, and evidence-based harm reduction. Strengthening national scientific bodies and emergency preparedness systems will also ensure that Argentina remains fully sovereign in its public health decision-making.

Argentina does not need to decide today whether to stay or leave the WHO. It only needs to put the organization on notice that membership is no longer unconditional. By engaging selectively, aligning with the United States, and preserving the option of withdrawal, Argentina positions itself to influence the future of global health governance rather than being shaped by it. This strategy safeguards both sovereignty and flexibility in a rapidly changing international environment.

11: MEDIA: FROM SPEAKING TRUTH TO POWER TO LICKSPITTLES OF STATE POWER

On 3 April 2023, the *Australian*'s US correspondent Adam Creighton published an opinion article blaming the wall of vaccine infallibility on media silence on its many failings. The article was republished by Brownstone on 4 April and, as of the time of writing in July, it was still on the list of the most popular articles on its site. When I first started discussing the rise in excess deaths in Australia in August 2021 (see chapter 5 above), a couple of Australian reporters talked to me about it but their editors were not interested in following up. That is just one small yet telling indication of how a combination of incuriosity and the desire to avoid even truthful reporting in case it fed vaccine hesitancy has caused long-term damage to media credibility in its primary mission to report honestly on major stories without fear or favour in a balanced and objective coverage.

The pandemic of journalistic malfeasance[76]

Matt Hancock was the UK Health Secretary in 2020 when the pandemic struck. A lockdown hawk and a moral pygmy, he was the author

[76] Brownstone Institute, 15 March 2023, https://brownstone.org/articles/the-pandemic-of-journalistic-malfeasance/

of draconian restrictions imposed on business, social, educational, and recreational activities in England in a rolling series of lockdowns.

He was forced to resign on 26 June 2021 after CCTV images captured him kissing and groping Gina Coladangelo, a senior aide he had hired, at the entrance to his office at a time when such intimate contacts were forbidden outside established relationships. The footage was promptly leaked to *The Sun*. Both Hancock and Coladangelo were married with children at the time but separated from their families in the ensuing scandal and have been living together since.

Hancock then decided to write a memoir and hired journalist Isabel Oakeshott as a co-author. Pandemic Diaries: The Inside Story of Britain's Battle against Covid was published in December 2022. The misleading title (now there's a surprise) notwithstanding, the book was not based on a contemporaneous diary but on Hancock's recollections supplemented by his records of communications.

As part of the collaboration and with the false security of a non-disclosure agreement, Hancock handed over to Oakeshott the entirety of his WhatsApp communications with all the key players involved in making policy to manage the Covid pandemic. She gave all 100,000 of the text messages to *The Telegraph* which has been publishing a series of reports and commentaries under the generic title The Lockdown Files since 28 February.

Oakeshott explained her decision to break the non-disclosure agreement by saying the country and the people deserve urgent answers to the flawed crisis management. They cannot afford to wait for the official inquiry report years down the track with the real risk of a whitewash.

The MSM journalists' lack of professional curiosity

Had the media done their job, I would not have felt compelled to embark on what turned out to be an epic voyage of discovery about pandemic policies. In thinking back over the still scarcely believable experience of the last three years, I've been combing through ideas and thoughts.

I started filing away in 2020. I have a Word document with the working title "Where have all the liberals gone" dated 23 May 2020. Another from 28 May has the title "Where have all the journos gone." It was published the next day, albeit with a different title, in the left-of-centre online Australian daily commentary *Pearls and Irritations.* Referencing official claims on the deadliness of the virus and the putative justifications for lockdowns, I wrote:

> *Almost all journalists seem to have lost their cynicism towards claims by the authorities and instead become addicted to pandemic panic porn. The measures taken have been extreme, more even than has been done during a war and more than was attempted during earlier, deadlier flu epidemics....*
>
> *A critical and sceptical profession would have put the government's and modellers' claims under the blowtorch and subjected them to withering criticism for the magnitude of errors by which their predictions have been off. Instead they have mostly joined the adoring multitudes in showering praise on the magnificence of the emperor's new robe. Or, to change the metaphor, it is as if the Wicked Wizard of Wuhan (WWW) has cast an evil spell over the whole world and turned it into an enchanted forest with humans confined to limited spaces and the other creatures roaming freely, no longer terrorised by homo sapiens.*

In an article published in the online Australian right-of-centre daily commentary *The Strategist* on 5 June on coronavirus winners and losers, I listed the media as among the losers: "an inquisitive, detached and critical press should have asked tough questions on justifications and evidence. Instead, most of the media became pandemic porn addicts." In an article in *Spectator Australia* in April 2021, finally, I noted that coronavirus had produced a "blizzard of bogus journalism."

I mention these not to pat myself on the back. Rather, it's because reading the Lockdown Files has left me seething with ice cold rage. (Or is "white hot" the stronger expression? Funny language, English.) As Janet Daley comments, we went "from disinterested journalism to Pravda in a single bound." And as Jeffrey Tucker so elegantly put it: "What is amplified and what is buried [by the MSM] is an editorial decision, not a reflection of reality." They amplified the superstitious fear and buried scientific scepticism in a double distortion of reality.

On 25 January 2020, unbelievable as it now seems, Donald Trump tweeted his thanks to China's President Xi Jinping: "China has been working very hard to contain the Coronavirus. The United States greatly appreciates their efforts and transparency. It will all work out well."

Two days later, noting Trump's remarks, Siobhán O'Grady wrote in *The Washington Post* that only a draconian government could institute such tough measures to restrict people's activities. She quoted Yanzhong Huang from the Council on Foreign Relations that China's extreme measures were "an emotional response." Often, they are not based on evidence and can cause serious side effects that are exacerbated by an unquestioning media that parrots the state's talking points. No s**t, Sherlock.

It didn't take long for the US media to flip and smear individuals and politicians who questioned lockdown and go after countries (Japan, Sweden) and states (Florida, Georgia, Iowa, South Dakota) that refused to lock down, while lavishing praise on Andrew Cuomo's performance in New York. YouTube removed a video of a US Senate committee hearing, and of the roundtable discussion by Governor Ron DeSantis with Trump's coronavirus adviser Scott Atlas and the authors of the Great Barrington Declaration (GBD), despite Florida's comparative success among US states on most key pandemic metrics based on their advice.

And still Dana Milbank wrote in the *Post* on 3 March a mocking piece on the GBD authors: "There is no known cure for long covidiocy." The glib retort would be to query if perchance he was looking in the mirror when the "long covidiocy" smear occurred to him. The more substantial response would be for someone to draw his attention to the Lockdown Files in the UK and ask: Who among his fellow-American journalists has done the Watergate-era equivalent investigations, in which the *Post* played the starring role, in relation to the pandemic?

Oakeshott has been criticised by some British journalists—Nick Robinson, Cathy Newman (who was so comprehensively yet courteously taken down in a viral interview with Jordan Peterson in January 2018 that has been viewed by more than 44mn people), Kay Burley—for having betrayed trust and confidentiality.

Spare me.

They would do better to engage in some soul-searching on the infinitely greater damage done to their profession by the way they joined the drumbeat of ever harder and serially longer restrictions dictated by data-free voodoo science. I doubt I was the only one to stop watching/listening to TV and radio news entirely just to avoid being triggered into extreme irritability at the fear porn being peddled by catastrophising reporters.

The WhatsApp messages were part of the official policy-making process and should be in the public realm by law. They properly belong to the people and not the politicians: written by ministers and aides who are all paid by and accountable to taxpayers, using official communications devices, to make decisions that affected everyone. By what ethical principle was the government keeping them hidden?

Oakeshott has acknowledged breaking a non-disclosure agreement. So what? The public interest is paramount and that too with a sense of urgency. With each new day's fresh batch of revelations, the critical murmurs seem to have died down as the enormity of the toxic dysfunctionality and malfeasance sinks into the public consciousness.

To be sure, an official inquiry has already been set up. However, the UK's experience with official inquiries into controversial government policies and actions is not very reassuring on the timeline of the hearings and publication and content of the final report.

The Bloody Sunday inquiry was set up in 1998, finished hearing evidence in 2004, but did not publish its damning report until 2010. The Chilcot Report was reasonably good on how the UK got into the Iraq War, but took more than seven years from 2009 to 2016. The Hutton inquiry into the suicide of British scientist David Kelly produced its report within six months but was a complete whitewash. I still remember my sense of total incredulity at the first news reports on the inquiry report.

How much material will be redacted and how much published by the official Covid inquiry? What will be the balance between a whitewash and an honest and robust analysis and recommendations with bite? Inquiry Chair Baroness Heather Hallett, a former High Court judge, insists she is "determined" to reach conclusions, make recommendations as soon as possible and not produce a whitewash.

Yet, the public hearings have not yet started, with the first ones scheduled for 13 June, and not a single witness has been called so far. With no less than 62 barristers instructed by the chair, it will not come cheap. The bill for the inquiry had climbed to £113 million in March 2023 based on the 37 public contracts awarded to date.

Against the backdrop of glacial progress by official inquiries and their capture by an establishment that is as desperate to defend its legacy as it is skilled at doing so (just go back in time and watch episodes of *Yes Minister* and *Yes, Prime Minister* again), the press has a duty to release information, accelerate debate and hold power to account while memories are still fresh and wounds are raw.

In an article for *The Telegraph*, Julia Hartley-Brewer—one of the few British journalists able to hold her head high for fearless pursuit of much of the nonsense of Britain's Covid policies—excoriates her journalistic colleagues. She asks if their questioning of Oakeshott's professional integrity is motivated by envy of a major scoop by a competitor (Toby Young calls it "the scoop of the decade"), or because it calls into question their own convictions on the essential soundness of government policies on lockdowns, school closures, masks, and vaccines.

They are more likely driven by anger at being shown up for their own intellectual laziness and lack of curiosity and investigative zeal in putting tough but necessary questions to policy pronouncements from the government for nearly three years. Instead, they cheered each fresh restrictive announcement and often demanded more, more stringent, earlier, and longer restrictions. Hartley-Brewer concludes: "Maybe if those journalists had bothered to ask the right questions in 2020 and in 2021, then we wouldn't have to search for the answers in the morass of Matt Hancock's WhatsApp messages in the here and now."

What might explain the media pusillanimity? With economic activity drastically curtailed, many media outlets became exceptionally dependent on government advertising revenue. In Canada and New Zealand, governments directly subsidised some parts of the media, worth CAD 600mn plus a supplementary $65mn "emergency relief" package and NZD 55mn, respectively.

In a pandemic era analogue of "If it bleeds, it leads," exaggerated catastrophism also brought bigger numbers of eyeballs to their sites, generating additional revenue. And possibly the echo chamber ended up terrorising the media class itself. It all added up to a woeful abandonment of journalistic curiosity, investigative entrepreneurship and willingness to challenge the state narrative.

Spectator Australia and SkyNews Australia were honourable exceptions to the media madness here in Australia, along with a few journalists at *The Australian* like Adam Creighton, Chris Kenny, and Steve Waterson. So too were GBNews in the UK and some individual journalists like Hartley-Brewer, Peter Hitchens, Allison Pearson, and Toby Young. The latter founded *The Lockdown Sceptic* (now *The Daily Sceptic*) which, along with *The Conservative Woman*, and Brownstone Institute in the US, helped vast numbers of people stay sane, if not alive, amidst the pressures of loneliness and despair.

Hitchens was another British journalist to call out lockdowns from the start. For his troubles he received a formal censure from the Independent Press Standards Organisation (IPSO). After the Lockdown Files began to be published, he wrote: "I intend to have a bronze medal struck, which I can wear on ceremonial occasions, recording this censure, intended as a rebuke and taken as an insult but which I will in future regard as an honour." Sounds about right.

The Bill Gates factor

A related question is the extent of influence of Bill Gates on media coverage of global health issues and the near-hagiographical reporting on his views on diseases. The Gates Foundation is reported to have given out $319mn to media outlets.

His modus operandi is to exaggerate the threat from a new disease, invest in new technology to combat the threat, hype its potential, see shares climb, sell at or near the peak, then admit that the threat did not materialise as badly as feared and express relief that it did not. And concede that the technology also failed to live up to expectations.

Writing in the *Spectator Australia* last month, Rebecca Weisser noted that Gates invested in BioNTech (which makes the Pfizer Covid-19 vaccine) in September 2019 with the share price at $18 and sold most of his shares two years later at $300 each, making a killing with a $242mn tax-free profit.

In February 2020, Gates warned that Africa's health services could be overwhelmed by the coronavirus, leading to ten million deaths. In April, Melinda Gates warned of dead bodies all over the streets of Africa. Towards the end of the year, Bill Gates wondered why Africa's Covid mortality toll was not as high as predicted. "One thing I'm happy to have been wrong about—at least, I hope I was wrong—is my fear that Covid-19 would run rampant in low-income countries." By March 2023, according to Worldometers, Africa's total number of Covid deaths was 258,000.

In a moderated conversation under the auspices of the Lowy Institute when Gates flew to Australia in January this year, he said (at around the 54:30 mark in this YouTube video of the event on 23 January): "We also need to fix the three problems of [Covid mRNA] vaccines .... The current vaccines are not infection-blocking. They're not broad, so when new variants come up you lose protection. And they have very short duration, particularly in the people who matter, which are old people".

Incidentally, Gates watched, from a front row seat, the Australian Open men's tennis final that was won by the world's best known unvaccinated athlete, Novak Djokovic. A penny for Gates's thoughts?

Regulator, heal thyself

Journalists were once a group that aspired to speak truth to power. My sorry conclusion is that too many today are people who regurgitate official lies to gain and maintain proximity to power. The tragedy of the fall of journalism-as-it-should-be is perfectly illustrated by the censures handed out to Hitchens, as mentioned above, by IPSO who also rebuked Toby Young for one column in *The Telegraph* in July 2020.

The latest example of the broadcast regulators coming down hard on the slightest misstatement from critical commentators is Ofcom pulling up Mark Steyn for the use of one wrong word—"definitive" instead of, say, "suggestive" or "possible"—in a GBNews broadcast on 21 April 2022.

As Dominique Samuels tweeted: "So Mark Steyn's comments were in breach of your 'broadcasting rules' but TV doctor Sara Kayat claiming [on ITV's *This Morning*] the Covid-19 vaccines were 100% effective, with NO counter opinion included, wasn't"? Precisely.

Disappointingly, GBNews let Steyn go. But the feisty commentator had his own say: "Ofcom is not an impartial arbiter, but rather a body that three years ago chose to take one side: the side of the state narrative. And when it did that, it killed honest discussion on TV and radio." Promising to take his appeal to a real court of law to expose Ofcom, he echoed Hitchens: "I wear my Ofcom death sentence with pride."

Thanks to the Lockdown Files, we now have "definitive" proof that much of Covid policy was cruel and inhumane, made on the hoof, driven by dogma and self-interest, without the requisite evidence and sometimes even against scientific advice, to foment fear, avoid picking arguments with political opponents, promote personal and party agendas, etc. It failed to stop the spread of Covid but has inflicted substantial and lasting damage.

How often did the media regulators pull up and formally censure ministers, newspapers and broadcasters for false claims in support of lockdowns, masks and vaccines? Liberal democracy operates in the belief—nay, the conviction—that a free press is an essential prop of free societies and that probing media scrutiny delivers better policy outcomes while also acting as a check on abuses of power.

On 11 March, *Der Spiegel*, hailed by *The Economist* as "one of continental Europe's most influential magazines," became the first MSM that I am aware of to publish a mea culpa by one of its columnists, Alexander Neubacher:

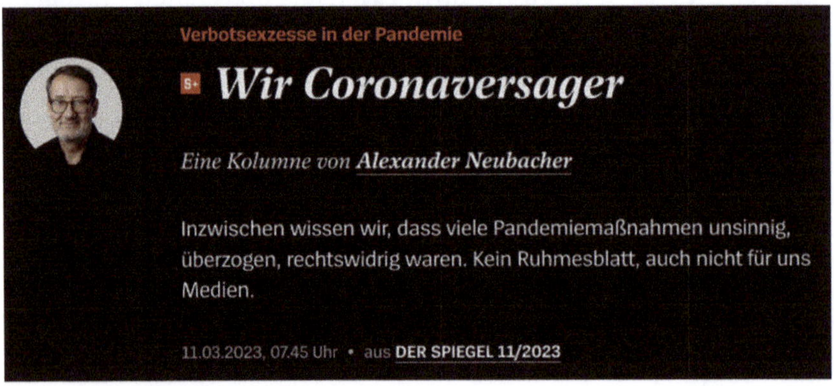

Verbotsexzesse in der Pandemie

S+ **Wir Coronaversager**

Eine Kolumne von **Alexander Neubacher**

Inzwischen wissen wir, dass viele Pandemiemaßnahmen unsinnig, überzogen, rechtswidrig waren. Kein Ruhmesblatt, auch nicht für uns Medien.

11.03.2023, 07.45 Uhr • aus **DER SPIEGEL 11/2023**

Google translation:

Ban excesses in the pandemic

Our corona failures

We now know that many pandemic measures were nonsensical, excessive, and illegal. No glory sheet, not even for us media.

In light of what we now know, is it unfair to ask: How many deaths and preventable injuries and illnesses might have been avoided but for the intimidation of robust media questioning and reporting by Ofcom and IPSO? If they are not prepared to address this double standard they risk shredding their own credibility.

Media complicity in policing the opinion corridor[77]

Like the Overton window of political possibilities, what the Swedes call the "opinion corridor" channels the range of acceptable speech. Among the many startling aspects of the topsy-turvy world that we have lived through since early 2020 is the extent to which the media and social media, often with the active collusion and indeed under requests-cum-instructions from national governments and international organisations, denied space and voice in their columns, letter pages and online commentary to questioning and criticism of the official narrative.

This is darkly ironic, for the net health, mental health, economic, educational and social outcomes would have been far better if the media had performed their traditional role of subjecting official claims to critical scrutiny and provided a platform to a range of responsible and credentialled commentary.

The *Australian* is the country's leading and most influential centre-right daily in print. Of course, because it is part of Rupert Murdoch's global media empire, people with left-of-centre political views routinely dismiss it as far-right (centre-right doesn't exist in their lexicon.)

Yet, it is rare in the Australian media landscape for being prepared to publish competing perspectives and thus shows greater viewpoint diversity than, say, the state-funded broadcaster the ABC.

---

[77] Brownstone Institute, 26 May 2023, https://brownstone.org/articles/media-complicity-in-policing-opinion-corridor/

More importantly, in the quality and depth of their analysis, several of its columnists are a cut above their competitors in the print media and often worth reading despite, or perhaps even more because, often arguing a case with which readers may strongly disagree.

* * *

Since the above article was written, Senator Alex Antic's probing questions led to official confirmation that in less than three years, the federal government intervened 4,213 times to restrict or censor posts about the pandemic on digital platforms. Moreover, echoing the growing understanding about the lead role played by the national security apparatus in the US pandemic response, these requests to the Australian media came from the Department of Homeland Security.

Mark Zuckerberg admitted on 10 June 2023: "Just take some of the stuff around Covid … A lot of the kind of establishment on that...asked for a bunch of things to be censored that, in retrospect, ended up being more debatable or true... It really undermines trust."

Fact-Checker, check thyself[78]

In two articles on this site on 13 November and 18 March, Andrew Lowenthal explained the intimate connections in the Virality Project between the US government, Stanford University, and Big Tech, to enforce Covid orthodoxy via the Censorship Industrial Complex. A similar collusion has operated in Australia but not, as far as we know, as an initiative of the security state.

This is the ABC RMIT Fact Check Unit. It is hosted jointly by the Royal Melbourne Institute of Technology (RMIT) that is mostly a publicly funded institution and the public broadcaster the Australian Broadcasting Corporation (ABC) that is entirely funded by the state.

---

[78] Brownstone Institute, 30 March 2024, https://brownstone.org/articles/fact-checker-check-thyself/

It describes itself rather grandiosely as a partnership that combines "academic excellence and the best of Australian journalism to inform the public through an independent non-partisan voice." This boast has helped to provide plausible cover for enforcing the orthodoxy of the medical establishment that suffers from the delusion that it is the single source of medical scientific truth.

The self-important pretentiousness was punctured this week. During a radio interview with 2GB host Ben Fordham on 18 March, businessman Dick Smith said, "No country has ever been able to run entirely on renewables—that's impossible." He said this in the context of advocating for nuclear power to be added to Australia's energy mix.

The fact check

ABC RMIT Fact Check promptly investigated this and adjudged that "experts consulted by RMIT ABC Fact Check suggested Mr Smith's statement doesn't hold up."

In a follow-up interview on 2GB on 25 March, Smith was angry. "The whole document is full of misinformation and lies, it's designed to discredit me. Absolutely disgusting," he told Fordham. He demanded immediate corrections from the taxpayer-funded broadcaster's fact-check unit and threatened defamation action otherwise as the verdict was damaging his credibility.

US columnist Michael Shellenberger, who played a central role in breaking the Twitter Files story, said: "The Australian government is demanding that X, Facebook, and other social media companies censor content that its fact-checkers say is inaccurate. But now, one of the government's main fact-checker groups has been caught spreading misinformation about renewables and nuclear." X owner billionaire Elon Musk joined in, posting that "Having government 'fact-checkers' is a giant leap in the direction of tyranny!"

Bizarrely, to support its negative verdict on Smith, the fact check quoted Stanford University's Professor Mark Jacobson to the effect that California had "been running on more than 100% WWS [wind-water-solar] for 10 out of the last 11 days for between 0.25 and 6 hours per day." Similarly, the fact check cited a forecast from the Australian Energy Market Operator that renewables will be able to meet the entire demand of the national electricity market by 2025, "albeit for short periods of time (for example, 30 minutes)."

This demonstrates gross reading comprehension problems. Or is it elementary maths? If California has been relying on renewables for between 0.25 and 6 hours per day, quite clearly that confirms Smith's claim, for renewables could not manage power needs for between 18 to 23.75 hours per day. In addition, Smith claimed subsequently, California can draw on its own and two other states' nuclear power as base-load backup power to renewables. Nor does a 30-minute capacity indicate the ability to meet Australia's electricity demand 24/7 for 365 days a year.

The proliferation of fact-checkers

The fact-check industry came into its own during the Covid years, gained in popularity, and proliferated in numbers of organisations and individuals. However, they typically operated with little transparency and clarity on the credentials of the fact-checkers and their qualifications to adjudicate between world-renowned experts making competing claims. After all, contestation is normal in scientific discourse. Anything that cannot be questioned but relies on authority alone is dogma, not science.

A good example of this syndrome was provided to this site on 27 March by Peter Gøtzsche, co-founder of the Cochrane Collaboration and Professor of Clinical Research Design and Analysis at the University of Copenhagen, who has published more than 97 papers in the "big five" medical journals (JAMA [*Journal of the American Medical Association*], *Lancet*, *New England Journal of Medicine*, *British Medical Journal*, and *Annals of Internal Medicine*).

Gøtzsche had produced a video of a conversation he had with Professor Christine Stabell Benn, "one of the most outstanding vaccine researchers in the world." On their own *Broken Medical Science* site, the video (published last October) is described thus:

In this episode, Peter C Gøtzsche discusses with Professor Christine Stabell Benn the research that has shown that live, attenuated vaccines reduce total mortality by much more than their specific effects would predict; that non-live vaccines increase total mortality; that the order in which the vaccines are given is important for mortality; what the harms are of the Covid-19 vaccines; and why they are overused.

After reading Martin Kulldorff's story in the *City Journal* on 11 March of how he was fired by Harvard University, Gøtzsche decided to test YouTube and put up the video on 24 March. It was taken down within an hour for violating its medical misinformation policy. They appealed but having "reviewed your content carefully," YouTube "confirmed that it violates our medical misinformation policy." Gøtzsche was very impressed that YouTube fact-checkers were able to conduct a careful and thorough review of a 54-minute conversation, involving two internationally eminent medical experts, in less than an hour.

Is it any wonder that fact-checkers were quickly discredited for several reasons. They took official claims by governments and the WHO as authoritative and true. This produced some hilarious flip-flops as the narrative on Covid changed with respect, for example, to the likely origins of the coronavirus in Wuhan's wet market or the research laboratory in the Wuhan Institute of Virology located just a few kilometres away. Also with respect to claims that the vaccines stop infection, transmission, and death.

Second, fact-checkers were shown to have a pronounced left-liberal bias. Third, their modus operandi turned out to be to ask different experts for their reactions to the claims under investigation and then side with the experts who aligned with their own bias. Fourth and most importantly, when challenged in court Facebook's defence in December 2021 was that fact-check pronouncements were protected "opinions" under the First Amendment.

Thorsteinn Siglaugsson was wickedly accurate in sketching the typology of fact-checking techniques. Create a straw-man argument that can be easily knocked down. Assert that a claim is not supported by evidence, is questioned by other experts, lacks context, is misleading, or is only partly true, etc. Engage in ad hominem attacks against the person rather than with their evidence and argument.

ABC RMIT Fact Check, check your own facts

Smith makes the point that the fact-checker never contacted him. He could have told them he was talking about the total energy requirements, not just electricity requirements. Professor Jacobson told Fact Check that four countries draw 100% of their electricity power requirements solely from renewables: Albania, Bhutan, Paraguay, and Nepal.

The first thing to note is that even the electricity consumption per capita of the four countries is substantially lower than that of Australia as an advanced industrial economy (Figure 11.1).

Figure 11.1: Energy use per capita in Albania, Bhutan, Nepal, Paraguay, and Australia

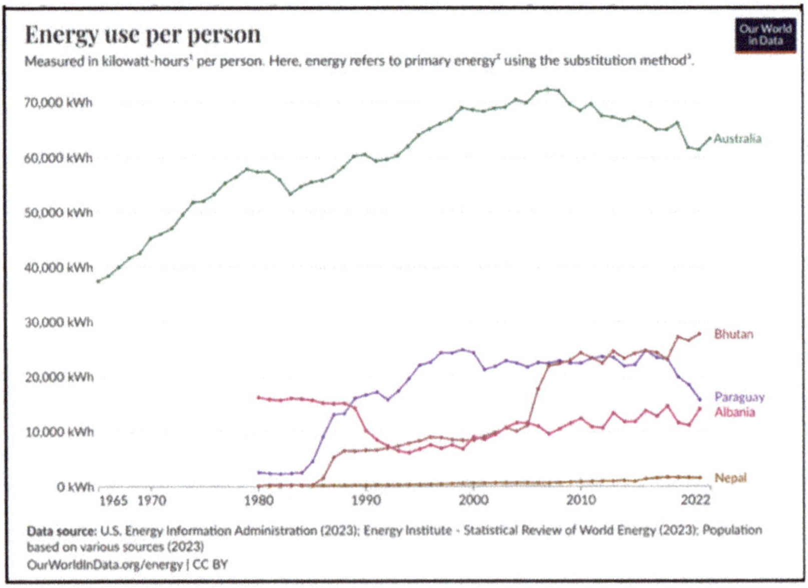

Second, none of the four countries is an island continent without the option of connecting to a geographically wider energy grid to make up for shortfalls national energy needs. In 2021, 24.1% of Albania's, 27.6% of Nepal's, and 10.1% of Paraguay's energy needs were met from imports.

Third, according to Our World in Data, the share of electricity production from renewables for Paraguay was 99.88% in 2021, and for the remaining three was 100%. But power for the electricity grid made up only 22, 41, 13, and 38 percent of the total energy consumption of Albania, Bhutan, Nepal, and Paraguay, respectively.

Figure 11.2 shows the energy mix of three countries using data from the International Energy Agency (Bhutan's is not available from that source).

Figure 11.2: Total energy supply by source, 2021

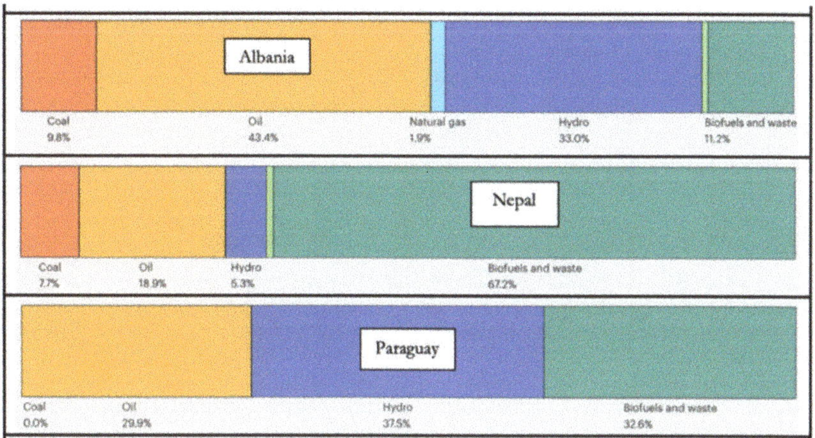

Source: International Energy Agency

Nepal

I'd like to look in more detail at Nepal, for a simple reason. I was born and grew up in the state of Bihar just 20-30km from the border with Nepal which is an open border for citizens of the two countries. Consequently I am intimately familiar with life and communities on both sides of the border. Like people in northern Bihar, many Nepalese lack access to electricity and rely heavily on wood, agricultural waste, and dung with high CO_2 emissions for their daily cooking and heating needs.

Similarly, on both sides of the border fossil fuels power the majority of transportation and diesel generators are commonly used as a power source to offset unreliable grid electricity supply. Speaking of which, a common complaint from local Indians is that Nepal imports a lot of the electricity produced in India even though India's own power requirements are not fully met.

In other words, the ABC RMIT Fact Check conclusions were misleading, lacked context, and made false claims about what Dick Smith had said in his interview. Good to see that despite repeated insistence that it was standing by its work, late on March 26 the Fact Check unit apologised to Smith and amended its report.

But this does rather beg the question. Having stood by their verdict for over a week, ABC buckled upon receiving a letter from Smith's lawyers. He is both a public figure with access to media and politicians and very wealthy. The founder of the successful Australia-New Zealand retail chain Dick Smith Electronics, his state honour includes the highest level of civilian recognition, the Companion of the Order of Australia (AC), awarded in 2015. Ninety-nine percent of Australians lack his reach and ability to issue credible legal threats and risk penury. Consequently his win is unlikely, on its own, to end the ABC's attitude problem rooted in arrogance, hubris, and complacency.

12: COVID AND CLIMATE CATASTROPHISATION

The Covid-19 pandemic is not the only recent example of an issue where alarmism has been fomented to command public and policy attention, demand urgent action, and impose severe restrictions on existing lifestyles and activities. Indeed the most prominent example that has been running a scare campaign for decades is climate change.

Covid, climate and the corruption of science and policy[79]

We can be confident that all true believers of The Science™ of climate change have taken careful note of the lessons offered by the coronavirus pandemic for managing the "climate emergency." Thus Carl Bildt, the former prime minister (PM) of Sweden: "The pandemic offers important lessons for managing future challenges, particularly climate change" which "warrants urgent attention."

---

[79] Amalgamation of: "Let's apply Covid scepticism to climate change," *Spectator Australia*, 4 June 2022, https://www.spectator.com.au/2022/06/lets-apply-covid-scepticism-to-climate-change/; "Covid, climate and the corruption of science and policy," *Spectator Australia*, 11 June 2022, https://www.spectator.com.au/2022/06/covid-climate-and-the-corruption-of-science-and-policy/; and "Learning from Covid, be wary of catastrophising climate models and activists," Resistance Press, 26 March 2023, https://resistancepress.com/article/learning-covid-be-wary-catastrophizing-climate-models-and-activists

The two agendas share ten items in common that should leave us worried, very worried.

Hypocrisy

The first is the hypocrisy of the exalted elites who preach to the deplorables the proper etiquette of abstinence to deal with the emergency, and their own insouciant exemption from a restrictive lifestyle. When the world's top leaders met at the G7 summit in Cornwall in 2021, they copped a lot of merited criticism for this sin. They social distanced and masked up for photo-ops but hobnobbed in close proximity *sans* masks in partylike atmosphere in private: one law for me, a member of the entitled elite, and another law for thee of the deplorable plebs. PM Scott Morrison was happy to attend as a guest despite having banned the rest of us from leaving Australia.

In the following years we witnessed the surreal spectacle of Britain's Parliament interrogating disgraced former PM Boris Johnson on allegations that he serially broke the lockdown rules he had imposed on everyone else—but not questioning the anti-scientific stupidity of the rules themselves. The partygate scandal continued to dog Johnson. The upsetting aspect of this was not the trivial details of partying after work with colleagues. Rather, it is proof that the very people who wrote draconian rules and gave the police full licence to crack down brutally, even for the most absurd, unhealthy, cruel and heartless rules, knew the rules to be nonsense. The photos of Johnson and aides partying were politically toxic because of the searing images of a masked Queen sitting alone at her husband's funeral.

At the UN climate talkfest in Glasgow, they could not accommodate all the private jets at one airport. Not to forget footage of Joe Biden's gas guzzling planes and limousines in Europe last year. There are multiple examples of the disconnect between what the "progressive" elites preach and practice. Bristol Mayor Marvin Rees was the UK's first city mayor to declare a climate crisis. On 28 May 2022 the BBC reported he had flown over 7,000km each way for nine hours to

Vancouver to deliver a 14-minute TED talk calling for urgent climate action, creating over 2,000kg of CO2.

Similarly, in the US too any number of photos show former president Barack Obama, California Governor Gavin Newsom and progressives' darling Alexandria Ocasio-Cortez living it up maskless on glittering occasions while serving staff had to be masked. A particularly notorious example was Newsom and his cronies without masks in the appropriately named French Laundry restaurant at a time when this was verboten, being served by fully masked staff.

Prince Harry and Meghan Markle have been widely mocked for jetting around the world to warn people about global warming. When Harry travelled to Sicily in July 2019 for an A-list climate gathering organised by Google, he was among 114 delegates who put on a "hypocritical display of mega yachts, private jets and conspicuous consumption while billions live in energy poverty," Alberta's Premier Jason Kenney tweeted. Swedish child-prophet Greta Thunberg's highly publicised sea voyage to New York from Europe in 2019 raised questions on the carbon footprint in the construction of the "zero-carbon" carbon-fibre racing yacht. Some members of her sailing crew returned to Europe by plane, while others flew across the Atlantic to sail the vessel back.

I wonder if anyone has done a calculation of the total carbon footprint of each annual Davos gathering where CEOs, prime ministers and presidents, captains of industry, Hollywood glitterati and other celebrities fly in on private jets, are driven around in gas-guzzling limousines and preach to us on the critical urgency of reducing emissions? I understand the hookers do quite well during that week, so perhaps there is a silver lining.

Mismatch of models and data

A second common element between Covid and climate change is the mismatch between models that inform policy and data that contradict the models. The long track record of abysmally wrong catastrophist predictions on infectious diseases from the Pied Piper of Pandemic Porn Professor Neil Ferguson is, if anything, exceeded by the failures of climate change alarmist predictions.

Calls for urgent climate action based on the language of "edging towards 'tipping points'" have been made over many years. At some point the Intergovernmental Panel on Climate Change (IPCC) morphed from a team of scientists into activists. The most recent example of the drum roll of "The end is nigh and this is absolutely your last chance to avert the end of the world from climate collapse" is yet another Chicken Little Sixth Assessment Report from the indefatigable IPCC. "There is a rapidly closing window of opportunity to secure a liveable and sustainable future for all," the report warns us. UN Secretary-General António Guterres called it a "survival guide for humanity."

A one-time climate action journalist-turned-sceptic, Michael Shellenberger, describes the UN as a "Climate Disinformation Threat Actor." Atmospheric scientists and former IPCC members Richard McNider and John Christy note that climate modelling forecasts have "always overstated the degree to which the Earth is warming compared with what we see in the real climate." One of the real signals of CO2-induced warming is in the deep atmosphere at 75,000 feet. Satellite and balloon data had shown only one-third the warming (0.7^{0}C) predicted by climate models.

"The end is nigh"!

An important reason for both Covid and climate catastrophism is the spreading of fear and panic in the population as a means to spur drastic political action. Both agendas have been astonishingly successful. Polls have consistently shown the hugely exaggerated beliefs about the scale of the Covid threat. On climate change, the gap between the stringent actions required, the commitments made, and the actual record thus far is used to create panic. The notion that we are already doomed promotes a culture of hopelessness and despair perhaps best epitomised in recent times by Thunberg's cry of "How dare you" steal my dreams and childhood with empty words.

A few examples of serially alarmist predictions that look silly by now:

- In 1982, UNEP Executive Director Mostafa Tolba warned of an irreversible environmental catastrophe by 2000 without immediate urgent action. This was repeated by another senior UNEP official in 1989.
- In 2004, a Pentagon report warned that by 2020, major European cities would be submerged by rising seas, Britain would be facing a Siberian climate and the world would be caught up in mega-droughts, famine and widespread rioting.
- In 2007, IPCC chair Rajendra Pachauri declared: "If there's no action before 2012, that's too late." He added ahead of the Bali climate meeting: "This is the defining moment."
- In 2009, NASA scientist Jim Hansen said President Barack Obama had only four years (i.e., his first term) to save the world from climate catastrophe.
- Most hilariously, in Montana, the Glacier National Park installed "Goodbye to the glaciers" plaques, warning: "Computer models indicate the glaciers will all be gone by the year 2020." Come 2020, all 29 glaciers were still there but the signs were gone, taken down by embarrassed park authorities.
- In January 2019, Ocasio-Cortez warned the world will end in 12 years if we fail to address climate change. Don't be surprised if around 2030, the point of no return is stretched out a bit farther once again and governments are called upon to take immediate urgent action because, of course, we are at the very edge of a tipping point.

It's hard to overstate the damage such failed predictions have caused to the climate change narrative. Used as a tactic to grab policymakers' attention, over time it gets trapped in the crying wolf syndrome.

Follow the science™

In addition to hypocrisy, models-data mismatch and fear porn, both Covid and climate change policies claim to be based in The Science™. The fabled 97% scientific consensus was in relation to the simple and trivial proposition that "the earth is warming due to human activity." That doesn't tell us how dominant human activity is as a cause of global warming relative to natural variability over long time cycles; the rise in temperature that will mark a point of no return for the stability of the earth's environment; and "tipping points" that will push the ecosystem into a self-exacerbating cycle of rapid collapse. Gradually The Science™ was captured by climate activists who acted as gatekeepers to restrict entry to climate science departments to the faithful and used peer review to reject contrarian articles. By this means the claim of "consensus" became self-validating.

This has proven harder with Covid, not least because the policy interventions defied settled science. We now know that Anthony Fauci and Francis Collins, from their perch atop the infectious diseases research funding agencies, orchestrated the takedown of the Great Barrington Declaration and smeared its three credentialled authors from Harvard, Oxford and Stanford universities as "fringe" epidemiologists. Yet, as of June 2023, the Declaration had been signed by 937,000 people worldwide, including 63,000 medical practitioners and public health scientists. In addition, there is now a flood of articles being published that show the lack of demonstrable public health outcomes from lockdowns against measurable collateral health, mental health, educational, social and economic damage; and the inefficacy of other measures like masks and vaccines alongside possible long-term harms from them as well. This has produced a palpable lessening of confidence in the authority of scientific experts across the board.

Silencing dissent

For appeal to scientific authority to work better, scientific consensus is very helpful. Yet, driven by intellectual curiosity, questioning existing knowledge is the very essence of the scientific enterprise. For the claim to scientific consensus to be broadly accepted, therefore, supporting evidence must be exaggerated, contrary evidence discredited, sceptical voices stilled and dissenters ridiculed and marginalised.

The rapidly consolidating Censorship-Industrial Complex covered both agendas until Elon Musk began releasing the Twitter Files to expose what was happening. This refers to the extraordinary censorship and suppression of dissenting voices, with extensive and possibly illegal collusion between governments and Big Tech—and, in the case of the pandemic, also Big Pharma and academia. Even truth was no defence, for example with accounts of vaccine injuries, if their effect was to promote narrative scepticism. The social media Big Tech censored, suppressed, shadow banned and slapped labels of "false," "misleading," "lacking context" etc. to content at variance with the single-source ministries of truth. "Fact checking" was weaponised using fresh young graduates—with no training, skills or capacity to sift between authentic and junk science—to put such judgmental stamps on pronouncements from world-leading experts in their field.

A nanny state to keep us all safe

Another shared element is the enormous expansion of powers for the nanny state that bosses citizens and businesses because governments know best and can pick winners and losers. Yet in both agendas, policy interventions have over-promised and under-delivered. The beneficial effects of interventions are exaggerated, optimistic forecasts are made and potential costs and downsides are discounted.

Lockdowns were supposedly required for only two-three weeks to flatten the curve and vaccines, we were promised, would help us return to pre-Covid normality without being mandatory. Similarly, for decades we have been promised that renewables are getting less expensive and energy will get cheaper and more plentiful. Yet increased subsidies are still needed, energy prices keep rising, and energy supply gets less reliable and more intermittent.

Moral framing

Moreover, in both cases growing state control over private activities is justified by being framed as minor and temporary inconveniences in the moral crusade to save the world and save granny. Moral framing has been used to discount massive economic damage resulting from Covid and climate change interventions. Alongside the substantial and lasting economic damage caused by savage lockdowns to businesses and the long-term consequences of a massive printing of money, the obstinate persistence of excess deaths is painful proof of collective public health self-harm.

Similarly, the world has never been healthier, wealthier, better educated and more connected than today. Energy intensity played a critical role in driving agricultural and industrial production that underpin the health infrastructure and comfortable living standards for large numbers of people worldwide. The pursuit of Net Zero by an early finite date requires policies that will result in degrowth and deindustrialisation. Instead de-risking strategies might serve peoples' short and long-term welfare better.

Widening inequality between the jet setting laptop Zoom class and the plebs

In a biting but accurate comment, Sarojini Naidu said it required a lot of money to keep Gandhi in the style of poverty he demanded. Similarly, a lot of money is required to support Covid and climate policy magical thinking where governments can solve all problems by throwing more money that must neither be earned nor repaid.

In both Covid and climate change, government policies have served to greatly widen economic inequalities within and among nations with fat profits for Big Pharma and rent-seeking renewable industries. Lockdowns led to the rise of the laptop class that could work from home because the working classes kept essential services like food distribution and garbage collection going. Australia's newest political phenomenon in the May 2022 elections, the Teal MPs, perfectly encapsulate the triumph of luxury politics where the costs of the rich suffused in the golden glow of virtue are borne mostly by the poor. I am so looking forward to the new government bringing an end to cycles of droughts, bushfires and floods.

Attempts to assess the balance of costs and benefits of Covid and climate policies are shouted down as immoral and evil, putting profits before lives. The precautionary principle has been flipped in both agendas and morphed into the slogan "abundance of caution" to justify the demonstrable collateral harms imposed now in order to forestall greater collective harm predicted in the future if no action is taken now, for it will be too late on the morrow or the morning after the disaster.

But neither health nor climate policy can dictate economic, development, energy and other policies. High income countries enjoy incomparably better health standards and outcomes because of their national wealth. All governments work to balance multiple competing policy priorities. The ideological exclusion of nuclear helps the push for renewables just like the rejection of cheap repurposed pills helps the vaccine push.

What is the sweet spot that ensures reliable, affordable and clean energy security without big job losses? Or the sweet spot of affordable, accessible and efficient public health delivery that does not compromise the nation's ability to educate its young, look after the elderly and vulnerable and ensure decent jobs and life opportunities for families?

Balance of responsibility between industrialised and developing economies

For post-industrial societies, climate action will require cutbacks to living standards as subsidies rise, power prices go up, reliability comes down, and jobs are lost. Poor countries will have to scale back ambitions to climb out of poverty. Should China, the world's biggest emitter today, apologise for achieving the fastest poverty reduction rate for the biggest number of people in history? Should a billion more Chinese, Indians and others have stayed poor and destitute over the last four decades, so Westerners could feel virtuous-green?

The rise of the international technocracy

The final common element is the subordination of state-based decision-making to international technocrats. This is best exemplified in the proliferation of the global climate change bureaucracies and the promise—threat?—of a new global pandemic treaty whose custodian will be a more powerful World Health Organisation. In both cases, the dedicated international bureaucracy will have a powerful vested interest in ongoing climate crises and serially repeating pandemics.

A look back from Canadian wildfires to Australian bushfires and floods[80]

Reports and videos of the smoke and haze from the intense wildfires enveloping Canada and drifting down south into the US bring back vivid memories of Australia's two-month long bushfires (in the Australian vernacular: Canberra is the country's bush capital) three and a half years ago, and floods last year. And so does the claim that the fires and floods validate the apocalyptic warnings and the ensuing impassioned debate over how much this is evidence of a climate emergency owing to anthropogenic global warming.

Guterres warned on 23 March that the damage from climate change is making the planet "uninhabitable." The environment is breaking down, with consequences that include intensifying heatwaves, droughts, floods, wildfires and famines. Others add forced migration and wars to the downstream consequences to heighten

[80] Brownstone Institute, 22 June 2023, https://brownstone.org/articles/a-look-back-from-canadian-wildfires-to-australian-bushfires-and-floods/

the panic porn. This is why, Guterres urges, 2023 should be the year of "transformation, not tinkering." Instead, governments remain trapped in incremental measures. Consequently, Guterres repeated on 15 June: "We are hurtling towards disaster, eyes wide open ... It's time to wake up and step up."

Whoa! Time out for a reality check.

Scientific uncertainty

To start with, as has been the case for three years in relation to Covid, the emphasis on scientific consensus reformulated into The Science™ engages in the strategy of suppression-by-denial of uncertainties and contestation of the gravity and urgency of the threats faced, the causal pathways and relative weightings of the different drivers that influence climate change in a timeframe of millennia, and the mix of alternative policy interventions like adaptation and mitigation to address the challenge.

The complexity of climate systems is due to nonlinear equations involving many different variables across time on land, sea, and air, as well as the interactive linkages among multiple subsystems like the atmosphere, oceans, glacier ice, permafrost, land surface, etc. The relative potency of the different drivers of climate change variability—such as CO2 emissions, solar variability, ocean circulation patterns, volcanic eruptions, and Milankovitch cycles of planetary orbital variations—is not known with any degree of precision. Geological records show that warming and cooling periods go through extended cycles with no apparent pattern to the intensity, severity, and timing of the cycles.

I have argued since March 2020 that Covid-19 is a serious but not an existential global health crisis. Similarly, it is possible to question the extent of the contribution of fossil fuels to climate change without necessarily denying that it does so. The uncertainties and contentions lie in the all too crucial details. In an article last year in *Health Physics*, three scientists from the University of Massachusetts

Lowell challenged the thesis that most of the increase in CO2 atmospheric concentration since 1850 has been from the anthropogenic fossil fuel component. They found that from 1750 to 2018, "the percentage of the total CO2 due to the use of fossil fuels … increased from 0% in 1750 to 12% in 2018, much too low to be the cause of global warming."

Empirical data contradicts catastrophising models and claims

Second, and again as with Covid, observational data can also be at variance with climate model predictions. The mathematical precision of the latter hides the reality of assumptions inputted into the models by bias-confirming humans which determine the scenarios that are produced. In the preceding section, I listed several predictions that have already been falsified, thereby satisfying Karl Popper's criterion for pseudoscience.

A reconstruction for southeast Greenland showed that temperatures have risen and fallen since 1796. If rising CO2 concentrations are a driver of Arctic warming, the nineteenth and twentieth centuries should have been noticeably colder than today. Instead, the study found there were warming and cooling episodes throughout 1796–2013; decadal periods in the 1800s were occasionally warmer than in 2013; and there was more sustained warming in the 1920s and 1940s than during the twenty-first century.

Similarly, an article in *European Geosciences Union* on 16 May by three climate scientists from Leeds University noted that from 2009–19, a reduction in the area of ice sheet on the Antarctic Peninsula and West Antarctica has been outweighed by area growth in East Antarctica and the large Ross and Ronne-Filchner ice shelves, for a net increase of over 5,000 square km. Some ask if, instead of a continuous rise in temperatures, there is not a limit to the heating effect from CO2 emissions on the atmosphere, not unlike evidence that the virus infection rate had its own natural limit after which it peaked and fell rather than climbing infinitely. Others speculate that there may be natural self-healing mechanisms to check uncontrolled climate extremes that keep the earth in balance over long cycles of history.

Figure 12.1: The global annual death rate from all natural disasters

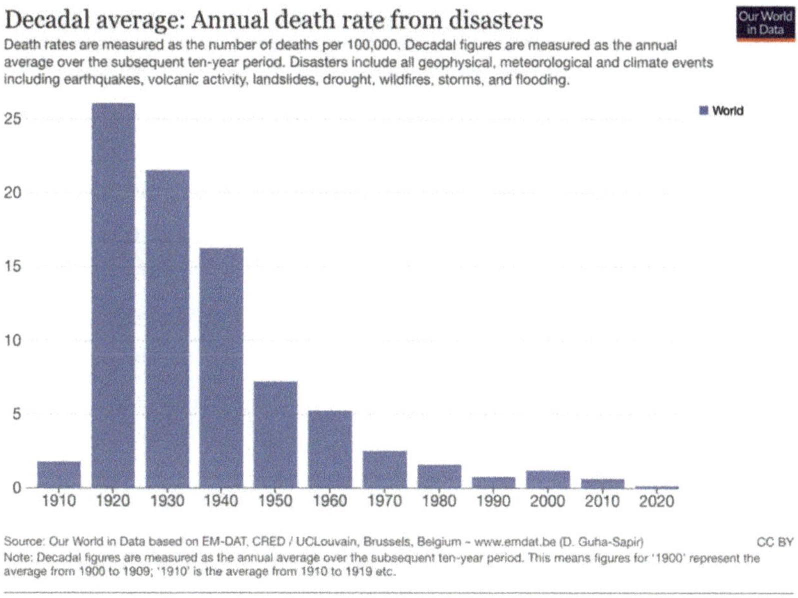

The recent Canadian wildfires, with the heavy smoke blanketing huge areas of the US as well, generated more catastrophising hysteria than light, just like the bushfires in Australia in the 2019–20 summer. The instant blame game points the finger at climate inaction. At 6.37 in the morning of 8 June, President Joe Biden tweeted that Canada's "record wildfires … are intensifying because of the climate crisis." Prime Minister Justin Trudeau followed at 9:21: Canada is experiencing "more and more of these fires because of climate change." And these are the guys who want to establish government mis- and dis-information boards? Their apparently irresistible urge to catastrophise ignores the inconvenient data that the mortality impact of all-cause natural disasters has experienced a steep decline since the 1920s–40s (Figure 12.1).

The Netherlands-based Clintel Foundation published a paper on 9 May arguing that the IPCC's Sixth Assessment Report ignored peer-reviewed literature which shows disaster losses have decreased since 1990 and that the death toll from extreme weather has fallen by 95% since 1920: "The strategy of the IPCC seems to be to hide any good news about climate change and hype anything bad." The disaster-addicted panel needs to invite a broader range of views inside its deliberations tent, they advise.

Yet another mostly ignored reality is that emissions from forest fires are much higher than the reductions resulting from government regulation. Research from University of California experts last year found that wildfire emissions in just one year in 2020 were twice as high as the state's greenhouse gas reductions from 2003 to 2019. Another study found that in 2021, emissions from burning boreal forests in North America and Eurasia were almost double that from aviation fuel. This means that reducing fuel loads (the dry, combustible wood that builds up on forest floors) that have accumulated owing to poor forest management is the better emission reduction strategy than focussing solely on fossil fuel reduction. Pressure from environmental activists to focus more on reactive fire suppression rather than proactive fire prevention strategies is harmful to long term emissions control. That is, prescribed burns that clear out the debris on forest floors could reduce CO2 emissions by more than mandating offshore wind farms and EV automobiles.

As we saw with Covid, the data is often cherry picked around the narrative, in particular the temporal benchmarks. If we look at the acreage burned in the US over the last 30 years, for example, there is a visually dramatic increase from just under three to around ten million acres per year. However, it has fallen steeply from a high of over 50 million acres per year since the 1920s.

The situation in Canada too is similar. According to a study by the Fraser Institute of trends in the 1959–2019 period, "there was a sharp increase in destruction caused by forest fires in the first half of this period, and a general decline in the second half." Around 7.6 million hectares were burned at peak in 1989, falling to 1.8 million hectares in 2019. The *Globe and Mail*'s editorial board argued on 26 July 2021 that prescribed burns improve a forest's overall health while fire suppression leads to "forests susceptible to massive blazes" from the kindling deadfall on the floor.

Debating bushfires and floods down under

Sydney was smothered in thick choking smoke that burning summer. Smoke from surrounding fires—from our house we could see the flames licking the sky just beyond the airport—gave Canberra the world's worst air quality index of 4,758 on 1 January 2020, more than twenty times above the official hazardous threshold of 200. Yet, Canberra's hottest day on record that month at 44^{0}C was no more proof of the scientific reality of global warming than Delhi's coldest December day on record (30th) was a refutation of it.

Amidst the blackened skies and burning landscapes of Australia's many fires that southern summer, the lazy response from some, for example the editorial board of the Financial Times, was to blame climate denialism for the natural disaster. Prime Minister Scott Morrison was sharply criticised for climate delinquency.

Although localised anger from the bushfire victims was understandable, much of the broader critique was misplaced. It showed wilful ignorance of Australia's bushfire-prone history, downplayed the responsibility of state governments for prudent forest management practices, overlooked the long lead times between emissions and climate change, sidestepped the weak links between global warming and specific weather events, and exaggerated Australia's impact on global temperatures.

Which one of these doesn't find an echo in North America at the moment? Yet the reality is that the wildfire hazard has become less serious in both countries (Figure 12.2).

Aboriginal communities have lived in Australia's harsh climate and terrain for tens of thousands of years. Recent research has documented the sophisticated system of land and bush management practices they employed to sustain and regenerate forests. The use of fire was an important part of this cycle.

Figure 12.2: The annual rates of deaths and economic damage from wildfires in Australia and Canada, 1910–2020

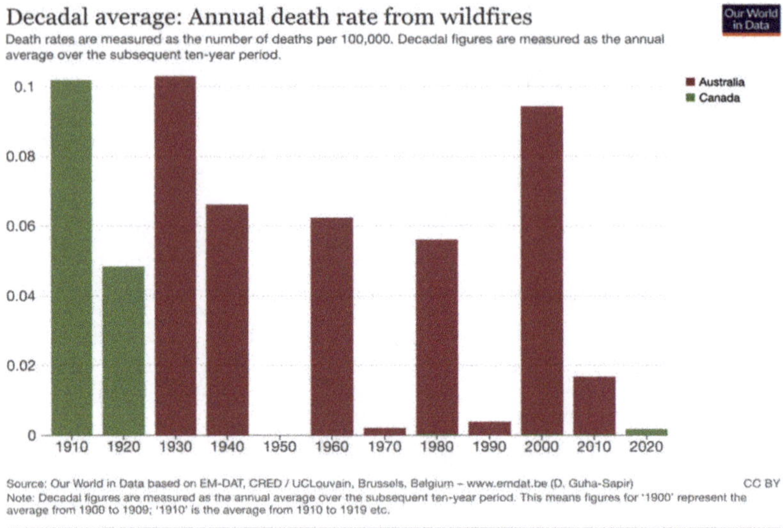

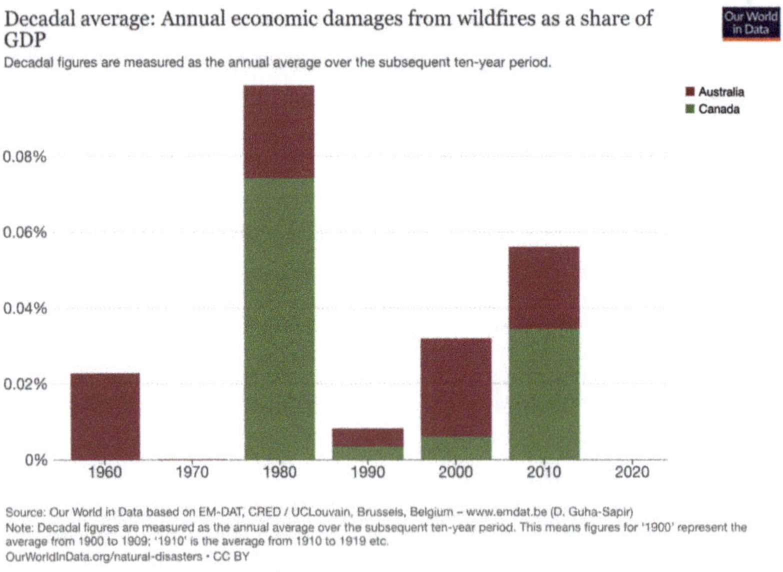

The UK Met Office published a perusal of 57 peer-reviewed scientific papers which noted that fire weather translates to fire activity only with natural or human ignitions (lightning, arson, carelessness) and "burned area is insensitive to fire weather in regions [including Australia] where fuel stocks or human suppression are the key fire limitations."

In a complementary brief, a Technical Report in 2015 from the Commonwealth Scientific and Industrial Research Organisation, the Australian government's peak scientific research body, noted that at any given place, fire potential depends on four "switches":

- Ignition, either human-caused or from natural sources such as lightning;
- Fuel abundance or load (a sufficient amount of fuel must be present);
- Fuel dryness, where lower moisture contents are required for fire; and
- Suitable weather conditions for fire spread, generally hot, dry and windy.

Queensland-based fire researcher Christine Finlay has long warned that reduced burning of fuel loads during the winter could increase the frequency of firestorms in the summer. Finlay, who studied the history of bushfires from 1881 to 1981 for her PhD, shows that bushfire-reduction operations since 1919 have been departing from traditional indigenous practices such as low-intensity cool-weather burning. And, according to her data, there is a direct correlation between the increased frequency and size of fires since 1919 and the accumulation of catastrophic levels of fuel load.

Controlled burning—which is conducted over large areas and under favourable wind and temperature conditions—is cheap and highly effective in reducing the incidence of bushfires as well as the likelihood that they will spread uncontrollably. And, unlike drastic efforts to reduce GHG emissions, it does not threaten livelihoods and living standards.

Bushfires have both structural and direct causes. Australia's average surface temperatures have increased by about 1.5^{0}C since the early 1900s. In a continent dominated by dry eucalypt landscape and hot temperatures, anthropogenic global warming might have aggravated the background conditions for fires to occur more readily, more often, in more places and for the fire season to last longer.

However, local weather patterns are little determined by complex and dynamic global variables and current emissions will influence climate conditions decades into the future, not this year or next year. The most authoritative international report only weak links between human-induced climate change and droughts, bushfires, floods and hurricanes. If Australia had achieved net carbon neutrality by 2019, that would have made no difference to that season's fires.

There are some things the Australian federal and state governments can do now and on their own to reduce the fire toll. Fire management authorities identify the direct causes of individual fires as arson, careless use of fire, lightning, etc. Arsonists must be apprehended and prosecuted and the public better educated on the risks.

Figure 12.3: Floods in Australia—Decadal average: Annual death rate and economic damage as a share of GDP (percent)

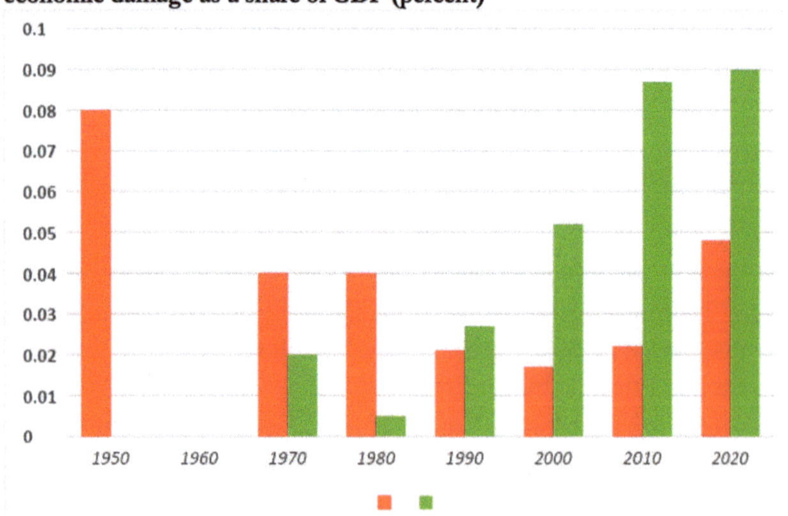

Source: Chart drawn by author using data from Our World in Data.

Climate alarmism got a second life a year later as massive floods hit eastern Australia. We moved to the Northern Rivers region of New South Wales in December 2021, just in time to be greeted in our new home by the floods as the whole area was badly flooded in February–March 2022. Again, however, not for nothing is Australia known as the land of droughts, fires and floods and, contrary to the trap of ahistorical presentism into which most media commentary fell, the death rates from periodic floods have not risen hugely over the decades (Figure 12.3). However, the economic damage has worsened and this probably reflects rising prosperity with more expensive farms and dwellings than in earlier times. A major contributory factor to the floods also is the unfortunate history of granting planning permission for residential developments in floodplains.

Yet, like the different metrics regarding wildfires, with floods also one can pick the area flooded, the number of people killed, or the scale of the property, crop, livestock and economic losses, and the per capita vs. aggregate statistics.

The third echo of Covid is in the way it falls into the trap of prioritising climate action to the neglect of other public policy goals and the cost-benefit calculation is reduced to shouting slogans which, if questioned, degenerate swiftly into abuse and demands for cancellation. In both cases, pressures to intellectual conformism and restrictions on freedom of expression and scientific inquiry in questioning the prevailing "progressive" benchmarks corrupt science into a cult. Why is it illegitimate, immoral and positively evil to be reluctant to cut back on comfortable lifestyles in the high income countries and aspire to the same in the poorer countries, that have been made possible and will be easier, respectively, by fossil fuel energy use?

The deadliest natural disasters are not related to climate change

Figure 12.4: Annual global death rates from wildfires and earthquakes, 1900–2020

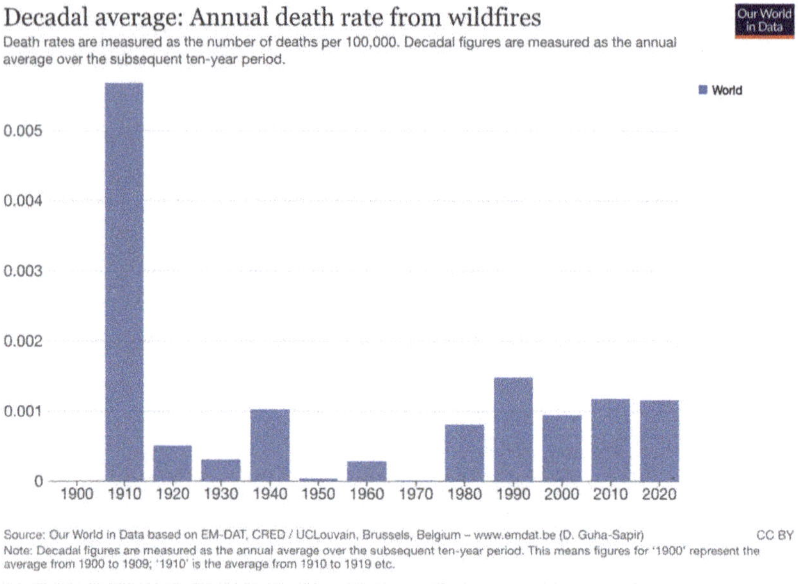

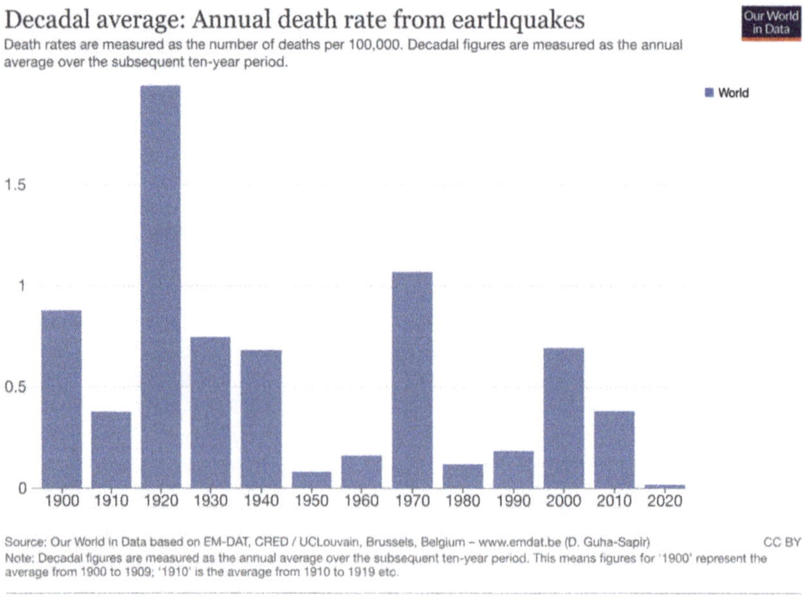

However, conflating man-made global warming with weather disasters betrays wilful ignorance of Australia's long history of bushfires (Figure 12.4). There have been several deadlier heatwaves and fires in Australia's short history even since European settlement, for example in January 1896 with 200 deaths across Australia in three weeks, and again in January 1939 with 71 deaths in the state of Victoria.

Some of the worst "natural" disasters resulted from human decisions. The primary blame for the Ukrainian famine of 1932–33 that killed 13% of the population lay with Stalin's policies. Similarly, Mao Zedong's ideologically-driven farming policies contributed to the great China famine in 1959–61 that killed tens of millions. In recent decades the natural disasters with the worst mortality impacts have been earthquakes and tsunamis (as on Boxing Day 2004 in the Indian Ocean that killed a quarter million people) which are not related to climate change.

In my living memory the worst drought that caused widespread famine in Bihar, my home state, (and in the eastern districts of adjacent Uttar Pradesh) was in 1966–67. The national grain production fell by one-fifth. Bihar's annual grain production declined from 7.5 million tonnes in 1964–65 to 4.3mn in 1966–67, causing a steep rise in the price of essential foods. I recall driving through unfamiliar countryside and striking up a conversation with some local farmers. When we inquired about how they were faring, they said they had hardly had any rain since the late first Prime Minister Jawaharlal Nehru's ashes had been scattered over the countryside as per his requests (in 1964).

The last really big famine in India as a whole was the great Bengal famine of 1943, in which, according to Nobel Laureate Amartya Sen's calculations, nearly three million of Bengal's 60 million people died over 3-4 years (Poverty and Famine*: An Essay on Entitlement and Deprivation*, 1981, chapter 6, "The Great Bengal Famine," p. 52).

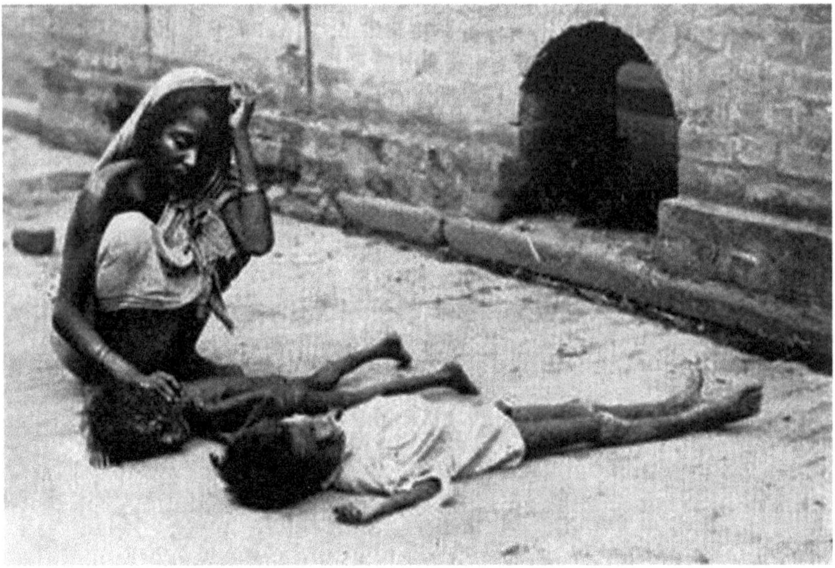

Source: "Dead or dying children in a Calcutta Street," *The Statesman*, Calcutta, 22 August 1943 (public domain).

Madhushree Mukherjee in her 2010 book *Churchill's Secret War: The British Empire and the Ravaging of India during World War II*, blames Winston Churchill for aggravating the severity of the famine by rejecting pleas from British officials governing Bengal to unload Australian wheat in Calcutta. Churchill insisted it must all go to British troops in Europe. Opposition parliamentarian Shashi Tharoor (a friend and colleague from UN days) and author of *Inglorious Empire: What the British Did to India* (2017), sharply criticised the celebration of the British wartime leader in the 2017 film *Churchill.*

Extreme cold is far deadlier than extreme heat

According to a 2014 study by the CDC, around 2,000 US residents died each year from 2006–10 from weather-related events: respectively, 63, 31 and 6% from cold, heat, and floods, storms and lightning. In 2021, a team from Monash University in Australia published the findings of the world's largest 45-country study spanning five continents on climate-related mortality from 2000–2019 in *Planetary Health*, a Lancet journal. Of the 5.1 million annual deaths from extreme temperatures (9.4% of all global deaths), 90.4% died from cold (Figure 12.5).

Yet, the press release from Monash spruiking the study, honed in on rising deaths from heat over the period and linked it to a 0.26°C rise in temperatures per decade. This despite the fact that cold-related death had fallen by 0.51% and heat-related deaths risen by 0.21%, representing a big net fall of 0.3% (15,200) in total weather-related annual deaths. Unsurprisingly, the Guardian headline also took the doomsayer approach: "Extreme temperatures kill 5 million people a year with heat-related deaths rising, study finds."

Figure 12.5: Cold weather dominates extreme weather-related mortality around the world

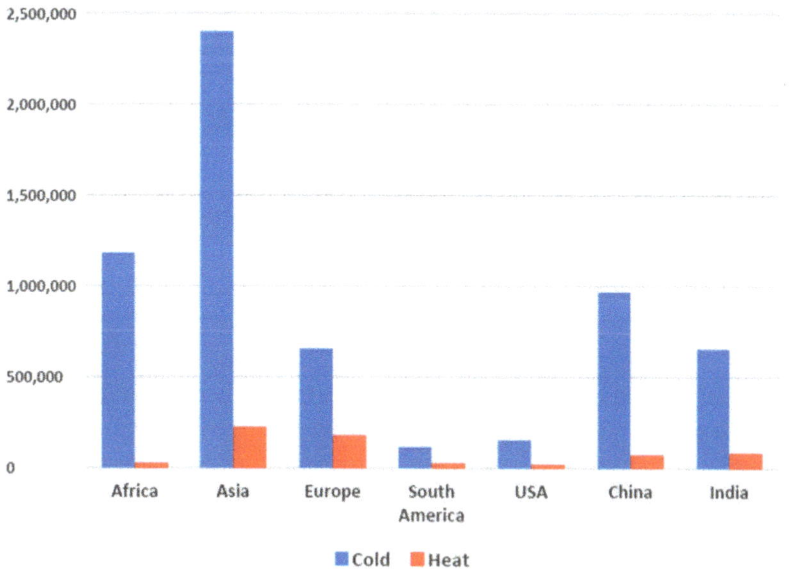

Source: Drawn by author from data in Qi Zhao, *et al.*, "Global, regional, and national burden of mortality associated with non-optimal ambient temperatures from 2000 to 2019: a three-stage modelling study," *Planetary Health* 5:7 (July 2021).

The Economist ran a story on 10 May that "expensive energy may have killed more Europeans [68,000] than Covid-19 last year." As with Covid, the brunt of climate action pain is borne by the poor and working class people. Speaking of Covid, as if damage from prolonged school closures and mask and vaccine mandates wasn't enough, 3,000 teachers in Oakland California went on strike recently demanding climate justice. Thanks to alarmist teaching in schools, more than half of British teenagers are convinced the world will probably end during their lifetime.

The limited impact of Australian and Canadian action on climate change

Climate action to lower the risks of bushfires can only be done globally. With between 1-1.4% of world CO2 emissions, Australia's and Canada's direct climate impact for good and bad is limited. The big four emitters are China, the US, India, and Russia, in that order, accounting for nearly 60% of global emissions (Figure 12.6).

Figure 12.6: Annual CO_2 emissions

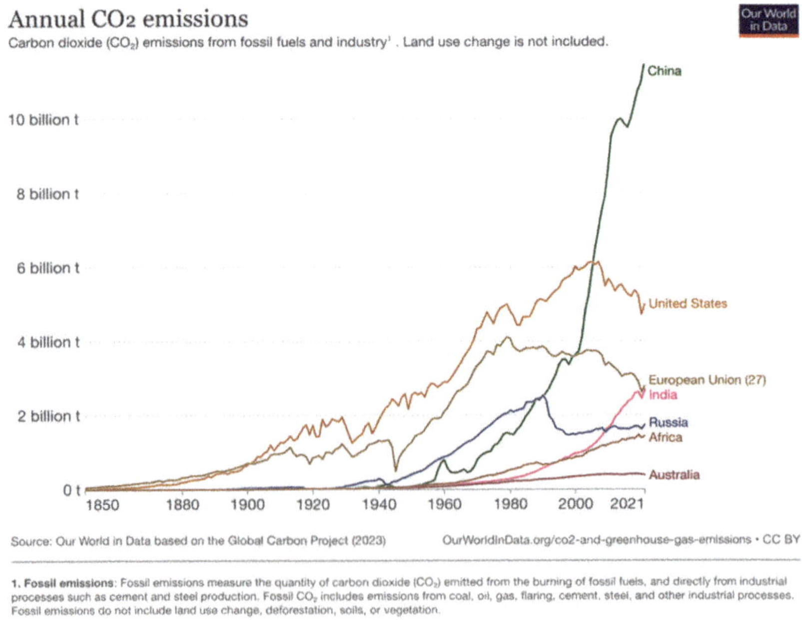

Advanced modern economies like Australia and the US have far better disaster preparedness infrastructure and skills and can limit the deadly toll more effectively than developing countries. Energy was a critical component of their industrialisation that today gives them such capacity.

Table 12.1: Changing share of annual CO_2 emissions, 1850–2021 (percent)

Country/Region	*1850*	*1900*	*1950*	*1985*	*2021*
Africa	0.0	0.1	1.6	3.3	3.9
China	0.0	0.0	1.3	9.8	30.9
EU-27	27.5	36.5	21.3	18.8	7.5
India	0.0	0.6	1.0	2.0	7.3
USA	10.0	33.9	42.3	22.9	13.5

Source: Our World in Data.

Figure 12.7: Energy use per capita

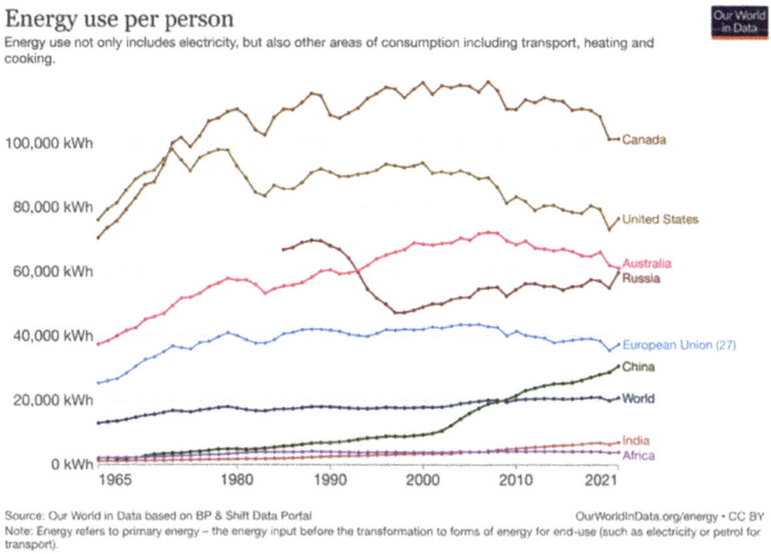

For developing countries, disaster preparedness requires transitioning to a modern economy, for which industrialisation is necessary. Industrialisation requires greater energy intensity to build high-quality dwelling, transportation, public health and education infrastructures. Figures 12.7 and 12.8 show the correlation between energy consumption and GDP growth. India's annual per capita energy consumption is only one-third the world average; Americans, Australians and

Canadians use between 9 to 15 times as much electricity per person. This explains the apparent paradox that the share of the industrial economies is significantly higher in the cumulative total of emissions even though China and India are among today's big emitters (Figure 12.9).

Figure 12.8: GDP, 1965–2020

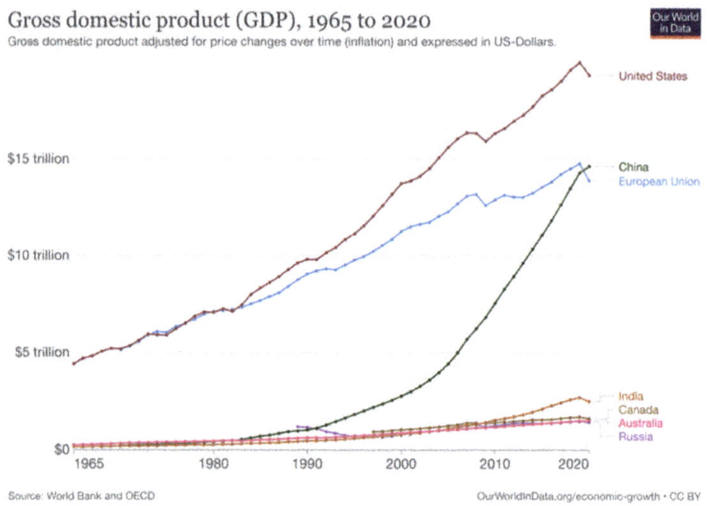

Figure 12.9: Annual CO_2 emissions by region

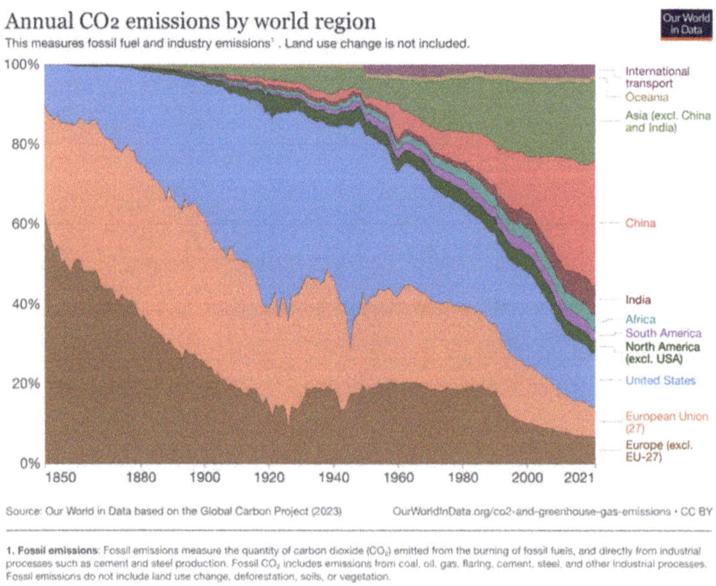

A country's growing intensity of energy use as it industrialises explains why cutbacks to the emission limits of developing countries require longer lead times and global climate agreements have reflected the different treatments of industrialised and developing countries. Such nuances are difficult to explain to a wider public not very interested in blame-shifting for historical and per capita emissions. They see that aggregate emissions from China and India are 34 and 7 times more than Australia's, respectively, and refuse to back tougher emission cuts by Australia.

The tide may be turning against climate alarmism

Fossil-fuelled based energy provided the power for the explosive lift-off of the masses from the subsistence lifestyle that had condemned them to nasty, brutish and short lives. Mimicking the surge in the growth of the democratisation of access to education, health and improving family finances with successive generations, China, India and other parts of the non-Western world have adopted, in accelerated overdrive if possible, the strategies of the industrial revolution to break free from their own misery-ridden lives.

We saw in the Covid era a restoration of the feudal world of class division between the Zooming laptop class and the working class deplorables. Part of that was the hypocrisy of the ruling class who brazenly flouted the very rules they imposed on everyone else, mingling merrily, *sans* masks, with partygoers from the world of financial, political and cultural privileges, even while the serving staff were compelled to wear masks as a condition of their employment.

Similarly, the Davos crowd fly in to their jamborees on private jets and are chauffeured around in gas guzzling limousines when they assemble annually to hector us deplorables to abandon our cars and flights. In May, a Briefing Paper from the World Economic Forum advocated for a 75% reduction of automobiles by 2050.

Against the weight of the folly of serially repeating historical evidence on picking winners, governments seem determined to coerce citizens out of reliance on existing cars into dependence on electric vehicles. Inevitably, because the market is unable to incentivise the switch to EVs, generous public subsidies have been offered. Who can be confident of the relative subsidies to Big Oil and Big Green, or the money flowing from them to fund climate denialism vs. climate alarmism?

EVs experienced a series of bad car days recently in the UK: their resale value has been dropping twice as fast as petrol cars; the number of free chargers dropped by nearly 40% because soaring energy costs made them uneconomic; and the one-third heavier battery weight means some bridges and upper storey parking lots, including in apartment complexes, could collapse under the strain of too many cars.

To cap it all, the brilliant comedic actor Rowan Atkinson of Blackadder, Mr. Bean and Johnny English fame, wrote in *The Guardian* on 3 June that he feels he was duped into buying electric. Unbeknownst to most of us, he has an electrical engineering degree and owns a fleet of cars. If we measure emissions at the end of the exhaust pipe, EVs are super. If, however, we look at the life cycle of cars, from all the components (for example, nickel) to the manufacturing process, the mix of fuels producing electricity, the impact of the heavier batteries and bigger tyres, and the waste disposal of all the bits and parts, then not so much. Keeping the petrol car for a few years more may be more climate friendly choice.

While the West is wedded to the fantasy Net Zero target and sin bins coal as a four-letter word, China's CO2 emissions increased by 4% in the first quarter of 2023 compared to last year. Meanwhile Britain fired up coal plants after recent heatwave made the solar panels too hot to work efficiently! Furthermore, as the fossil fuel share of energy generation falls, the claim that renewables can supply power on a reliable basis is being exposed as a myth. Consumers (including yours truly just this week) are getting notices of rapid power price surges to explode the related myth that renewables mean cheaper power. Many American communities are pushing back against the ballooning wind and solar projects scarring rural landscapes. Perhaps Fraser Nelson is right and the tide really is turning against climate alarmism as reality bites ordinary folks.

The Clintel group's World Climate Declaration, issued by several high profile scientists on 18 February and signed by 1,500 scientists by mid-June, insists that there is no climate emergency. It informs us that warming has natural as well as anthropogenic causes. The rate of increased warming is also slower than predicted by inaccurate climate models. It calls on scientists to be concerned more with science and less with politics to openly address uncertainties and exaggerations in predictions, while urging politicians to weigh costs against imagined benefits and prioritise adaptation strategies based on proven and affordable technologies.

This sure doesn't sound radical and conspiratorial. But it may prove a step too far for Net Zero politicians who were recently condemned by Alexandra Marshall in the *Spectator Australia* as "liars, scoundrels and morons." Asides from that, of course, they are likely to be among the nicest people you will ever meet.

Postscript

An article published in the *Journal of Hydrology* in May 2023 found that "small- and medium-size precipitation systems both exhibit *significant decreases* during 2001–2020 …. The large-size precipitation systems exhibit nonsignificant increasing trends during 2001–2020" (emphasis added). This adds to the finding of an earlier study covering a longer timeframe, published in *Hydrology and Earth System Sciences* in 2020, that owing to "the intensification of disaster reporting, people think that rainfall events have become more intense or frequent recently. However, … the fact is that the highest frequency of record rainfall events occurred in the period 1960–1980; later the frequency was decreased remarkably." Demetris Koutsoyiannis concludes: "None of the figures in none of the continents and none of the sources of data provides support on the intensification allegation." Instead, "the observational data … could support the opposite hypothesis, namely that of extreme rainfall deintensification."

Net zero lawfare[81]

Ah, the progress achieved by social justice progressives. Mass immigration: the devaluation of Western civilisation, delegitimisation of Western culture, demoralisation of white males, sexual assault of white females and retribalisation of once cohesive nations. Gender affirmation: the abandonment of girls and women's safety, dignity and equality in toilets, changerooms, prisons and sports. Net zero: the deindustrialisation of the West and the impoverishment of its people. The fanatic pursuit of renewables—more accurately described as unreliables—has led to environmental vandalism of the iconic Kosciuszko National Park by the Snowy 2.0 pumped storage project, while in the UK families' property rights can be overridden by for profit-renewable developers in the push for increased solar power generation.

On 21 June, I commented on how international organisations are taking over an increasing range of functions from the governments of states, posing threat both to national sovereignty and to democracy with national bureaucrats working in tandem with international technocrats—the lanyard class—to overrule citizens' choices. This followed a previous article six months ago warning about the threat posed by judicial overreach as unelected and unaccountable judges displace elected governments as the real rulers. Little did I know how soon both theses would be validated by a curious ruling (not a formal judgment) from the International Court of Justice (ICJ).

Over the past two decades, climate activists have essentially adopted a smug 'we've won' tone on a three-part 'scientific consensus'

---

[81] *Spectator Australia*, 9 August 2025, https://www.spectator.com.au/2025/08/net-zero-lawfare/

on adverse impacts of rising CO2, human activity being primarily responsible for the rise in emissions and the imminence of climate catastrophe without urgent drastic action. All three parts have come under attack in recent times. Many serious scientists have always been sceptical of the 'science is settled' claim on the unique rise in harmful emissions caused by the fossil-fuel-driven industrial revolution. More and more have begun to speak out on the growing panic over a climate emergency. Their response to climate catastrophisation can be summarised succinctly as 'Rubbish!', albeit expressed in more polite and scientifically neutral language. The doom merchants have a three-decade-long catastrophic record on predictions of catastrophes. The World Climate Declaration issued two years ago has been signed by 2,000 experts from 60 countries, including over 160 Australians. In the meantime there has been public awakening and rising resentment and firming opposition to the questionable assumptions, significant harms and outright futility of climate targets encapsulated in the slogan 'net zero'—in an age when slogans are mistaken for sound and fully costed policy. Consequently many Western governments have begun to backtrack, none more so than the Trump administration that also recognises the strategic folly of climate polices that have demonstrably failed to end global reliance on fossil fuels, added to energy costs while making supply increasingly less reliable, and transferred wealth and industrial might to China.

Faced with growing expressions of scientific doubt, public backlash and policy reversals, climate activists have switched from trying to persuade governments to weaponising the courts to force compliance with their agenda. Article 92 of the United Nations Charter describes the ICJ as the UN's 'principal judicial organ' and all member states are automatically parties to the ICJ. Chapter IV of its Statute, which is annexed to the UN Charter, deals with advisory opinions. Article 96 of the Charter stipulates that the General Assembly may request the ICJ 'to give an advisory opinion on any legal question' or authorise another UN body to seek one.

In September 2021, inspired by the youth group Pacific Island Students Fighting Climate Change, Vanuatu launched a campaign for an advisory opinion. On 29 March 2023, the UN General Assembly requested an advisory opinion from the ICJ on the legal obligations and liability of states on climate change. On 23 July, the court published its advisory opinion. Relying primarily on IPCC reports which 'constitute the best available science on the causes, nature and consequences of climate change' and on the widespread acknowledgment of the adverse effects of climate change across the UN system, the court concluded that climate change is 'an urgent and existential threat'. The court justified its conclusion on states' commitments to both environmental (Kyoto Protocol, Paris agreement, UN Framework Convention on Climate Change) and human rights treaties: the 'adverse effects of climate change' such as rising sea levels, drought, desertification and natural disasters, 'may significantly impair the enjoyment of certain human rights', including 'the right to health'. Applying a stringent standard of due diligence, the court held that a state does incur legal responsibility if it 'fails to take all measures which were within its power to prevent the significant harm'. The 'obligation to prevent significant harm to the climate system and other parts of the environment… *applies to all States, including those that are not parties to one or more of the climate change treaties*' (my emphasis). Thus in the 15 judges' unanimous opinion, climate obligations are legal, substantive and enforceable, not just aspirational. Previously vague obligations have been elevated to binding duties under customary international law to prevent significant environmental harm and cooperate internationally to uphold fundamental human rights in the face of escalating climate risks. Failure to do so leaves a country exposed to claims for restitution from those who have been harmed.

Ironically, such an opinion from the ICJ is itself not binding but merely advisory. However, it will shape climate governance around the world in myriad ways in the years to come in academia, courts, bureaucracies and civil society. Vanuatu's special envoy on climate change, Ralph Regenvanu, believes that the ICJ opinion will shift discussions from one of 'voluntary commitments' to reduce emissions, to one about binding obligations under international law. It will embolden activist courts and judges around the world who are committed to the climate crusade. The logic underpinning the advisory prepares the ground for individual liability, speech restrictions and legal intimidation. The opinion comes across more like an activist manifesto than a sober judicial pronouncement.

All governments engage in policy trade-offs involving economic goals, development assistance and energy security that triangulate emissions, affordability and reliability. Who exactly will enforce this opinionated reasoning on the geopolitical heavyweights like China, Russia and America? On 29 July the US Department of Energy issued a report that rejects the core tenets of climate alarmism, notes that US policies will 'have undetectably small direct impacts on the global climate', and insists that the dominant energy systems deserve to be celebrated for their role in 'the rise of human flourishing over the past two centuries'. Accordingly, the US is set to revoke many restrictive climate regulations in the push for continued global energy dominance. The previously smug mainstream media has reacted with fury. A *New York Times* article on 31 July quoted climate scientists who attacked the report for using 'cherry-picked' data to support a 'scattershot collection of oft-debunked skeptic claims' in 'a coordinated, full-scale attack on the science'.

To have attracted such flak, the DOE report must be over the target.

13: STATE POWER AND COVID CRIMES

The Covid years witnessed the biggest expansion of state power in the history of Western democracies, accompanied by the most serious curtailment of civil liberties, political freedoms and individual rights. In the process, people and commentators overlooked two abiding verities. Once governments have acquired more powers, they rarely surrender it back to the people voluntarily. And any new power that can be abused, will be abused, if not today by current agents of state, then sometime in the indeterminate future by their successors.

Lockdowns and masks[82]

The three major controversies over pandemic management for the past three years have been lockdown measures, universal masking recommendations and mandates, and Covid vaccines.

The last was a pharmaceutical intervention using revolutionary new technology. The first two were radical departures from the existing scientific and policy consensus as encapsulated in official documents from the World Health Organisation (WHO) and in several national pandemic preparedness plans. They established the willingness of the state to dictate every aspect of people's lives, down to the most ridiculous and absurd details.

[82] Brownstone Institute, 2 January 2023, https://brownstone.org/articles/state-power-and-covid-crimes-part-1/

For example, people were told when they could shop, the hours during which they could shop, what they could purchase, how close they could get to others, and which direction they could move in by following arrows on the floor. Governments also stepped into nation' bedrooms at home to dictate with whom people could and could not be intimate: a ukase that notoriously turned Professor Neil "Lockdown" Ferguson himself into Professor Pantsdown.

Lockdowns thus proved the extent to which people would comply with state directives without deploying independent critical thinking and, like frogs in boiling water, their almost total lack of concern about the gradually increasing degree of infringements of civil liberties and personal freedoms.

Compliance with often idiotic rules was ratcheted up to another level still with mask recommendations-cum-mandates, with one additional notable feature. Governments were able to mobilise members of the public to exert peer pressure and societal coercion to enforce compliance, backed by often brutal police coercion against pockets of resistance and protest.

In retrospect, it's doubtful if the degree of state and social coercion deployed to increase vaccine uptake would have been possible without the ground having first been prepared with lockdowns and masks.

Lockdowns

Lockdowns were a euphemism for a wholesale shutting down of all social and most economic activities and locking up entire populations under de facto house arrest. They were imposed on and off for two years with the goalposts of justification shifting from flatten the curve in 2-3 weeks to protect the health system, wait for the vaccine and stop the new variant.

They were based neither on good science and best-practice medicine, nor were they commensurate with the age-stratified threat from the novel coronavirus to individual and public health. By contrast the health, mental health, social, educational and economic harms caused by the lockdowns have locked in generational poverty and inequality within and among states.

The Neil Ferguson-led Imperial College London models of Covid mortality that panicked governments into unprecedented extreme countermeasures turned out to be several factor fold higher than empirical outcomes. A peer-reviewed study published in the *European Journal of Clinical Investigation* by Eran Bendavid, Christine Oh, Jay Bhattacharya and John Ioannidis in January 2021 failed to find "clear, significant beneficial effect" of stringent lockdowns "on case growth in any country."

That remains the case to this day either when looking at countries or at US states.

Early data—from China, Italy, Spain, the *Diamond Princess* cruise ship—told us in February–March 2020 already that the most vulnerable were elderly people with existing serious health conditions. All the data since then has been entirely consistent with this and it was also underlined in the Great Barrington Declaration in October 2020: "We know that vulnerability to death from Covid-19 is more than a thousand-fold higher in the old and infirm than the young. Indeed, for children, Covid-19 is less dangerous than many other harms, including influenza."

On 16 November, *The Guardian* reported that Europe faces a "cancer epidemic" because one million cancer diagnoses were missed because of lockdowns. In the UK, which experienced the highest proportion of lack of access to healthcare in Europe during the pandemic, there were almost 9,000 excess cancer deaths by mid-November 2022 since the start of the pandemic. Meanwhile Sweden, the object of much abusive analysis in the MSM in most of 2020, was fully vindicated in 2022 with one of the lowest all-cause mortality rates—the metric most resistant to being gamed to fit a narrative bias—in Europe.

Masks

Once lockdowns were firmly in place as public policy, the next previously discredited and discarded nonpharmaceutical intervention to come on the policy agenda was facemasks for the general population in indoor and outdoor community settings. A 14-year-old British student named Jack Watson was able to spot the many inconsistencies, contradictions and absurdities of lockdown and mask restrictions for schoolchildren. A 1920 study of mask-wearing during the Spanish flu concluded that it had not shown sufficient effectiveness to "warrant compulsory application for the checking of epidemics."

It's worth quoting in full paragraph 4.15 from the *UK Influenza Preparedness Strategy 2011* that succinctly encapsulated the scientific and policy consensus:

> *Although there is a perception that the wearing of facemasks by the public in the community and household setting may be beneficial, there is in fact very little evidence of widespread benefit from their use in this setting. Facemasks must be worn correctly, changed frequently, removed properly, disposed of safely and used in combination with good respiratory, hand, and home hygiene behaviour in order for them to achieve the intended benefit. Research also shows that compliance with these recommended behaviours when wearing facemasks for prolonged periods reduces over time.*

This conclusion was reaffirmed in the WHO report published in September 2019 that summarised the best available studies to date: "Ten RCTs were included in the meta-analysis, and there was no evidence that face masks are effective in reducing transmission of laboratory-confirmed influenza" (p. 26).

An Australian Department of Health document in July 2020 advised that facemasks are most likely to be effective for source control when worn by an infected person, if worn correctly and consistently (no touching the front of the mask, no pulling it down intermittently—both extremely common real-world behaviour!), but less effective in protecting uninfected people.

Facemasks is the issue on which my trust in the US Centers for Disease Control and Prevention (CDC), which exercises an outsized influence globally, was broken irreparably. The CDC tweeted that during the March–July 2020 period, "universal mask use helped reduce Covid-19 cases, hospitalisations, and deaths" in Delaware. It was telling the truth, but not the whole truth.

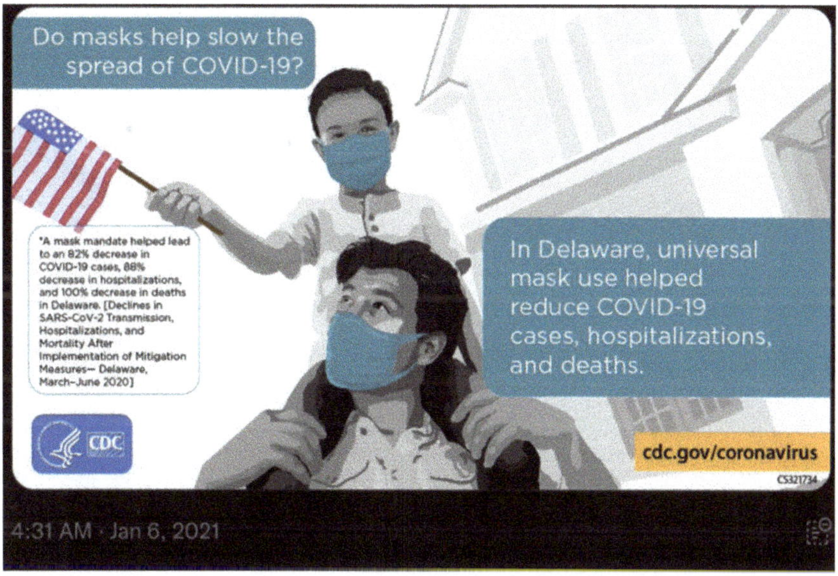

The mandate was introduced on 28 April when Delaware had 235 cases (7-day moving average). On 30 June cases had indeed fallen to 89. But they began to climb again in autumn and on 12 December Delaware had 826 cases: nearly four times as many as when the masks were brought in (Figure 13.1). Fair enough, you might say, like many others the CDC failed to anticipate the seasonal surge. Except the tweet was sent out on 6 January 2021. This is not a well-intentioned mistake overtaken by events but deliberate dishonesty.

Figure 13.1: The CDC's false claims on Delaware's mask mandate success, 6 January 2021

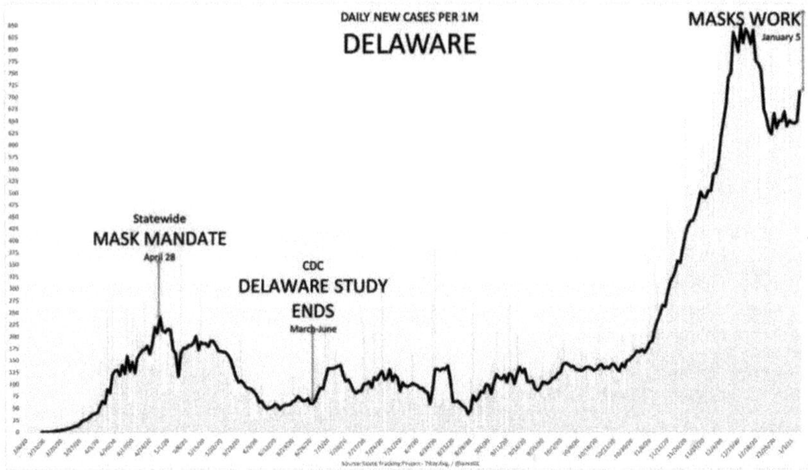

Anthony Fauci too shed credibility with his notorious and numerous flip-flops on masks. His attempts to claim the noble lie as his primary motivation for the changing stance, saying he was trying to prioritise masks for healthcare workers and prevent a public run on them, only deepened perceptions of shiftiness.

Firstly because in fact his initial scepticism accurately reflected the existing consensus and secondly because he was repeating the same argument in a private email to a friend as well. Missouri Attorney General Eric Schmitt tweeted after Fauci was deposed in November that the good "America's doctor" was not able to cite a single study to support his pro-mask health advice. Incidentally, during the deposition Fauci responded to questions with "I don't recall" an astonishing 174 times. A likely explanation for his convenient amnesia is he knows that the truth is not his ally.

Masks dehumanise us and are a potent force for stoking mass fear. In December, a hundred doctors, paediatricians, clinical psychologists and academics wrote an open letter to the UK Government warning that requiring masks in schools breached WHO guidelines and were creating a "climate of fear." Masks should "play no part in the life of healthy children," they said. In autumn 2021, Scotland introduced mask mandates for schools but England did not, yet weekly cases in both showed broadly similar infection curves.

One of the most valuable sets of observational data is the brilliant series of comparative charts produced by Ian Miller in *Unmasked: The Global Failure of Covid Mask Mandates* (2022). The most significant result of the community-wide mask recommendations was twofold: the highly and instantly visible prop perpetuated and locked in the reign of fear and it demonstrated broad compliance with the effort of governments to exercise population-wide social control.

Vaccines[83]

The real-world effectiveness of Covid vaccines has not matched the hype of the 95% efficacy claimed in manufacturer trials on the basis of which they were granted emergency-use authorisation. They've proven disappointingly leaky with a surprisingly swift waning of effectiveness, necessitating boosters every few months.

In many cases vaccine rollouts coincided with an upsurge in infections, substantiating the concerns expressed by many experts that a mass vaccination campaign in the middle of a pandemic will drive the evolution of vaccine-escape variants and generate self-perpetuating waves of infections from the mutating variants.

A study from Oxford University in June showed the infection risk increased by 44% in the double-vaccinated in England. An analysis in July by El Gato Malo showed that US states with higher vaccination rates were experiencing higher Covid hospital admissions. By the end of 2022 the vast majority of Covid deaths in many countries were among the vaccinated and boosted.

[83] Brownstone Institute, 3 January 2023, https://brownstone.org/articles/state-power-and-covid-crimes-part-2/

This has discredited officials and health experts from President Joe Biden on down who claimed that the vaccines would prevent infection, onward transmission, severe illness and (initially)/or (as a fallback justification) death. Hence their early but by now abandoned claims about the pandemic of the unvaccinated.

By contrast, by the end of 2022 stories, like the video documentary Anecdotals, which simply give voice to the vaccine-injured, and studies alleging a wide range of serious side effects and injuries from the vaccines were challenging the official narrative of the vaccines being safe and effective.

Neither safe nor effective was the growing chorus instead. On 25 November 2022 the physician-scientist Dr Masanori Fukushima from Kyoto University warned that "the harm caused by vaccines is now a worldwide problem" and that "given the wide range of adverse events, billions of lives could ultimately be in danger."

There is nothing objectionable in principle to harnessing revolutionary new mRNA technology to improve public health. Major medical advances in the past have been made possible by technological breakthroughs. But a revolutionary technology increases the testing burden for ensuring safety, even while a raging pandemic heightens the urgency of accelerated vaccine development and manufacture. If granted emergency use authorisation to cater to the second demand, prudence strengthens the imperative to rigorous monitoring of short, medium and long-term side effects in numbers and severity.

This is where authorities have fallen short and caused significant long-term damage to public confidence in the major institutions. Attempting to force-vaccinate the whole world with a new and untested technology was the height of irresponsibility and ignoring the mounting evidence of serious adverse events amounts to criminal negligence.

The best, if not the only true measure of the whole of society impact of an epidemic or pandemic is excess mortality. Norman

Fenton and Martin Neil subjected worldwide excess mortality data to linear regression models and found no significant link between excess deaths in 2022 and (a) Covid cases in 2020, (b) long Covid, (c) lockdown stringency, or (d) healthcare quality. But they did find "a statistically significant linear relationship between countries that are highly vaccinated and excess deaths." Elliot Middleton calculates that in 2020, Covid deaths (meaning not all were *from* Covid) accounted for 42% of all excess deaths in the US.

Remember, this is before the announcement of a vaccine breakthrough and therefore the excess mortality toll is not affected by the count of vaccine-injured. Thus, although Covid deaths comprised a substantial portion of the total toll, the lockdown component was still higher—and policymakers should have known this at the time in 2020 itself but chose to ignore it despite multiple warnings from credible sources.

Ziva Kunda's influential 1990 article "The Case for Motivated Reasoning" has nearly ten thousand citations. Her thesis was that motivation shapes reasoning. Reliance on a biased set of cognitive processes means that people are more likely to arrive at conclusions they want to arrive at, by using the strategies for accessing, constructing and evaluating tools and data that are the most likely to yield the conclusions they desire. Very hot [cold/dry/wet] this year? Climate science tells us it's because of climate change and therefore the current weather conditions validate the science. Infected by Covid after the sixth jab? Be grateful for the six doses as otherwise you would most likely have died.

As the saying goes, you cannot reason people out of beliefs that they arrived at without the use of reason.

In December, a new "hindcasting" paper from the Commonwealth Fund made claims for vaccine success that were simply too inflated even to be plausible: 3.3mn lives, 18.6mn hospitalisations and 120mn infections averted just in the US alone in 2021–22! It was picked up and reported by the MSM. Unsurprisingly, the conclusions are derived from "a model pretending to be data" that cannot be replicated. It's an internal self-referential circular argument in which the conclusions are contained in the assumptions whose details are not made public.

The authors hold that "The reported "mild" nature of Omicron is in large part because of vaccine protection." Without vaccines, they estimate that Omicron's infection fatality rate (IFR) would have been 2.7 times higher than for the original variant.

Alex Berenson writes this is: "The dumbest, most dishonest argument for Covid jabs thus far, long after pretty much universal agreement that vaccines stop neither infection nor transmission but are, at best, modestly effective for a short transient period." According to Our World in Data, Omicron has killed around 450,000 people worldwide (including the US) in the 8-month April–November 2022 period inclusive, despite the majority of the world's people being unvaccinated. Collating the empirical outcomes from Our World in Data and Worldometers, at the end of the year, Africa's double-vaccinated were 27.5% of the population, compared to 69% in the US and 66.9% in Europe. Their respective cumulative Covid deaths per million people (DPM) were <0.01, 1.00 and 0.71. Only 4 of 47 European countries have DPM below 1,000. By contrast, only 6 of 58 countries in Africa have DPM *above* 1,000, and of these six, five have higher vaccination rates than the African average.

Yet, we are expected to believe that somehow, the vaccines miraculously saved one million Americans in that 6-month timeframe.

Away from the tautological conclusions of models, there is little reliable data to show clinical benefits of Covid vaccines in preventing hospitalisation and death and much evidence to the contrary.

Japan is among the latest countries to offer evidence of the "immunity debt" phenomenon (Figure 13.2). Japan is a country where owing to congested conditions, and perhaps out of concern for the elderly in one of the world's oldest societies (over 65s make up almost a third of the population), mask-wearing has long been a common cultural feature in the November–February winter months.

This was done whenever someone had the sniffles, or else feared catching the cold. It was a sign of consideration for others. Compliance therefore is not an issue for the government and by all accounts, since the pandemic facemasks have become a ubiquitous feature of public life in Japan.

Figure 13.2: Japan's immunity debt comes due

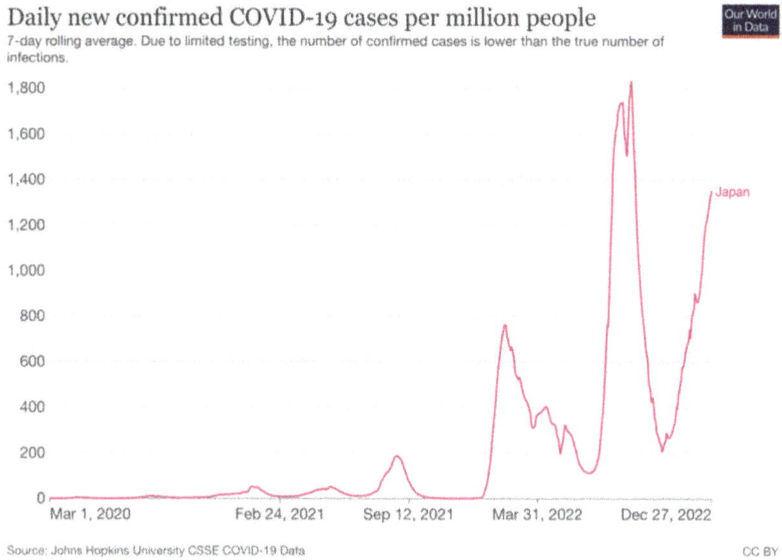

Vaccine requirements were slower to be introduced there but they seem to be making up for lost time. I am due to travel to Japan later this month and one of the entry requirements is three doses of the vaccine or else a PCR test within 72 hours of departure. In 2020 Japan was heavily criticised for tardiness in not taking the novel virus seriously enough to impose restrictions.

Figure 13.3: Covid deaths/mn people in Japan and Denmark, June–December 2022

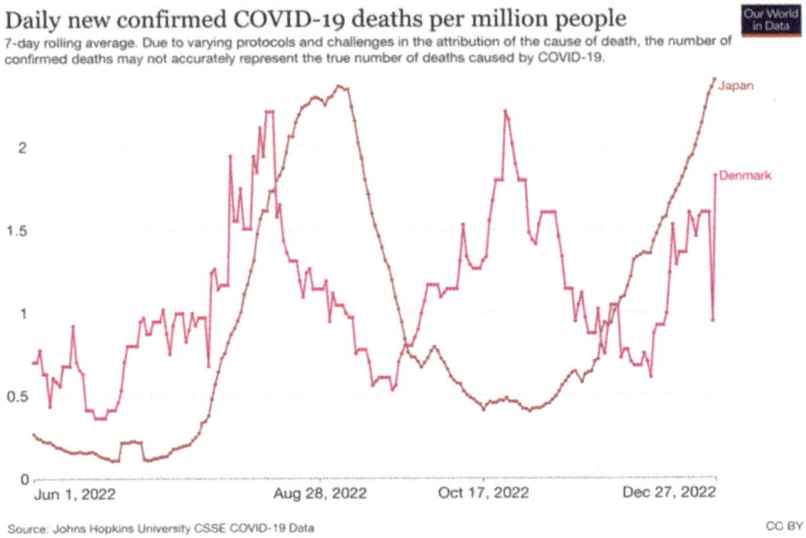

In an article for *The Japan Times* in January 2021, I pointed out that given their relative performances, instead of attacking Japan, the most locked down countries should envy its results. Ironically, with heavier restrictions and vaccine mandates, Japan's Covid metrics have deteriorated substantially. Figure 13.3 compares it to Denmark where, it will be recalled, authorities dropped vaccine recommendations for under-18s from 1 July and for under-50s from 1 November. Sweden and Norway swiftly followed suit.

Will the penny drop in Japan, where their own data shows they did hugely better before going down the route of heavier restrictions and higher vaccine coverage? That perhaps, just possibly, pharmaceutical and nonpharmaceutical interventions might be driving sustained waves of the virus? Don't hold your breath. Japan's ability to look reality firmly in the eye, turn around, and walk resolutely in the opposite direction is no less impressive than in the Western democracies.

Japan isn't alone. The graphic illustration of the ineffectiveness of Covid vaccines in preventing the infection and mortality tolls can be shown with several countries. All these charts (Figures 13.2–13.9) prove the pointlessness of vaccine certificates. In Japan, the total number of Covid deaths until 80% of the population was vaccinated on 9 December 2021 was 18,370. In little over one year since then, the death toll has climbed by another 37,858. That is, more than twice as many have died with Covid in the twelve months since 80% of people were fully vaccinated than in the 19 months until then.

Figure 13.4: Vaccination coverage in Australia, Israel, Japan and USA

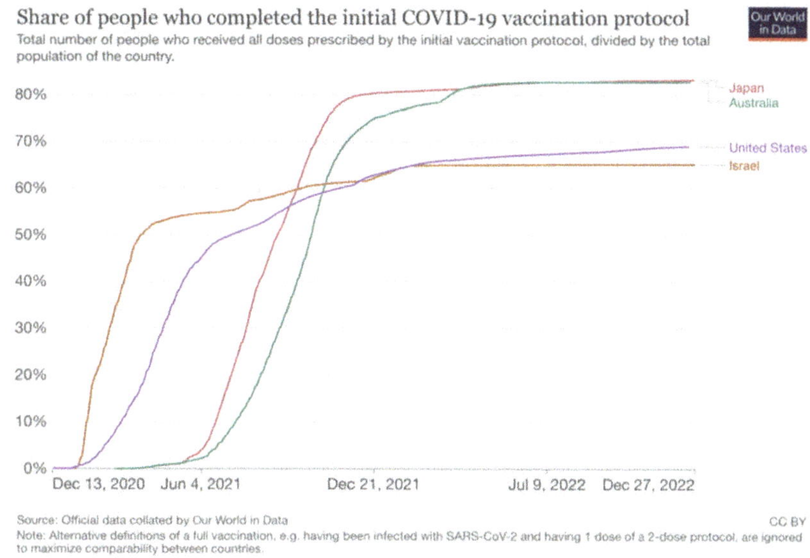

Israel's vaccination drive hit 50% of the population on 28 March 2021, on which date its Covid death toll was 6,185. Another 5,838 Israelis had died with Covid by 28 December 2022, meaning nearly half the total Covid dead came after half the population was fully vaccinated. Israel and Palestine are one example of different vaccination rates among adjacent communities (Israelis high, Palestinians low) having little impact on their death rates.

In the US too the 516,000 Covid deaths after reaching 50% double-vaccination coverage on 9 July 2021 represents 46% of all Covid deaths until 28 December 2022. Australia hit the 50% vaccination threshold on 11 October 2021, with the Covid death total being 1,461 on that date. The mortality toll was 16,964 on 28 December 2022. Thus more than times as many Australians died with Covid in the 14 months since 50% were double-vaccinated as in 19 months until then. For what it's worth, New Zealand's experience has been even worse. Its Covid death toll as at 28 December was 2,331, 78 times higher than 30 at 50% vaccination mark, and 57 times higher than 41 at 70% vaccination.

How anyone can look at the Covid vaccination and mortality metrics of New Zealand, Australia, and Japan and still hold fast to the "safe and effective" vaccine narrative is beyond comprehension. Instead, one more initially plausible hypothesis is that the behaviour of the Covid virus is vaccine-invariant, and a second hypothesis is that the vaccine may actually be driving infections, serious illness and deaths by some mysterious mechanism not yet identified by scientists—although some studies are starting to point the way.

Earlier, Gibraltar, Cambodia, (Figure 13.5) and the Seychelles were examples of countries where Covid infections spiked in 2021 despite substantial vaccination in their populations.

Figure 13.5: Cambodia's Covid vaccination coverage and cases/mn people

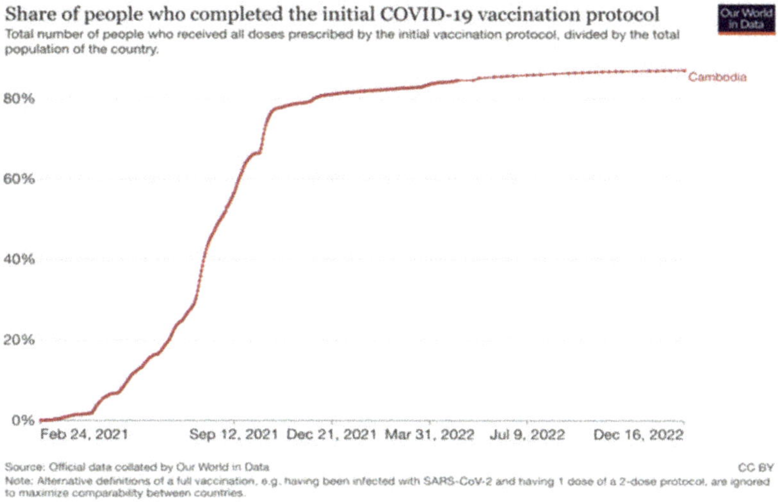

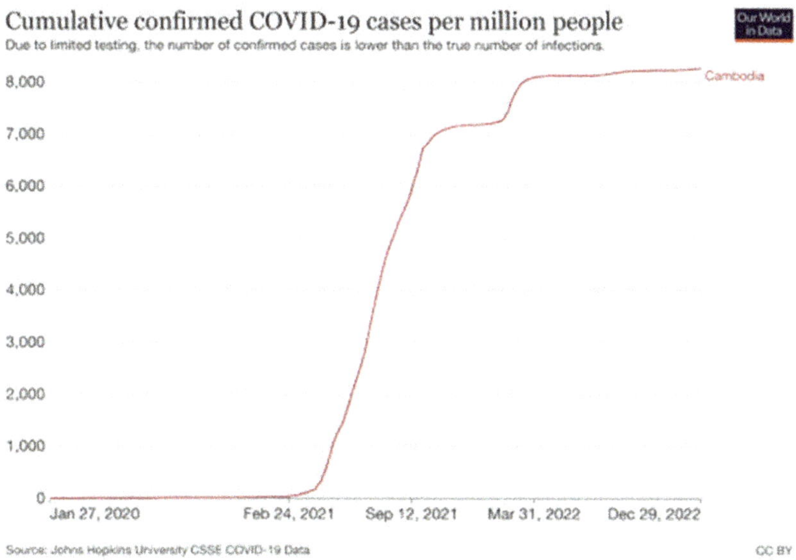

Figure 13.6: Covid deaths in Australia, Japan and Israel

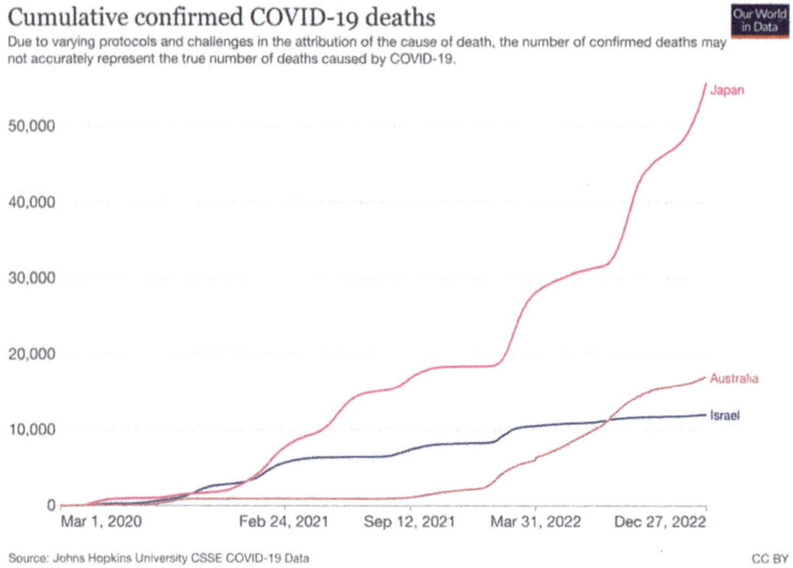

Figure 13.7: Covid deaths in USA

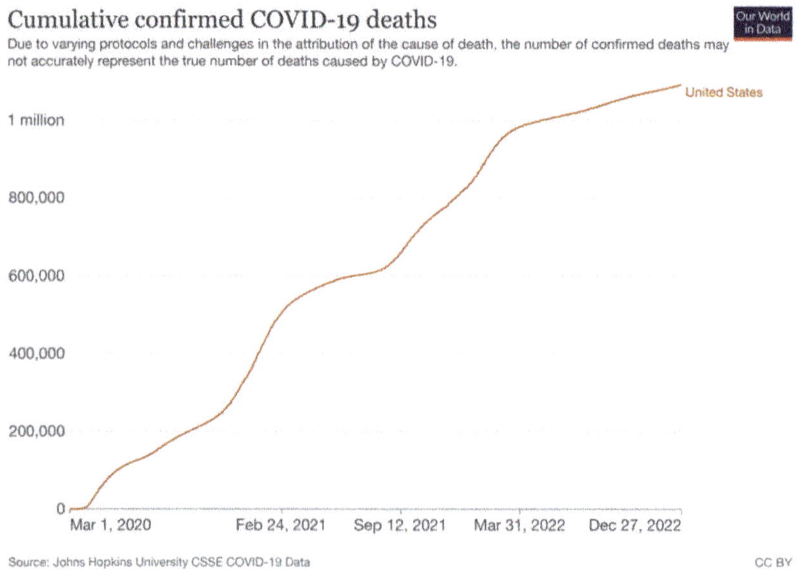

The weekly surveillance report from New South Wales (NSW) Health for the weeks of 18–31 December, published on 5 January, was the last one for the year. The next one will be published on 12 January but the reports covering the 52 weeks for 2023 will no longer include the vaccination status of people hospitalised, admitted to ICU or dead with Covid.

Until the week ending 21 May 2022, the reports lumped together the unvaccinated with those whose vaccination status was not known. Figures 13.8–13.9 therefore represent the entire data set for NSW Covid-related hospital and ICU admissions and deaths, from 22 May to 31 December 2022 inclusive, for which these statistics are available by vaccination status. It's worth noting that 83% of the state's total population was at least double-vaccinated, which accounted for 75.7% of Covid-related hospital admissions (slightly underrepresented) and 83.2% of deaths (almost exactly the same as population share).

Figure 13.8: NSW Covid metrics by vaccination status, 22 May–17 December 2022

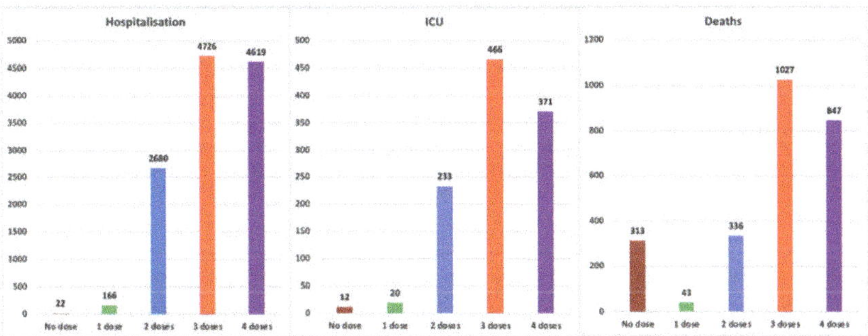

Source: NSW Health, *Weekly Surveillance Reports*.

Figure 13.9: NSW weekly Covid-related deaths by vaccination status, 22 May–17 December 2022

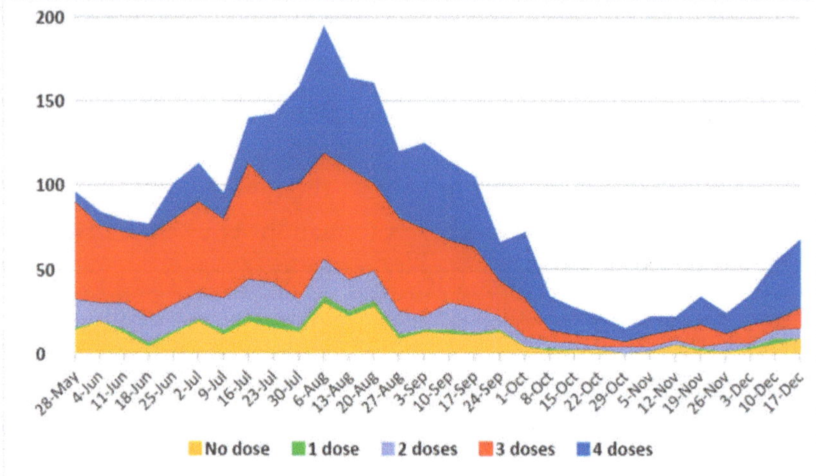

According to the federal Department of Health, by year's end 96.0% of Australian adults (16+) were double-vaccinated, 72.4% had received at least three doses and 44.2% four doses. For NSW the corresponding figures were 95.8, 70.5 and 45.6%. With all due respect (or not) to the Australian health bureaucrats, it is impossible to spin Figures 13.8 and 13.9 as graphic evidence for the vaccines being effective.

A study out in December 2022 in preprint of employees of the Cleveland Clinic in Ohio from 12 September to 12 December found that effectiveness of the new bivalent Covid vaccine—authorised by the FDA on the basis of trial results from eight mice—was only 30%. The real shock was discovering that infection rates increase incrementally with each successive dose of a Covid vaccine.

The infection rates among those vaccinated with three or more doses was three times higher than among the unvaccinated. The authors said: "The association of increased risk of Covid-19 with higher numbers of prior vaccine doses in our study, was unexpected." Prior infection is relatively more effective against reinfection.

Benefits-Harms analysis[84]

Last June, a paper by a team that included the *British Medical Journal* editor Peter Doshi concluded that data from the Pfizer and Moderna trials indicated their vaccines are more likely to put people in hospital from adverse effects than keep them out by protecting against Covid, by 2.4 and 6.4 people per 10,000, respectively. They concluded: "The excess risk of serious adverse events found in our study points to the need for formal harm-benefit analyses, particularly those that are stratified according to risk of serious Covid-19 outcomes such as hospitalization or death."

Another peer-reviewed study, published in the *BMJ Journal of Medical Ethics* on 5 December, looked at the net benefit-harm ratio of a third vaccine for 18–29 year olds (that is, university students). According to its findings, for every one Covid hospitalisation prevented in this group by an mRNA booster shot over a six-month period, 18.5 serious adverse events would occur, including 1.5-4.6 booster-associated myopericarditis cases in males (typically requiring hospitalisation).

Because the net harm to healthy young adults is not outweighed by public health benefits "given modest and transient" vaccine effectiveness against transmission, "university booster mandates are unethical."

The existing standard metric in 2020 for allocating finite health resources was cost-benefit analysis using quality adjusted life years (QALY) for measuring health outcomes. Yet hardly any government seems to have performed such analyses or, if they did, bothered to publish them. As governments rarely shy away from promoting an analysis that supports their official line, it's a safe assumption that they

[84] Brownstone Institute, 4 January 2023, https://brownstone.org/articles/state-power-and-covid-crimes-part-3/

knew that the obsession with Covid health outcomes as the single measure of success was a gross distortion of public policy priorities.

It led many into the blind alley of an eradication strategy and Zero Covid policy—an ambition that even China has been compelled to abandon under the force of circumstances. The abandonment of QALY was necessary to reject the reality—let's call it data or evidence denialism—that the disease burden of Covid-19 had an extremely steep age gradient.

In an article in *Spectator Australia* on 24 October 2020, I wrote:

> *... the biggest tragedy will be across the developing world over the next decade, with over 100mn more people pushed into extreme poverty, tens of millions of additional dead from increased infant and maternal mortality, hunger and starvation with more poverty and disrupted crop production and food distribution networks, sharp cutbacks in immunisation and schooling, and destruction of the informal sectors of the economy in which daily wage earners earn a pitiful living. Most countries will also need to prepare for potential spikes in mental health problems and suicides from the fear generated by exaggerated alarmism as well as the loneliness, isolation, financial ruin and despair caused by the lockdowns.*

One of the most contagious but almost completely preventable serious viral diseases through timely childhood vaccination is measles. As a consequence of the serially prolonged shutdowns, around 33mn children missed out on either the first or the second dose of the vaccine compared to 2019.

This was the first fall in the number of measle vaccines given since 2014. According to an article in *The Lancet* in January 2022, 24 measles vaccination campaigns in 23 countries were postponed in 2020. This increased the risk of the disease for over 93mn people, mostly of course among poor people in poor countries. Nigeria,

India, Indonesia, Afghanistan, Pakistan, Ethiopia and Brazil were among the worst affected.

According to a report in *The Telegraph* (UK) on 27 December, measles is all set to be an imminent global threat next year, thanks both to the lockdown-induced disruptions to existing immunisation campaigns and to the rise in vaccine hesitancy spreading from scepticism about Covid vaccines to older established vaccines—another consequence that was also predicted.

Vaccine scepticism is showing up in public opinion polls in the US. A Rasmussen poll published on 7 December found 32% were not vaccinated, 7% had suffered a major side effect but a massive 57% were concerned about major side effects. People believed vaccines are effective at stopping infection by a 56-38 majority, which is quite a sizable cohort of doubters, especially among Republicans.

Michael Gunner, Chief Minister of Australia's Northern Territory, went into an anti-vaxxer meltdown on 22 November 2021: "If you're out there in any way, shape or form campaigning against the mandate, then you are absolutely anti-vax."

In other words, even though I warned that lockdowns would seriously damage existing critical immunisation efforts and coercion to improve Covid vaccine take-up would increase cross-vaccine hesitancy, I was an anti-vaxxer. Got it.

There are suspicions of possible spikes in miscarriages, stillbirths and neonatal deaths (from birth to 29 days) in Israel in 2021 that coincide with vaccines for pregnant women. Ditto a decline in Sweden's birth rate. Dr James Thorp, an obstetrician-gynaecologist who spoke at Senator Ron Johnson's Roundtable on Covid vaccines on 7 December 2022, said that he had observed "a substantial increase" in infertility, miscarriage, foetal death and foetal malformation since vaccination. Similar anecdotal claims of substantially elevated miscarriages following vaccination were made by Dr Luke McLindon in Brisbane, drawing on experience in his own fertility clinic.

However, the Royal Australian and New Zealand College of Obstetricians and Gynaecologists reiterated there was no evidence of negative impact on fertility or increased risk of miscarriage, stillbirth or other adverse pregnancy outcomes from the Covid vaccines and the risks arising from Covid infection were greater.

Yet, now even the *New York Times* is reporting that vaccines have a significant effect on menstrual cycles. But, being the *Times*, the report is slanted towards erratic cycles in "gender-diverse people." The two most revealing parts of the article are the highly critical comments from a swarm of angry readers, and this statement: "The increased transparency around menstrual changes or other side effects of vaccination could also have another benefit: reducing people's vaccine hesitancy."

Who knew?

Little wonder Florida Governor Ron DeSantis is seeking a grand jury investigation into "any and all wrongdoing" with respect to Covid vaccines. It could be a manoeuvre to pry loose more information from pharmaceutical companies about the vaccine' trial results and their potential side effects.

Empirical population-wide data—distinct from individual-level benefits for limited periods in the high-risk groups—have hinted for some time that multiple doses of Covid vaccines have fallen far short of expectations in real-world effectiveness. Far too many countries have shown a positive correlation between uptake of boosters and infections.

A recent peer-reviewed study in *Science Immunology* by a group of German scientists indicates that the third and subsequent doses of mRNA vaccines could be weakening the immune system, increasing the risk of infection and of prolonging and making the illness more serious. This could help to explain the rolling waves of infection in the highly vaccinated countries.

A familiar hypothetical moral dilemma poses the question: is it morally permissible to save one million lives by killing and harvesting the cells of one infant? By 17 December 2022, 19 children had died in the UK from Strep A disease: a doubly higher child death toll than from Covid (8) in 2020. Professor Susan Hopkins, chief medical adviser at the UK Health Security Agency, said the surge in scarlet fever caused by Strep A infection was three times higher than normal for the season and was creating panic among parents.

This was likely caused by the immunity debt resulting from not exposing preschool kids to circulating pathogens owing to lockdown-induced isolation from other children. Professor Carl Heneghan, director of Oxford University's Centre for Evidence-Based Medicine, commented: "At some point the immune deficit brought about by lockdowns has to be repaid."

In addition, by December 2022 around one quarter of British teenagers were suffering from mental health problems. The same phenomenon is the most likely explanation for the 25% rate of respiratory infection among German children.

Sweden, the lonely outlier as governments embraced toughening lockdowns in a panicked cascade from early 2020, has been the standout OECD performer over the past three years on most data sets on excess mortality.

A pity then that the Swedes did not award the Nobel Prize for medicine to one of their own, chief epidemiologist Anders Tegnell, as much for the courage of his scientific convictions in standing against the herd as for providing the world with the most instructive control group of all against the anti-scientific idiocy of lockdowns. Alternatively, the Norwegian committee could have awarded him the Peace Prize for the refusal to mandate massive human rights violations.

Insurance data from Germany showed an upsurge in sudden, unexpected deaths from 6,000 to 14,000 per quarter since the vaccines began to be administered on 27 December 2020. Meanwhile Australia's raw numbers put excess deaths at 16% compared to historical averages, according to official figures from the Australian Bureau of Statistics from 1 January to 30 September 2022. Of the 19,986 excess deaths, 8,160 were with Covid, meaning 59% of the excess deaths have non-Covid causes.

The Actuaries Institute, Australia's peak actuarial body, added its voice for an urgent investigation of the "incredibly high" 2022 excess death rate. In the US, CDC data show American' life expectancy had fallen from 78.8 years in 2019 to 76.4 in 2021. Since the average age of a Covid death is higher than the average life expectancy—81.5 according to one calculation—this suggests a significant rate of non-Covid mortality among younger cohorts.

An educated guess would point a finger of causation at lockdowns and vaccines as among the factors to be investigated.

Michael Tomlinson makes another interesting observation by looking at the big-picture "wood" of all-cause mortality over the last few years. The long-term curve shows "a trend of five declining peaks and progressively flattening curves, so the overall picture is one of gradual subsidence, which is only to be expected as immunity builds up." The post-vaccination mortality decline was almost identical with the pre-vaccination decline, again showing the interventions-invariant characteristic of the virus. His conclusion after looking at "the greatest surge in the research literature in living memory"?: "In the rearview mirror, the effect of government interventions on excess mortality should hit us in the face —but it doesn't."

Tipping points in vaccine narrative?

There are signs that some pivotal countries might be at tipping points in the dominant narrative of safe and effective vaccines. Eminent British cardiologist Aseem Malhotra, an early promoter of Covid vaccines, now describes this as "perhaps the greatest miscarriage of medical science we will witness in our lifetime."

The equation just doesn't compute for healthy non-elderly people when the numbers needed to vaccinate in order to prevent one death are weighed against the numbers who suffer serious adverse effects. In a two–part peer-reviewed article published in the *Journal of Insulin*

Resistance on 26 September, Malhotra concluded: "There is a strong scientific, ethical and moral case to be made that the current Covid vaccine administration must stop until all the raw data" has been released and "subjected to fully independent scrutiny." He called on the medical and public health professions to "recognise these failings and eschew the tainted dollar of the medical-industrial complex." On 12 December a group of British doctors joined him in calling for an official investigation of mRNA vaccines.

On 28 December Dr John Campbell, whose YouTube channel has 2.6mn subscribers, issued a call for a pause in the vaccination campaign "until a full, population scale risk/benefit analysis is carried out, and published for free and open peer review." He also called on the health authorities to review the intramuscular injection technique used in the delivery of mRNA vaccines, specifically, to check if aspiration was being carried out to ensure the tip of the syringe needle doesn't go into a blood vessel. As a sad comment on the madness gripping the world, he made the call on his Rumble channel rather than risk his lucrative YouTube account being suspended.

Andrew Bridgen MP delivered a comprehensive indictment of the vaccine narrative in the UK Parliament on 13 December. Referencing Malhotra, he noted that despite many criticisms, "there has so far not been a single rebuttal of Dr. Malhotra's findings in the scientific literature." He pointed to the nearly half-million yellow card reports of adverse effects, "more than all the yellow card reports of the past 40 years combined." As indeed has been the experience in the US. Yet in the past, he pointed out, vaccines had been "completely withdrawn from use for a much lower incidence of serious harm."

In Australia a similar tipping point came with the submission to a parliamentary inquiry from Dr Kerryn Phelps, a former president of the Australian Medical Association and a high profile former MP, about vaccine injuries suffered by her wife and, less seriously, herself. It was great to have someone of her stature and visibility state: "Regulators of the medical profession have censored public discussion about adverse events following immunisation, with threats to doctors not to make any public statements about anything that "might undermine the government's vaccine rollout" or risk suspension or loss of their registration."'

Phelps reiterated the old-fashioned consensus that the burden of proof has been shifted to the vaccine-injured "rather than the neutral scientific position of placing suspicion on the vaccine in the absence of any other cause and the temporal correlation with the administration of the vaccine."

Her elevated public persona means her "coming out" has given voice to countless others who have suffered vaccine injuries in silence and provides cover to others to speak publicly, thereby breaking what Dr Christopher Neil rightly calls "AHPRA's culture of fear," referring to the medical regulator the Australian Health Practitioner Regulation Agency. Neil, a cardiologist, himself lost his job in a Melbourne hospital for refusing the jab.

Australian doctors have also called on governments to stop silencing doctors, let them help their patients make decisions based on informed consent and conduct investigations into mRNA vaccines. In fact, in Victoria, 500 health professionals had come together in the Australian Covid Medical Network to sign an open letter back in October 2020 calling on the state government to end lockdowns.

Five techniques[85]

Already by early- and mid-2020, hard data should have rung alarm bells on the doomsday narrative being peddled by modelers like Neil Ferguson of Imperial College London of catastrophic mortality counts without lockdown.

---

[85] Brownstone Institute, 5 January 2023, https://brownstone.org/articles/state-power-and-covid-crimes-part-4/

Data were readily available from the *Diamond Princess* cruise ship (712 of 3,711 elderly people on board were infected and 14 died), Sweden, the *USS Theodore Roosevelt* (736 of the 4,085 young and fit sailors who disembarked tested positive, 6 were hospitalised and 1 died) and the *Charles de Gaulle* (60% of 1,767 crew members tested positive, 24 were admitted to hospital and two to ICU, with no reported deaths)

Why then did the so-called health and infectious diseases experts keep calling for lockdown? Noah Carl posits three answers: benefits were concentrated in elites (the laptop class) demanding lockdown while costs were widely dispersed; the benefits were immediate while the costs were downstream (delayed screenings and checks for treatable illnesses if detected early, immunity debt, cancelled childhood immunisation programs, out of control public debt, inflation, educational harms, etc); and benefits were more easily and immediately measurable than costs and harms.

Frightening and Terrifying the Populace

With help from the media, social media and police, people were frightened, shamed and coerced into submission and compliance with arbitrary and increasingly authoritarian government edicts. The intense and unrelenting propaganda unleashed on the people by governments using sophisticated tactics of psychological manipulation and enthusiastically amplified by the media was astonishingly successful in a remarkably short time.

In a six-nation poll of advanced industrial democracies (UK, USA, Germany, France, Sweden, Japan) published in mid-July 2020, people overestimated coronavirus cases by between 2 and 46 times the confirmed cases (11-22% of the population), and Covid-19 deaths by between 100 to 300 times confirmed deaths (3-9%). The compliance rate for wearing masks ranged between 47% in the UK and 73% to 84% in the US, France, Germany and Japan for indoor public spaces, and between 63% to 84% in public transport.

The outlier was Sweden, with 14% and 15% compliance in the two settings. Even though Sweden's Covid metrics are widely known by now not to be worse than those of the others, governments and public health authorities are still in denial on the ineffectiveness of wearing masks as an infection control measure.

Faced with a national medical emergency, implementing radical policies in blind panic is not as good as sending the reassuring message: "We've got it, no need to worry. She'll be right." Instead governments actively spread and amplified fear. Massaging people's opinions in order to ensure compliance with radical new measures became a more important task of government than managing the country calmly through the crisis.

In the 1950s, US psychologist Albert Biderman developed a coercion chart based on eight techniques to extract confessions from American POWs: isolation, monopolisation of perception, humiliation and degradation, exhaustion, threats, occasional indulgences, demonstrating omnipotence, and trivial demands.

All have been used to impose public health fascism ('Faucism" was a popular neologism) by the unethical weaponisation of fear. In *A State of Fear: how the UK government weaponised fear during the Covid-19 pandemic*, Laura Dodsworth comprehensively exposed how fear was brandished by behavioural scientists to control citizens.

The Orwellian-sounding Scientific Pandemic Insights Group on Behaviours (SPI-B) came up with the equivalent of "PsyOps" on citizens by such means as co-opting the media to increase the sense of personal threat "using hard-hitting emotional messaging" and promotion of "social disapproval."

Frederick Forsyth compared the covert tactics to frighten Britons into compliance with the tactics of the former Soviet Union and East Germany to scare East Berliners into supporting the Berlin Wall for keeping them safe against the menace from the West. Almost 50 psychologists and therapists asked the British Psychological Society to investigate " to promote compliance with a contentious and unprecedented public health strategy.

On 14 May 2021, *The Telegraph* published a report that scientists who had advised the UK government on how to ensure compliance with coronavirus policy directives by increasing public fear now admit their work was "unethical," "dystopian," and even "totalitarian." One member of SPI-B said they were "stunned by the weaponisation of behavioural psychology" and "psychologists didn't seem to notice when it stopped being altruistic and became manipulative."

Yet, UK media regulator Ofcom said nothing about state brandishment of fear using taxpayer-funded propaganda. Instead on 23 March 2020 it issued a directive that any report on Covid with content that "may be harmful" would face statutory sanctions. Accuracy of criticisms was no defence. On 27 March it warned against broadcasting "medical or other advice which ... discourages the audience from following official rules and guidance."

The German government also allegedly commissioned scientists to create a model to justify preventive and repressive public health measures. In Australia, Queensland's chief health officer Jeanette Young's logic on school closures was also fear-fuelling: "it's about the messaging." Canadian David Cayley commented that masks promote the "ritualisation of fear."

Sacralisation of lockdowns

In the first year of the pandemic, a team from Otago University in New Zealand (my former university) published an interesting study that provided some explanation for the strong public support for lockdown measures. This support came despite known or predicted collateral harms, including loss of livelihoods, elevated mortality from neglect of other diseases and ailments, "deaths of despair" from greater loneliness, and police abuses.

The answer, they said, is the moralisation of restrictions in pursuit of a Covid eradication strategy. People did not take kindly even to mere questioning of the restrictions. With many governments deploying state propaganda to the full to instil fear of the disease and shame all effort to question restrictions, the moralisation deepened into sacralisation.

This offers a plausible explanation for why people who so warmly embrace the moral framework of diversity, inclusion, and tolerance (the DIE framework) in social policy settings ended up supporting vaccine apartheid for those hesitant to get jabbed by shots with worryingly thin efficacy and safety trials before approval for public use.

Vilification of scientific dissent

Even after the data made it indisputably clear that SARS-CoV-2 was not a once in a century but closer to once in a decade disease outbreak, and that the virus curve was going to follow its own trajectory untethered to policy interventions, authorities were too heavily invested in the narrative and continued to pretend the virus was far more lethal, non-discriminatory and infectious than in reality.

They concentrated all messaging in their own single points of truth and to maintain public support, they demonised and denigrated legitimate scientific debate on the lethality of the virus, the effectiveness and ethics of lockdowns, masks and vaccine mandates, and the harms inflicted by these interventions.

This effort would have faced many more challenges but for the prior success in turning the debate from a scientific discourse into a moral imperative and the successful enlistment of media and social media to the effort.

Crushing public dissent and protest

"Social" distancing is deeply dehumanising. Isolation robs people of social support; exhaustion and fatigue weaken mental ability and physical capacity to resist; monopoly perception eliminates information at variance with compliance demands. The shocking arrest of Zoe Buhler in Victoria was a very public demonstration of omnipotence in inflicting degradation and humiliation, as was forcing women to wear masks during labour.

Enforcing 5km travel limits, and mask mandates on solitary fishermen and farmers driving tractors in lonely paddocks, made sense as the enforcement of trivial demands to develop habitual compliance. Obedience is doing what you are told, regardless of right and wrong. Resistance is doing what's right, heedless of consequences.

The opening sentence of the Universal Declaration of Human Rights affirms "the inherent dignity and the equal and inalienable rights of all members of the human family" as "the foundation of freedom, justice and peace in the world." Putting "inherent dignity" before "inalienable rights" was deliberate. Take away people's dignity and you take away their humanity, enabling the state to commit atrocities at will and sustain a long-term abusive relationship with citizens.

State propaganda whipped up public emotions with public shaming and social ostracism of sceptics and recalcitrants. This helps to explain why and how science was turned on its head by replacing scepticism with cult-like absolutism: if you cannot question, that's dogma and propaganda, not science. This hit peak stupidity with Fauci's narcissistic claim that attacks on him were really "attacks on science."

Media bribery and bullying

Many media outlets became financially beholden to governments for massive advertising that promoted the lockdown, mask and vaccine narrative. Some also had "global health reporters" embedded with money from the Gates Foundation. The NZ government set up a NZ $55mn subsidy scheme over three years (2020/21–2022/23) called the Public Interest Journalism Fund. Jacinda Ardern's government further reinforced New Zealand's collective moral fervour by proclaiming its doctrine of the health ministry as the "single source of truth" on anything to do with coronavirus, including public health interventions. Canada set up a five-year $600mn federal fund in 2018 to help media outlets that was supplemented with a $65mn subsidy as "emergency relief" in 2020, whose recipients were not publicly identified.

The media fanned the flames of fear through a relentless daily diet of panic porn. For example on 10 February, after Iowa lifted all pandemic restrictions, a *Washington Post* headline said: "Welcome to Iowa, a state that doesn't care if you live or die." Opinion polls in the US, UK, Ireland and France showed the tsunami of false beliefs about the numbers infected and killed, their average age and Covid's rank among all causes of death.

"A climate of fear is preventing experts from questioning the handling of the pandemic, with reputations smeared, jobs lost and even families threatened," said Lucy Johnston. Harvard epidemiologist Martin Kulldorff lamented that instead of reporting "reliable scientific and public health information about the pandemic," the media "have broadcast unverified information, spread unwarranted fear [and] promoted naïve and inefficient counter measures such as lockdowns."

The four faces of state power[86]

The ease with which the majority of people slipped into compliance with lockdown restrictions was a distressing surprise. The acceptance of facemasks in community and children's school settings was a disappointment. Government' success in turning Western liberal democracies into citizen-informant states was both shocking and dispiriting.

[86] Brownstone Institute, 6 January 2023, https://brownstone.org/articles/state-power-and-covid-crimes-part-5/

In Australia this led many to ruefully recall a quip from the late Clive James. The problem, he said, is not that too many Australians are descended from convicts, but from prison guards. Except citizens enthusiastically becoming informers on family, friends, neighbours and colleagues was not uniquely Australian but a common phenomenon across the Western world (and also some but not most others).

All institutional checks on overreach and abuse of executive power—every single one of them, from legislatures to the judiciary, human rights machinery, professional associations, trade unions, the Church and the media—turned out to be not fit for purpose and folded just when they were most needed. Waystations on the journey to where we are today with a biosecurity-cum-biofascist state include the national security, administrative and surveillance states.

National security state

The liberal democratic state reconciles two principles that can be in tension: rule by the majority and protection of minorities. It does so by requiring the government to obtain consent of the people through regular elections conducted on the basis of universal adult suffrage, but at the same time placing limits on the exercise of state power, prioritising individual rights and providing institutional bulwarks against the state encroaching on citizen' rights.

During the Cold War the Manichean framing of the worldwide struggle against the dark forces of communism led to the rise of the national security state in which limitations on state powers began to be steadily, and sometimes stealthily, lifted. The size and powers of the military-intelligence complex were progressively expanded and individual rights and freedoms were circumscribed.

Acting abroad in violation of core American values—extrajudicial assassination of foreign enemies as determined by secretive processes, overthrow of elected regimes deemed hostile to US interests, military and economic assistance to friendly dictatorships—was also institutionalised.

Administrative state

The administrative state had a mainly internal focus and facilitated the circumvention of the traditionally separated executive, legislative and judicial spheres. In that sense and to that extent this represented encroachments on constitutional governance. Agencies and departments displaced duly enacted legislation with regulations and replaced judicial processes with administrative determinations.

Think of the ability of tax authorities to confiscate private property without court orders and, in the last three years, powers given to police to impose heavy instant fines and the manner in which the Trudeau government froze the bank accounts of not just the protesting truckers, but of anyone who had donated even modest amounts to the Freedom Convoy.

When administrative agencies can create, adjudicate and enforce their own rules with no need for parliaments and courts, the administrative state has arrived, prompting David E. Lewis to ask: "Is the Failed Pandemic Response a Symptom of a Diseased Administrative State?"

Surveillance state

Meanwhile, the reach of technology had steadily expanded the ability of the state to snoop on people. It took the exposures of Edward Snowden to awaken us to the extent to which we now live in a digitised surveillance state. Some governments, and by no means only totalitarian regimes, require telecommunications, social media and home entertainment technologies to be intercept-compliant and filter and censor content on official request. This gives governments a measure of control not simply over our acts but also our speech and thoughts.

Biosecurity-cum-biofascist state

"Tech tyranny" reached its apotheosis during the pandemic with the unholy polygamous marriage between Big Government, Big Pharma,

Big Tech and Big Media/Social Media. Only the naive would believe that governments would now willingly, let alone voluntarily, roll back their vastly expanded powers to control people's behaviour, speech and thoughts.

The respected news agency Associated Press conducted a year-long investigation into the mass surveillance technology that was installed on people's phones for contact tracing to keep their community safe from the coronavirus. On 21 December, it reported:

> *From Beijing to Jerusalem to Hyderabad, India, and Perth, Australia ... authorities used these technologies and data to halt travel for activists and ordinary people, harass marginalized communities and link people's health information to other surveillance and law enforcement tools. In some cases, data was shared with spy agencies.*

Have the pandemic management responses, deploying military-grade propaganda and psychological manipulation, been national security countermeasures and not public health directives all along, as argued by Philip Altman and his team? This thesis was argued in Brownstone articles in November–December by Debbie Lerman and Jeffrey Tucker.

Daily Sceptic editor Will Jones asked similarly if the pandemic was orchestrated as a trial run for checking the infrastructure and preparedness for responding to a biological attack. There's some evidence to suggest that a pandemic plan from 2007 was put into action when the opportunity arose in 2020. Jones followed up by noting how the UK deployed counterterrorism units to crush scientific and social media dissent on lockdowns and vaccines.

I am in no position to evaluate these claims. But securitisation of the pandemic response is the one thing that would explain the extraordinary efforts to enforce the stringent measures pending the development of vaccines, and then the remarkable shortcuts taken to roll them out under rushed trials, with no long-term efficacy and safety data, and downplaying the explosion of (greatly underreported) serious adverse events.

Finally, how to explain the appointment of Sir Jeremy Farrar as the WHO chief scientist in 2023, other than as brazen gaslighting of the public? Both hailed and reviled as the UK's answer to Anthony Fauci as among the most influential pro-lockdown advisers, he was one of the original authors to dismiss the lab-leak theory in a coordinated campaign of misinformation.

On 30 January 2020, he tweeted: "China is setting a new standard for outbreak response and deserves all our thanks." His words had closely echoed that of the WHO director general himself. Combined with the pursuit by a powerful coalition of Western countries of an expansive global pandemic treaty that would greatly strengthen the role of the WHO director general and regional directors to compel countries to implement its directives, this is yet another strand in the institutional infrastructure of a health permacrisis that has cut deep inroads into citizen' liberties in recent years.

This is the year when we will learn if Covid illiberalism will begin to be rolled back or has become a permanent feature of the political landscape in the democratic West. Although the head says to fear the worst, the eternally optimistic heart will still hope for the best.

The rise of the public-private partnership in tyranny[87]

The slogan cuius regio, eius religio (whose the reign/realm, his the religion) was adopted in Europe in the mid-16th century to end the religious wars. It was an agreement among the monarchs that he who governs the territory decides its religion. Faith therefore was not a matter of individual choice of beliefs, values, morality, and rituals. Rather, the subjects bowed to the superior power of the sovereign as his faithful followers.

---

[87] Brownstone Institute, 7 September 2023, https://brownstone.org/articles/the-rise-of-the-public-private-partnership-in-tyranny/

Adherents of other religions either fled to more congenial kingdoms or else risked being robbed of all property and perhaps even killed. In time, however, Church and state reached amicable separation and learnt to live in peaceful coexistence.

Looking around at the Western world today, it seems as though people, led by their political, intellectual, and cultural elites, are intent on reversing the gains of the Industrial Revolution, discarding the fruits of the Enlightenment and erasing long-established empirical knowledge with regard to basic biology.

It seems the state in some countries might be enforcing its own new religion of belief systems and values articulated by a small elite that self-identifies as progressive social justice warriors. In this cause they have recruited private-sector companies to function as the 21st century equivalent of feudal dukes and overlords to enforce the core beliefs and rituals of the state-decreed religion, sometimes with cult-like attributes.

In 2015 the University of California advised faculty and students to avoid causing offence by saying "There is only one race, the human race," because it denies "the significance of a person of color's racial/ethnic experience and history." More recently we had the example of a shock-inducing diversity workshop at Western University in Ontario, Canada with a slide giving as an example of microaggression the assertion that "the most qualified person should get the job."

As I continue to hold fast to both propositions, I guess I am beyond redemption. I console myself with the thought that Martin Luther King, Jr. would today be called out as a racist for his dream of a society where people are judged not by the colour of their skin but by the content of their character. The Western presentation also warned that "white silence, white privilege, and white shame leads to a lot of white complicity in white supremacy," which does rather suggest an obsessive compulsive disorder focussed on whiteness.

The zeitgeist encourages the demonization of everything European and the romanticization of non-Western cultures and history.

You can praise any culture in the world except Western but must blame only Western culture for all the world's ills. The Albanese government wants to insert a new chapter in Australia's constitution to create an Aboriginal body, called the Voice, to make representations to parliament and the government. The Liberal and National parties are opposed and opinion polls currently show more voters intending to reject than to endorse the constitutional amendment.

The latest Newspoll (3 September) for the *Australian* has No jumping ahead 53-38. This is a dramatic reversal from the 56-37 support for Yes in February. Support has fallen also for the Labor Party and Prime Minister (PM) Anthony Albanese.

Universities are meant to be the bastions of academic freedom and robust policy debate. Australia's university sector is essentially publicly funded. Not one university has taken a public position to oppose the Voice. But the senior leadership teams of several universities have put their full weight behind the Voice. Melbourne University, for example, did so on 7 March, months before anyone even knew the wording of the referendum question.

Nor have the universities' public information sessions to promote dialogue on the contested policy initiative demonstrated a balance of speakers to argue the merits of both sides. As James Allan, a law professor at Queensland University, wrote in the *Australian*, this is "not just a form of virtue signalling with other people's money; it comes close to being an improper use of taxpayer money."

Worse, the fear among academics that speaking publicly against the Voice could damage their careers has a chilling effect and promotes preemptive self-censorship. It's telling that the author of an article on this subject, writing for the *Spectator Australia*, chose to remain anonymous. My article in the *Weekend Australian* on 29 July elicited many supportive messages from university colleagues, along with regrets that they dared not voice their opposition publicly.

Corporations, on the other hand, engage in virtue signalling with shareholders' money. In Australia this includes Qantas, once publicly owned but now a private company. The airline is giving yes campaigners, but not opponents, free flights to travel the country in their promotional efforts and has painted several planes with the Yes slogan.

Yet, on 31 August, the Australian Competition and Consumer Commission, the consumer watchdog, launched legal proceedings against Qantas for defrauding the public by continuing to sell tickets for cancelled flights for up to two weeks after, and for delaying notification of cancelled scheduled flights to thousands of existing ticket-holders.

The airline has been exceptionally tardy in processing refunds for flights cancelled during the pandemic disruptions. The ACCC wants Qantas to pay a fine of over AUD 250 million. The airline is also hoarding half a billion dollars of unrefunded customer money from flights that were cancelled during the lockdowns. Thus, far from a virtuous corporate entity, Qantas has been severely infected with the culture of arrogance.

In some ways the biggest shock that genuinely has acted as a wake-up call for millions was the debanking of the well-known British politician Nigel Farage in June by Coutts Bank, a subsidiary of the National Westminster Bank. NatWest, as it is commonly called, is 39% owned by the British government after the public bailout of its predecessor Royal Bank of Scotland in 2008, which was renamed NatWest in 2020.

Having compiled an extensive, 40-page Stasi-style surveillance report on Farage, the bank concluded that his views did not align with their values as an "inclusive" organization (yes, really). Then its CEO—a Dame, no less—lied in a private briefing to a BBC journalist to claim he had lost his account for falling below its minimum threshold but was caught out in the lie and forced to resign—but with a generous payout.

In truth Farage was cast out because of wrongthink: for leading Brexit, supporting Donald Trump, and opposing Black Lives Matter (BLM). The defenestration was based on a dossier written seemingly by a pink conquistador that was a tawdry, political hit job.

Laughably, the reputational-risk committee that engaged in this Kafkaesque parody ended up destroying the reputation of the bank, whose clients have included Mafia bosses, dictators, and Russian oligarchs. Karma bites. (By the way, in Hinduism karma does not mean destiny independently of your actions. Rather, it means the opposite: you cannot escape but are destined to reap the consequences of your actions.)

The debanking scandal also highlighted the risk of the trend to a cashless society in the age of growing digitization. We have been seduced by the conveniences of digitized life oblivious, like frogs in boiling water, to the threats to privacy and, more critically, the enhanced capacity of corporate and state actors not just to engage in surveillance of our activities and preferences, but also to cut us off from financial life support.

From there to China's social credit system is but a short step. Canada gave us a foretaste of that with government-directed financial sanctions on the truckers' Freedom Convoy and anyone who had donated to their cause, no matter how modest the amount or how indigent their individual circumstances. Few governments or financial institutions seem at all bothered with the multiple inconveniences inflicted on the elderly by the rapid move to a cashless society.

The faddish causes to which corporates are increasingly attracted and which they support financially include the ESG (environmental and social governance) and DIE (diversity, inclusion, and equity) agendas. The Human Resources departments of public and private sector, media, and sporting institutions have been captured by proliferating numbers of DIE "experts" who increasingly rule the roost over staff engaged in merely the core mission of the institutions.

This includes signing on to the central tenets of the social justice agenda of critical race theory, an open-ended rainbow spectrum of gender identity, #MeToo, and BLM. Financial institutions and companies divesting from fossil fuel industries in pursuit of Net Zero is another example.

How about banks concentrate on banking services and Qantas on flying planes on time, without losing luggage and at reasonable prices?

The bigger picture is the rise of corporate fascism that fuses the power of the state, corporations (including media corporations), social media, and technology giants. This was most clearly evident in their concerted coercion on all matters related to Covid but clearly is poised to embrace pretty much all of social life.

Call it the public-private tyranny partnership. Traditionally coercion and tyranny have been the preserve of states, with citizen consent the exclusive preserve of liberal democratic states. The private sector has been the domain of choice and competition where the customer is always right. Now the citizen must hew to state-dictated morality and the customer must bow to the corporate moral compass.

Paraphrasing Mao Zedong, do morals grow from the dollar-encrusted barrels of corporate guns wielded by executives aided and abetted by their DIE staff? They who hold and use political, economic, and cultural power get to set and control the moral compass for society, and all must bow down to this, or else?

The puzzle is why public and corporate sector executives believe they have the qualifications, training, skills, and judgment to set the moral compass for society at large. This is especially so when their values are in fact out of alignment with the dominant values of the society in which they operate. They and their boards are chosen for their business and management expertise and competence to create value-added products and deliver services.

Their capacity to set ethical standards even for the company employees, let alone for their customers, is highly suspect. I am not aware of any university setting up a task force of eminent ethicists to set university policy on contested morals with regard to race, gender identity, and Covid-related mandates.

On what basis does an Australian university choose to honour the president of Ukraine with a Zoom public lecture but ban contacts with Russian scholars? And that too without consulting or in any way involving its in-house International Relations experts?

How then do we derisk society from the looming threat of corporate fascism? The scope for individual action is limited but not nonexistent. After PayPal closed down the account of the Free Speech Union in the UK, and of all activities associated with its founder Toby Young including the *Daily Sceptic*, I closed my PayPal account (this requires some perseverance).

Now when confronted with a PayPal portal for paying for a purchase from an Australian store or hotel, I call the provider and ask for bank details to make an electronic transfer, explaining my opposition to use a politicized financial service provider. If no alternative is available, I switch to another provider. For similar reasons, I no longer use GoFundMe and have stopped watching the Australian cricket team since they began taking the knee before every game. The choice for each one of us is to go along with the cancellation mob in order to get an easy ride, or to put up with added inconvenience in order to set things right again.

The more effective avenue for large-scale change, however, is through political choices. The cultural elites may well feel morally superior to the hoi polloi and console themselves with the thought that they are on the right side of history.

Meanwhile, though, they are decidedly on the wrong side of the people. By contrast, politicians like Giorgia Meloni, who became popular enough to become prime minister of Italy by appealing to family, faith, and country—values that do align with that of most voters—are derided and mocked as mere populists.

The governing Conservative Party in the UK has lagged 20 points behind Labour in the polls for months. Its best and perhaps only hope for shaking things up is to challenge the received truths in regard to racial justice, gender identity, and environmental agendas and revert to the Meloni formula, abandon Net Zero, end coercion in directing consumers away from stable and inexpensive sources of energy, reaffirm basic biological facts, protect women's rights to safe spaces and dignity, and end woke policing and cancel culture in all public institutions.

So far PM Rishi Sunak and his cabinet ministers have engaged in brave talk but failed to take urgent and demonstrably effective action. Were the Tories to succeed in reversing their sliding fortunes in the UK, the reverberations would be felt across the Western democratic world.

The Covid resistance deserves the Nobel Peace Prize[88]

Alfred Nobel's will (excerpt) (Paris, 27 November 1895) stipulates that the peace prize is to be awarded to the person who shall have done the most or the best work for fraternity between nations, for the abolition or reduction of standing armies and for the holding and promotion of peace congresses.

The nomination processes start in September each year and nominations must be submitted before 1 February of the year in which the prize is awarded. The Norwegian Nobel Committee is responsible for selecting the Nobel Peace Prize laureates. Among those eligible to submit nominations, I have done so several times in the past. From February to October, the committee scrutinises the list of candidates and progressively whittles it down, culminating in the announcement of the prize in early October and the award ceremony in Oslo in early December.

Inexplicably, none of my nominees won the prize. Rumour mills speculated that some came pretty close, but in the end no cigar. Disheartened, I discontinued my submissions. Last year I did consider nominating some of the world's leading organisations and individuals engaged in fighting the Covid lockdowns, mask, and vaccine mandates over 2020–23.

[88] Brownstone Institute, 16 February 2024, https://brownstone.org/articles/the-covid-resistance-deserves-the-nobel-peace-prize/

Because of my 100% perfect track record of failure, I decided this could be the kiss of death and in the end abandoned the idea. Nonetheless, I hope some of them have been nominated by others. Let me explain why, in the context of the history of this prize, they would be deserving candidates—but unlikely winners.

The Peace Prize has often departed from Nobel's explicit criteria

The strict criteria are sometimes put forward as the explanation for why Mahatma Gandhi was not awarded the prize. Be that as it may, after the Second World War, the Norwegian committee's definition of peace grew increasingly more expansive and flexible, embracing fields as diverse as environmental activism, indigenous rights, food security, and human rights. It gradually acquired the overtones of a political act or message with a messianic element of hope to nudge the world towards striving for the broader conception of peace favoured by the committee.

In relation to the founder's will, this produced some strange choices. There have been many eyebrow-raising laureates: those who waged war, others tainted with terrorism, and still others whose contributions to peace were tenuous (planting millions of trees), laudable though their campaigns were in their own right.

The 1973 joint recipients were North Vietnam's Le Duc Tho and US Secretary of State Henry Kissinger for ending the Vietnam War. In 1994 Yasser Arafat got the prize (jointly with Yitzhak Rabin and Shimon Peres) for efforts "to create peace in the Middle East." Yes, truly.

The 1970 laureate was Norman Borlaug for his role in the green revolution. In 2007 Al Gore and the IPCC were selected for their role in spreading awareness about "man-made climate change" (yes, the committee used this gendered language).

It is the many awards in relation to human rights, freedoms, and democracy promotion that are most relevant to why the committee should give careful consideration to the heroes of the Covid resistance.

Last year's Nobel Peace Prize was awarded to Nargis Mohammadi of Iran "for her fight against the oppression of women in Iran and her fight to promote human rights and freedom for all." The three 2022 laureates from Belarus, Russia, and Ukraine were recognised for their promotion of "the right to criticise power and protect the fundamental rights of citizens. They have made an outstanding effort to document war crimes, human right abuses and the abuse of power." In 2021, the joint winners from the Philippines and Russia were lauded "for their efforts to safeguard freedom of expression.'

In 2014, Pakistani Malala Yousafzai and India's Kailash Satyarthi (even the Nobel committee was hyphenating India and Pakistan!) received commendations "for their struggle against the suppression of children and young people and for the right of all children to education." The 2010 winner was China's Liu Xiabo "for his long and nonviolent struggle for fundamental human rights in China.'

In 2003, Iran's Shirin Ebadi got the nod "for her efforts for democracy and human rights. She has focused especially on the struggle for the rights of women and children." The 1991 laureate was Myanmar's Aung San Suu Kyi for her "struggle for democracy and human rights." In 1983, the committee awarded the prize to Lech Walesa for his "struggle for free trade unions and human rights in Poland.'

In the 1970s, the recipients included Amnesty International (1977) and Ireland's Sean MacBride (1974) for promoting and defending human rights around the world.

The 2009 award to newly elected US President Barack Obama "for his extraordinary efforts to strengthen international diplomacy and cooperation between peoples" was one of the strangest selections in the history of the peace prize. Reacting to Obama's award, I wrote at the time: "The Nobel Committee has embarrassed itself, patronized Barack Obama, and demeaned the Peace Prize. In choosing activism, it risks setbacks to pet causes it champions." (*Ottawa Citizen*, 14 October 2009).

With the award to Obama, the prize crossed the line from dubious or questionable to risible. Premature doesn't even begin to cover it. Remember, Obama was sworn in on 20 January 2009. So the individuals and organisations that nominated him between September 2008 and 31 January 2009 would have justified their choice with reference to his deeds and words almost entirely *before* he became president. The prize was "for awesomeness," for yes he can, not yes he did. As Hendrik Hertzberg wrote in the *New Yorker* (12 October): "At least at the Olympics the judges wait till after the race to give you the gold medal. They don't force it on you while you're still waiting for the bus to take you to the stadium."

Gasps of incredulity intermingled with snorts of derision, including among Obama admirers and supporters beginning to fret over his compromises on core promises and values. It devalued the work of most previous laureates and mocked the efforts of all who put in time, thought, and care in nominating over 200 individuals and institutions, many no doubt deserving of the prize.

It turned the prize itself into a joke, provided handy ammunition to Obama's domestic opponents while embarrassing many supporters, and risked making progress on several of his worthwhile initiatives more difficult. It also risked the perverse consequence of forcing Obama to brandish his public hawk credentials instead of releasing his inner dove. Ironically, Obama was awarded the prize at the very time that, kowtowing to the rising power that must not be offended, he became the first US president in almost two decades to refuse to meet the Dalai Lama (so he was willing to meet with the enemies but not the advocates of freedom?), a worthy previous laureate (1989).

The Covid resistance is worthy of serious consideration

Many previous laureates have thus been chosen for their advocacy and struggles for human, women's, and children's rights, including education.

Few readers of this site will disagree with the claim that lockdowns, mask edicts, and vaccine mandates amounted to the most egregious assaults on human rights, children's rights, civil liberties, personal and business freedoms, and democratic practices, affecting the biggest number of human beings in history.

The boundary between liberal democracy and draconian dictatorship quickly disappeared. The right to peaceful protest, a hallmark of democracy, was criminalised. In the Cambridge Freshfields Law Lecture on 27 October 2020, Lord Jonathan Sumption, the recently retired UK Supreme Court Justice, said:

> *During the Covid-19 pandemic, the British state has exercised coercive powers over its citizens on a scale never previously attempted… It has been the most significant interference with personal freedom in the history of our country. We have never sought to do such a thing before, even in wartime and even when faced with health crises far more serious than this one.*

People were told when they could shop, the hours during which they could shop, what they could purchase, how close they could get to others, and which direction they could move in by following arrows on the floor. We experienced the wholesale house arrest of healthy populations; violations of bodily integrity, "my body my choice," and informed consent principles; the spread of the surveillance, administrative, and biosecurity state; the treatment of people as germ-ridden disease carriers and biohazards; the sheer dehumanisation of people who just asked to be left alone; the cruelty of denying final goodbyes to dying parents and grandparents and the emotional closure of full service funerals; joyful celebrations of weddings and birthdays; state diktats of whom we could meet (and sleep) with, how many, where and for how long; what we could buy, during which hours and from where; and the theft of children's education and economic security by loading them with debt decades into the future.

All institutional checks on overreach and abuse of executive power, from legislatures to the judiciary, human rights machinery, professional associations, trade unions, the Church, and the media, turned out to be not fit for purpose and folded just when they were most needed.

In January 2022, Unicef reported on the devastating setbacks to children's education. Robert Jenkins, Unicef Chief of Education, said "we are looking at a nearly insurmountable scale of loss to children's schooling." There was a two-decade reversal in children's educational progress in the US. Japan experienced a jump in suicides by more than 8,000 between March 2020 and June 2022 compared to pre-pandemic numbers, mostly among women in their teens and 20s.

By February 2021, lockdowns had forced an estimated 500 million children around the world out of school, more than half of them in India. Dr Sunita Narain, Director General of the Centre for Science and Environment, said that similarly, more than half the world's additional 115 million people were pushed back into extreme poverty living in South Asia. India, she said, was all set to usher in a 375-million strong pandemic generation of children who were at risk of suffering long-lasting impacts like increased child mortality, being underweight and stunted, and educational and work-productivity reversals.

In October 2020, Sweden decided to lift all remaining "recommended" restrictions on over-70s. Health Minister Lena Hallengren explained that months of social isolation had meant loneliness and misery and a "decline in mental health likely to worsen the longer the recommendations remain in place." Part of the emotional stress load on the elderly caused by lockdowns resulted from the destruction of family life, the fundamental unit of human society. The forced separation of loved ones took an enormous toll on mental well-being, with measurable consequences for physical health. From the UK we had stories of elderly people refusing to go into rest homes. They'd rather die in pain surrounded by family at home, than face a lonely death cut off completely from family after leaving home.

Then came the vaccine mandates, for injections rushed to market under emergency use authorisation with limited trial safety and efficacy data. The efficacy rapidly waned, the risk-benefits equation for other than the elderly and the comorbid was always highly suspect, and their contributions to persistent all-cause excess deaths remains unexamined. Yet, people were manipulated and coerced into being jabbed on pain of dismissal from many jobs and excluded from public spaces.

In Australia, there was pervasive police surveillance of social media and public spaces, state control of economic activities, suspension of parliament to rule by executive diktat, instant heavy fines on police officers' whims, and martial law masquerading as medical law. Thousands of Australians remain stranded abroad, unable to come home because of government limits on daily arrivals. Returnees Sarah and Moe Haidar were not allowed to see or touch their 9-week premature baby in a Brisbane hospital, instead relying on FaceTime, until quarantine period was over.

A fully vaccinated Sydney grandmother was denied a permit to go to Melbourne to help care for her grandchildren while her daughter battled advanced breast cancer. In a country town, a pregnant woman posting on Facebook to support a peaceful protest against Victoria's lockdown was handcuffed and arrested in her house in the early morning, still in her pyjamas, in the presence of her family. A mother from across the border in New South Wales lost her baby after being denied treatment in Brisbane because Queensland hospitals were only for Queenslanders.

As I said, previous recipients of the peace prize have typically paid a heavy personal price for their defence of human, women's, and children's rights. Most of them demonstrated exceptional courage of conviction in their struggles. I was in the fortunate position of not having to pay any personal price for my opposition to Covid edicts but I know many people who suffered but courageously kept to their principled opposition to the biggest state-sponsored campaign against well-established rights and freedoms.

Some set up alternative news and commentary sites that created and grew new communities to share findings and thoughts and overcome the sense of isolation. Others spoke out despite threats, often carried out, of severe repercussions to jobs and lives. New organisations sprang up to counter the all-pervasive propaganda and censorship through the collusion of the state, the pharmaceutical industry, legacy and social media, and tech platforms. Canadian truckers organised a freedom convoy to Ottawa that captured world attention but petrified Justin Trudeau into harsh authoritarian countermeasures.

There should be no shortage of potential candidates for the peace prize to recognise their brave efforts to keep the flame of freedom flying through these dark times.

Why this is probably a false hope

In the context of the history of the Nobel Peace Prize since the 1970s, then, individuals and groups that have resisted the assault on people's rights are worthy of the prize this year. But the same history also shows that to the committee, dissidents against regimes and governments disliked by the West receive the recognition: China, Iran, Myanmar, Pakistan, Russia. Not so Western dissidents resisting their own governments.

Call me cynical, but if Julian Assange or Edward Snowden had exposed the same wrongdoings on the part of China, Russia, or Iran instead of the US, their chances of a Nobel Peace Prize would have been as steeply higher as the chance of an elderly person is of dying from Covid compared to that of a health teenager.

Writing in the *Daily Mail* in 2022, Andrew Neil, former editor of the *Sunday Times* (1983–94) and current chairman of the *Spectator* magazine, commented that Assange's Wikileaks had revealed:

> *War crimes covered up. Torture. Brutality. The rendition and incarceration of suspects without due process. The corruption of inquiries*

> *trying to hold it to account. The bribery of foreign officials to look the other way when America did bad things.*
>
> *All this by the self-styled greatest democracy in the world.*

Assange went to considerable trouble to redact material that could endanger any individual and no credible evidence has ever been produced to show that any individual was in fact harmed. Yet that remains the most commonly levelled charge against him, that he recklessly and knowingly put the lives of US personnel in danger. His prosecution by US authorities is clearly political, not criminal, meaning that it amounts to persecution.

It's hard to see the Norwegian Nobel Committee defying the suffocating Covid narrative that took over the Western world, with a very few honourable exceptions. Of course if they were to do so, that would really stir things up and help to dismantle the narrative. One can but hope for the best while expecting otherwise.

14: CONNECTING THE POLICY DOTS FROM NUCLEAR AND INTERNATIONAL CONFLICTS TO COVID INTERVENTIONS

I had worked as a policy analyst and adviser in international affairs for many decades as a global governance expert at the intersection of scholarship and policy. But I was not and am not a health policy expert. As a retired person when the pandemic was declared in 2020, I had the freedom and time to deepen my knowledge of pandemic policy and also the freedom to say what I wanted without fear of losing my job. Because I had been writing for many quality national and international newspapers for several decades, I had a platform to disseminate my views. Having first familiarised myself with some of the specialist vocabulary, I applied insights from my global governance background in the worlds of research and policy to Covid-19 policy interventions. A particularly striking feature of these cross-linkages is how they transcend the familiar liberal-conservative divide to demonstrate independent evidence-based critical thinking instead.

A Covid vocabulary[89]

When the novel coronavirus began to dominate world news in 2020 (the virus may already have been in circulation in 2019), a modest existing knowledge on pandemic policy, based in a background in

[89] *Spectator Australia*, 14 January 2023, https://www.spectator.com.au/2023/01/a-covid-vocabulary/

global governance, indicated that governments were departing radically from the existing scientific and policy consensus. Several well credentialled experts tried to say so but were dismissed as has-beens or fringe dwellers suffering from relevance deprivation syndrome. This was troubling.

Being retired, I had immunity against being fired. With time to do my own policy oriented research, I began digging deeper into Covid pandemic management as a policy challenge. And this meant familiarising myself with the language of health experts and a resulting expansion of my vocabulary. What follows is a description of the key new words I learnt over the last three years, but also words I've learnt to hate. With each step on the journey, confidence and trust in the public health clerisy fell further.

We began with the distinctions between (a) infection and case fatality rates and (b) pharmaceutical interventions like vaccines and drugs and nonpharmaceutical interventions like enhanced surveillance, testing and contact tracing; social distancing (a euphemism for anti-social behaviour like physical distancing); workplace and school closures; working from home; sanitisers and surface cleaning. This led to "lockdowns," another euphemism for shuttering all economic and social activity and locking up entire populations in their homes because the health experts said so despite the previous consensus against it.

As part of the public discourse on justification for the unprecedented lockdowns and possible timing for lifting the restrictions, officials and commentators fussed over the "R" number (how many more people on average will one sick person infect?) or the rate at which the virus was reproducing in order to assess if it was still growing or contracting. By 2022 the world had lost interest in this 2020 obsession.

As the debate between lockdown enthusiasts and sceptics heated up, the language deteriorated into name calling and "Covidian" and "Covidiot" were deployed as reciprocal insults. With masks we tried to understand the difference between and relative merits of face-cloths, surgical masks and N95 respirators; healthcare, outdoor and indoor settings; and why the medical consensus did an instant (that is, without any additional data or scientific studies) 180-degree turn on masks from being pointless to an extremely critical individual and community protection measure.

The existing standard metric in 2020 for allocating finite health resources, a cost-benefit analysis using quality adjusted life years (QALY) for measuring health outcomes, was similarly abandoned without explanation.

In 2021 we turned our attention to vaccines and the importance of numbers: absolute risk reduction, relative risk reduction, and (a) the number needed to vaccinate in order to prevent one additional infection or death for the specified group (e.g. elderly, young, children, industry or setting-specific employees) and (b) the number of "serious adverse events" that would result in that many vaccinated people within each target cohort as a critical "safety signal." We also had to grasp the distinction between vaccine efficacy in controlled clinical trials and vaccine effectiveness in the real world.

The equations just didn't compute. The famed 95% efficacy claimed in trials has produced empirical outcomes of 77% of all infections and 85% of all Covid deaths in New South Wales, from 22 May–31 December 2022 (the period for which data separated by vaccination status is available, as the practice is being discontinued in 2023), having been vaccinated at least once. Finally, in response to the increasingly esoteric (and desperate) justifications for the vaccination drives despite the empirical outcomes showing their poor performance, we began looking at all-cause "excess mortality" that is less susceptible to statistical and linguistic manipulation.

For example, in an informative and instructive analysis in *Spectator Australia*, Jason Strecker goes through the Australian statistics on excess deaths to comprehensively demolish the self-serving claims by federal and state politicians of how many lives they saved by their lockdown policies. You've gotta love this sub-heading from the *NY Times* subscriber-only newsletter (4 January): "Mass vaccination, though miraculously effective, didn't usher in a lower overall death toll." Which leads me finally to Merriam-Webster's word of the year concept of "gaslighting," by the mainstream media as much as by governments.

Moving to words I learnt to hate, "Follow The Science" was the dishonest slogan used to shut down legitimate scientific inquiry while implementing many unscientific and even some anti-scientific policies. "Staying Apart to Stay Together" was a too-clever-by-half effort to camouflage an oxymoron. "Two [three] weeks to flatten the curve'? Yeah, right. Three years later, it's our lives, spirits and economies that have been flattened. "Protect the health service'? No, it's the mission of the health service to protect us.

Sure enough, as the winter pressures return on the broken, dysfunctional yet sacralised National Health Service (NHS) in the UK that has in recent times spent massive amounts of money recruiting DIE (diversity, inclusion and equity) bureaucrats while firing frontline staff who refused the jab, the *Daily Mail* reported on 4 January that the government is drawing up plans to reintroduce Covid-era measures "to save the NHS." An online poll showed 65% of over 13,000 readers oppose any measure being brought back but, surprisingly, 22% support the return of facemasks. Another pet peeve was "We are all in this together" and equivalent like the virus doesn't discriminate, it's out hunting whoever it can find, etc. No, not really, not by risks, benefits nor burdens are we all in this together.

And finally, the concept currently in vogue: "abundance of caution," used to impose a negative test requirement for Chinese arrivals from 5 January 2023 despite medical advice to the contrary. This upends the precautionary principle as previously understood and implemented. The principle emerged in the 1970s as a formula to pout novel products and processes on hold until it could be demonstrated that they would not cause unforeseen harms. The onus was on industry to first prove no harm, for example the risk of toxic spillage or leakage, before taking any innovation to market. Instead the abundance of caution slogan is used to justify novel interventions to justify harms being inflicted because of the possibility of greater harms if no action is taken.

Furthermore, it substitutes a slogan for a policy and confirms the trigger-happy authoritarian instincts of the government to reimpose curbs on people's freedoms on the minister's whim, with no justification advanced in the form of a cost-benefit analysis. It speaks to the undying conceit of politicians that they can control viruses. And it highlights their complete abandonment of caution on the harms of government interventions, despite three years of worldwide evidence that the rise and fall of the virus curve has been policy-invariant, while the damage from the ill-conceived interventions has been severe and will be long lasting.

Wartime parallels: Iraq and Covid[90]

At the time of the Iraq war, I was a senior UN official yet publicly critical of the drive to war before and during the war, including in the pages of the esteemed *International Herald Tribune.* (The demise of that paper was a sad loss to the world of high quality international journalism.)

The resort to emotional blackmail by the warmongers, where critics of the impending war were tarred for standing shoulder-to-shoulder with the Butcher of Baghdad, was instructive. Of course, very soon "We, the critics" were amply vindicated.

The whole episode left me with two conclusions. First, the resort to emotional arguments and moral blackmail generally implies that they have little reasoned argument and evidence to support their case and are deflecting to bluster instead. Second, whenever we are presented with excitable exclamation marks (Saddam Hussein already has

[90] Brownstone Institute, 15 February 2023. https://brownstone.org/articles/wartime-parallels-iraq-and-covid/

weapons of mass destruction (WMD)! He can hit us with his WMD in just 45 minutes! Coronavirus could be more cataclysmic than the Spanish flu! The sky is falling!), it is a very good idea to substitute sceptical question marks instead:

- Why would Saddam do that?
- Where is your evidence?
- What is your end goal?
- Are the proposed means proportionate to that goal?
- What will be the human and economic cost?
- How long will this take?
- Will you recognise success?
- What is your exit strategy?
- What are the checks against mission creep?

Instead of such healthy scepticism to force a dose of reality and calm down the agitated excitement, the coronavirus panic has also shown a remarkable triumph of the Henny Penny (or Chicken Little) tunnel vision. Thinking back to that as the coronavirus madness took hold of the world in 2020, I was surprised at how close the fit was to the Iraq war analogy once I thought the whole thing through. The lockdown, mask and vaccine mandates in particular revealed seven disturbing echoes of the 2003 Iraq War syndrome.

The first parallel is with respect to threat inflation. In the "Foreword" to the "dodgy dossier" of September 2002, UK Prime Minister (PM) Tony Blair wrote: Saddam Hussein's "military planning allows for some of the WMD [weapons of mass destruction] to be ready within 45 minutes of an order to use them." This turned out to be disinformation that was vital to rally the party, Parliament and the nation behind the decision to go to war.

British intelligence services had informed Blair in April 2002 (a year before the war) that Saddam Hussein had no nuclear weapons and any other WMD would be "very, very small." The Chilcot Inquiry was told a decade later that Blair accepted this but converted to George W. Bush's way of thinking after a subsequent visit to the US president's ranch in Crawford, Texas.

Similarly, to gain public backing for the degree of state intrusion into peoples' private lives and control over nations' economic activities without precedent even in wartime, the immediacy, gravity and magnitude of the coronavirus threat had to be made apocalyptic.

SARS-CoV-2 is not remotely as lethal as the Spanish flu of 1918–19 that killed the fit and young as virulently as the elderly and infirm. It infected 500 million people (one third of the world's population) and killed 50 million, equivalent to around 250 million dead today. Our health systems are infinitely better than a century ago. Yet authorities did not close down whole societies and economies in 1918. In other deadly pandemic episodes also we suffered but endured.

To overcome these hesitations of history and experience, the threat from SARS-CoV-2 had to be inflated beyond all previous calamities in order to panic countries into drastic action. This was successfully done by Neil Ferguson's catastrophist Imperial College London model of 16 March 2020 that is by now widely discredited. It deserves to acquire a notoriety equivalent to Iraq's dodgy dossier and Ferguson's mortality estimates should be judged to be the equivalent of Blair's 45 minutes to being hit by Saddam's WMD.

The second echo comes from the thinness of evidence. The infamous Downing Street Memorandum of 23 July 2002 made it clear that the US administration was determined to go to war and military action was inevitable. For their part, however, British officials did not believe there was sufficient legal justification: there was no recent evidence of Iraqi complicity with international terrorism, Saddam's WMD capability was less than that of Libya, North Korea or Iran, and he was not a threat to his neighbours. It was necessary to create the conditions that would make an invasion legal, hence "the intelligence and facts were being fixed around the policy" and the US "had already begun "spikes of activity" to put pressure on the regime."

With Covid-19, similarly, instead of evidence-based policy, many governments resorted to policy-based evidence to justify lockdowns, masks and vaccines.

The third similarity is in the denigration of critics who had the temerity to query the evidence. Those who questioned the lack of evidence to invade Iraq were demonised as apologists for the Butcher of Baghdad. Those who asked for evidence to justify the biggest expansion of state power in Western political history were shamed as wanting to kill granny. Most recently we learnt of how a unit of British intelligence kept tabs on the writings of journalists like Toby Young and Peter Hitchens because of their critical stance on government policies.

The fourth parallel is in the dismissal of collateral harm as exaggerated, speculative, without evidence, motivated, etc. Yet evidence continues to mount on the many different pathways through which the Grim Reaper claims his growing mass of victims from the panicked responses to Covid.

The fifth echo is in the lack of a clear exit strategy. Instead of a quick victory in Iraq followed by consolidated democratic regimes in a stable region and an orderly withdrawal, the US found itself stuck in a quagmire and eventually went back home an exhausted and vanquished conqueror. Almost all lockdown governments are now struggling with public justifications to declare victory and lift the lockdown. Modellers still want none of it and the apocalyptic warnings keep coming back, despite mounting evidence of a policy-invariant gradual decline in the spike in cases and deaths around the world. Covid is now endemic. The cognitive dissonance in Covid policy has been starkly evident in the continuation of the travel ban on unvaccinated visitors to the US well after authorities had been compelled to concede vaccines had no appreciable impact on infection and transmission.

Another resemblance is mission creep. One big reason for the self-created exit trap is that the original mission of flattening the curve so the health system could cope with a slowed spread of the virus, steadily morphed into the more ambitious but impossible mission of eliminating the virus. Or, to change metaphors, the goalposts didn't just keep shifting. They were dug out and replanted in an entirely new paddock in an altogether different location.

Seventh and finally, like the US media in 2003, most mainstream media commentators across the democratic West abandoned critical inquisitiveness in 2020 to become cheerleaders for the "war on corona." Except the censorship and suppression of dissenting voices seems to have been far, far worse in the last three years than was the case in 2003, with possibly illegal collusion between governments and Big Tech.

My transition from nuclear to Covid[91]

Many people have expressed curiosity about my switch of interest from nuclear nonproliferation and (especially) disarmament to the Covid pandemic policies of lockdowns, masks and vaccines. This section attempts to explain the transition from one policy to the other in 2020.

The common elements linking the national security and public health policies are scepticism about the dominant narrative and beliefs underpinning countries that subscribe to the effectiveness of nuclear weapons and nonpharmaceutical and then pharmaceutical interventions to manage threats to national security and health, respectively; interrogating claims by political leaders and top officials against real-world data, historical evidence and logical reasoning; and analysing benefits against costs and risks.

In both cases the net conclusion is that the emperor—the nuclear emperor and the pandemic policy emperor—is naked.

[91] Brownstone Institute, 8 May 2023, https://brownstone.org/articles/my-transition-from-nuclear-to-covid/

Readers of this site will be familiar with these arguments in relation to the grievously misguided policy interventions to deal with the Covid disease. I'd like to reach back into my pre-Covid professional background to show the analogous shortcomings and flaws of national security policies that rely on nuclear weapons.

Myth one: The bomb ended the Second World War

The belief in the policy utility of nuclear weapons is widely internalised owing in no small measure to Japan's surrender immediately after the atomic bombing of Hiroshima and Nagasaki in 1945. Yet the evidence is surprisingly clear that the close chronology is a coincidence. Hiroshima was bombed on 6 August, Nagasaki on the 9th, Moscow broke its neutrality pact to attack Japan on the 9th, and Tokyo announced the surrender on 15 August.

In Japanese decision-makers' minds the decisive factor in their unconditional surrender was the entry of the Soviet Union into the Pacific war against the essentially undefended northern approaches, and the fear they would be the occupying power unless Japan surrendered to the United States first. This was analysed in great detail in a 17,000-word article by Tsuyoshi Hasegawa, professor of modern Russian and Soviet history at the University of California Santa Barbara, in *The Asia–Pacific Journal* in 2007.

Nor, for that matter, did the Truman administration believe at the time that the two bombs were war-winning weapons. Rather, their strategic impact was vastly underestimated and they were thought of merely as an incremental improvement on the existing weaponry of war. It was only after 1945 that the military, political and ethical enormity of the decision to use atomic/nuclear weapons gradually sank in.

Myth two: The bomb kept the peace during the Cold War

Nor was the bomb the decisive factor in the territorial expansion of the former Soviet Union across central and eastern Europe during the 1945–49 years when the US held an atomic monopoly. In subsequent years during the long peace of the Cold War, both sides were determined to protect their own spheres of influence on either side of the highly militarised North-South spine that divided Europe into the NATO and Warsaw Pact alliance structures.

Nuclear weapons are credited with having preserved the long peace among the major powers in the North Atlantic (the argument that holds NATO to have been the world's most successful peace movement) and deterred attack by the conventionally superior Soviet forces throughout the Cold War. Yet this too is debatable. There is no evidence that either side had the intention to attack the other at any time, but was deterred from doing so because of nuclear weapons held by the other side. How do we assess the relative weight and potency of nuclear weapons, West European integration, and West European democratisation as explanatory variables in that long peace?

After the Cold War ended, the existence of nuclear weapons on both sides was not enough to stop the US from expanding NATO's borders ever eastwards towards Russia's borders, in violation of the terms on which Moscow thought Germany's reunification and the admission of united Germany into NATO had been agreed. Several Western leaders at the highest levels had assured the last Soviet leader Mikhail Gorbachev that NATO would not expand even "one inch eastward."

In 1999 Russia watched helplessly from the sidelines as its ally Serbia was dismembered by NATO warplanes that served as midwives to the birth of an independent Kosovo. But Moscow did not forget the lesson. In 2014 the nuclear equation did not stop Russia from reacting militarily to the US-backed Maidan coup in Ukraine—that displaced the pro-Moscow elected president with a Westward-looking regime—by invading eastern Ukraine and annexing Crimea.

In other words, the more or less constant US–Russia nuclear equation is irrelevant to explaining the shifting geopolitical developments. We have to look elsewhere to understand the rebalancing of

US–Soviet/Russia relations over the past several decades since the Second World War.

Myth Three: Nuclear deterrence is 100% effective

Some profess interest in nuclear weapons in order to avoid nuclear blackmail. Yet there is not one clear-cut instance of a non-nuclear state having been bullied into changing its behaviour by the overt or implicit threat of being bombed by nuclear weapons. The normative taboo against this most indiscriminately inhumane weapon ever invented is so comprehensive and robust that under no conceivable circumstance will its use against a non-nuclear state compensate for the political costs.

This is why nuclear powers have accepted defeat at the hands of non-nuclear states rather than escalate armed conflict to the nuclear level, as in Vietnam and Afghanistan. President Vladimir Putin's serial threats in connection with Ukraine did not succeed either in intimidating Kyiv into surrendering, or in preventing Western countries from providing substantial and increasingly lethal armaments to Ukraine.

According to a careful statistical analysis of 210 militarised "compellent threats" from 1918–2001 by Todd Sechser and Matthew Fuhrmann in *Nuclear Weapons and Coercive Diplomacy* (Cambridge University Press, 2017), nuclear powers succeeded in just 10 of these. Even then the presence of nuclear weapons may not have been the decisive factor compared to their general military superiority. Non-nuclear states were successful in 32% of attempts at coercion, compared to just 20% success for nuclear-armed states, and nuclear monopoly gave no greater assurance of success.

Reversing the direction of analysis, countries whose possession of the bomb is not in doubt have been subjected to attacks by non-nuclear-weapon states. The bomb did not stop Argentina from invading the UK's Falkland Islands in the 1980s, nor the Vietnamese and Afghans from fighting and defeating the US and the Soviet Union respectively.

Lacking compellent utility against non-nuclear adversaries, nuclear weapons cannot be used for defence against nuclear-armed rivals either. Their mutual vulnerability to second-strike retaliatory capability is so robust for the foreseeable future that any escalation through the nuclear threshold really would amount to mutual national suicide. Their only purpose and role, therefore, is mutual deterrence.

Yet, nuclear weapons did not stop Pakistan from occupying Kargil on the Indian side of the Line of Control in 1999, nor India from waging a limited war to retake it—an effort that cost over 1,000 lives. Nor do nuclear weapons buy immunity for North Korea. The biggest elements of caution in attacking it are its formidable conventional capability to hit the heavily populated parts of South Korea, including Seoul, and, recalling China's entry into the Korean War in 1950, anxiety about how China would respond. Pyongyang's present and prospective arsenal of nuclear weapons and the capacity to deploy and use them credibly is a distant third factor in the deterrence calculus.

If we move from historical and contemporary cases to military logic, strategists face a fundamental and unresolvable paradox in ascribing a deterrent role to the bomb. In a conflict dyad involving two nuclear-armed countries, in order to deter a conventional attack by a more powerful nuclear adversary, the weaker state must convince its stronger opponent of the ability and will to use nuclear weapons if attacked, for example by developing tactical nuclear weapons and deploying them on the forward edge of the battlefield.

If the attack does occur, however, escalating to nuclear weapons will worsen the scale of military devastation even for the side initiating nuclear strikes. Because the stronger party believes this, the existence of nuclear weapons will induce extra caution but does not guarantee immunity for the weaker party. If Mumbai or Delhi were to be hit by another major terrorist attack which India believed had Pakistan connections, the pressure for some form of retaliation could overwhelm any caution about Pakistan having nuclear weapons.

Myth Four: Nuclear deterrence is 100% safe

Against the contestable claims of utility, there is considerable evidence that the world averted a nuclear catastrophe during the Cold War, and continues to do so in the post-Cold War world, as much owing to good luck as to wise management, with the 1962 Cuban missile crisis being the most starkly graphic example.

For nuclear peace to hold, deterrence *and* fail-safe mechanisms must work every single time. For nuclear Armageddon, deterrence *or* fail-safe mechanisms need to break down only once. This is not a comforting equation. Deterrence stability depends on rational decision-makers being always in office on all sides: a dubious and not very reassuring precondition. It depends equally critically on there being no rogue launch, human error or system malfunction: an impossibly high bar in the age of Kim Jong Un, Donald Trump and Vladimir Putin.

The number of times that we have come frighteningly close to nuclear holocaust is simply staggering. On 27 October 2017 a newly-formed organisation, the Future of Life Institute, gave its inaugural "Future of Life" prize, posthumously, to one Vasili Alexandrovich Arkhipov. If you have never heard of the NGO, the prize or the laureate, not to worry: you are in good company. Yet there is a good chance neither you nor I would have been around today to read and write this were it not for Arkhipov's courage, wisdom and calmness under pressure.

The date of the prize marked the 55th anniversary of a critical incident on which the fate of the world turned during the Cuban missile crisis of October 1962. On that day, Arkhipov was a submariner on duty near Cuba in the Soviet submarine B-59. Unknown to the Americans, whose entire quarantine strategy and enforcement of the blockade was motivated by the determination to prevent Soviet nuclear weapons from being brought into and stationed in the region (the sovereign status of both Cuba and the USSR be damned), there were already more than 160 Soviet nuclear warheads present in the area and commanders had been given the authority to use them in the event of hostilities.

US forces began to drop non-lethal depth charges just to let the Soviet crews know that the Americans were aware of their presence. But of course the Soviets had no way of knowing that the American intentions were peaceful and, not unreasonably, they concluded they were witness to the start of World War III. The captain of B-59, Valentin Savitsky, and another senior officer voted to launch a 10kt nuclear-tipped missile. Savitsky said, "We're gonna blast them now! We will die, but we will sink them all—we will not become the shame of the fleet," according to files in the US National Security Archive.

Unfortunately for Savitsky but fortunately for us, the protocol required the decision to launch to be unanimous among the top three officers on board. Arkhipov vetoed the idea, thereby proving that not all Soviet vetoes are bad. The rest is history that wouldn't have been otherwise. *That's* how close we came to Armageddon in the missile crisis of 1962.

There have been numerous other examples where the world came too close for comfort to a full-fledged nuclear war:

- In November 1983, in response to NATO war games exercise Able Archer, which Moscow mistook to be real, the Soviets came close to launching a full-scale nuclear attack against the West.
- On 25 January 1995, Norway launched a scientific research rocket in its northern latitude. Because of the speed and trajectory of the powerful rocket, whose stage three mimicked a Trident sea launched ballistic missile, the Russian early warning radar system near Murmansk tagged it within seconds of launch as a possible American nuclear missile attack. Fortunately, the rocket did not mistakenly stray into Russian airspace.

- On 29 August 2007, an American B-52 bomber carrying six air-launched cruise missiles armed with nuclear warheads made an unauthorised 1,400-mile flight from North Dakota to Louisiana and was effectively absent without leave for 36 hours.
- In the one-year period to March 2015 following the 2014 Ukraine crisis, one study documented several serious and high-risk incidents.
- A 2016 Global Zero study similarly documented dangerous encounters in the South China Sea and South Asia.
- As for near misses in an accident, in January 1961, a four megaton bomb—that is, 260 times more powerful than that used at Hiroshima—was just one ordinary switch away from detonating over North Carolina when a B-52 bomber on a routine flight went into an uncontrolled spin.

This selective catalogue of misperceptions, miscalculations, near misses, and accidents underscores the message of successive international commissions that as long as any state has nuclear weapons, others will want them. As long as they exist, they will be used again someday, if not by design and intent, then through miscalculation, accident, rogue launch, or system malfunction. Any such use anywhere could spell catastrophe for the planet.

The only guarantee of zero nuclear weapons risk is to move to zero nuclear weapons possession by a carefully managed process. Proponents of nuclear weapons are the real "nuclear romantics" (Ward Wilson) who exaggerate the bombs' significance, downplay their substantial risks, and imbue them with "quasi-magical powers" also known as nuclear deterrence.

The claim that nuclear weapons could not proliferate if they did not exist is both an empirical and a logical truth. The very fact of their existence in the arsenals of nine countries is *sufficient guarantee* of their proliferation to others and, some day again, use. Conversely, nuclear disarmament is *a necessary condition* of nuclear nonproliferation.

Thus the logics of nuclear disarmament and nonproliferation are inseparable. In the Middle East, for example, it simply is not credible that Israel can be permitted to keep its unacknowledged nuclear arsenal indefinitely, while every other state can be stopped from getting the bomb in perpetuity.

The normative boundaries between conventional and nuclear, regional and global, and tactical and strategic weapons, as also between nuclear, cyber, space, and autonomous weapon systems controlled by artificial intelligence, are being blurred by technological developments. These create the risk that, in an escalating crisis, second-strike capabilities are under threat because the command, control, and communications systems could be vulnerable as conventional and nuclear capabilities get hopelessly entangled.

For example, conventional anti-satellite weapons can destroy space sensors and communications that are critical components of nuclear command-and-control systems. Although more pronounced on the Chinese and Russian sides, their potential destabilising impact on deterrence stability is also of some concern to US and allied experts.

Nuclear weapons also add significant financial cost in an ever more competitive fiscal environment. Not only is there no diminution in the need for and costs of full conventional capabilities; there are additional costs in relation to the safety and security requirements that cover the full spectrum of nuclear weapons, material, infrastructure, facilities, and personnel. In addition, as Britain and France have discovered, investment in the essentially unusable nuclear deterrent can take funds away from conventional upgrades and expansion that are actually usable in some contemporary conflict theatres.

The cataclysmically destructive potential of nuclear weapons puts a premium on secrecy and underpinned the creation and expansion of the national security state that relies on claims to technocratic expertise of the scientific-bureaucratic elite. This too was a forerunner of the rise of the biosecurity state in which national security, public health institutions, and powerful corporations in the media, social media, and pharmaceutical sectors became seamlessly fused.

From the North Atlantic to the Indo-Pacific

Reflecting the Anglo–European dominance of global scholarship, the strategic studies literature has been preoccupied with Euro–Atlantic nuclear relations. Yet a prospective Russia–NATO/US war is only one of five potential nuclear flashpoints, albeit the one with the gravest consequences. The remaining four are all in the Indo–Pacific: China-US, China-India, Korean Peninsula, and India-Pakistan.

A simple transposition of the dyadic North Atlantic frameworks and lessons to comprehend the multiplex Indo-Pacific nuclear relations is both analytically flawed and entails policy dangers for managing nuclear stability. As China and the US struggle for primacy in the vast Indo–Pacific maritime space, will they fall into what Harvard University's Graham Allison calls the "Thucydides Trap" of a 75% historical probability of armed conflict between the status quo and rising powers?

The geostrategic environment of the subcontinent had no parallel in the Cold War, with triangular shared borders among three nuclear-armed states, major territorial disputes, a history of many wars since 1947, compressed timeframes for using or losing nuclear weapons, political volatility and instability, and state-sponsored cross-border insurgency and terrorism.

In the North Atlantic nuclear rivalry, submarine-based nuclear weapons deepen strategic stability by enhancing survivability and reducing successful first-strike possibilities. By contrast, the race to attain continuous at-sea deterrence capability through nuclear-armed submarines is potentially destabilising in the Indo-Pacific because the regional powers lack well-developed operational concepts, robust and redundant command-and-control systems, and secure communications over submarines at sea.

Strategic submarines (SSBNs) are the most stabilising platform for nuclear weapons deployment for assured destruction through second-strike capability. For this to be credible, however, they must be exempted from the usual practice of demating weapons from missiles and storing them in physically dispersed locations. This too weakens the arms race suppressing and crisis stability enhancing potential of China's and India's no-first-use policies.

Conclusion

The case for nuclear weapons rests on a superstitious belief of magical Realism in the utility of the bomb and the theory of deterrence. The extreme destructiveness of nuclear weapons makes them qualitatively different in political and moral terms from other weapons, to the point of rendering them virtually unusable. Like the emperor who had no clothes, this might well be the truest explanation of why they have not been used since 1945.

The hubris and arrogance of the nuclear-armed states leaves the world exposed to the risk of sleepwalking into a nuclear disaster. Remember, people are not aware of their actions while they are sleepwalking. This is of course the key argument also with respect to lockdowns, masks, and vaccines, that their net costs and damage greatly exceed their purported benefits.

Moreover, compared to the sophistication and reliability of the command-and-control systems of the two Cold War rivals, those of some of the contemporary nuclear-armed states are dangerously frail and brittle. Each additional entrant into the nuclear club multiplies the risk of inadvertent war geometrically and these would vastly exceed the dubious and marginal security gains of possession.

The risks of nuclear weapons proliferation and use by irresponsible states, most of whom are in volatile conflict-prone regions, or by suicide terrorists, outweigh realistic security benefits. A more rational and prudent approach to reducing nuclear risks would be to actively advocate and pursue the minimisation, reductions, and elimination agendas for the short, medium, and long terms identified in the Report of the International Commission on Nuclear Non-Proliferation and Disarmament.

15: ACCOUNTABILITY AND JUSTICE

As previous chapters have documented, significant harms were done to large numbers of people in many countries by the non-pharmaceutical and pharmaceutical interventions. Not all of this, perhaps not even most of this, can be attributed to good intentions under conditions of extreme urgency and unknown science, information and data. The highest level decision-makers, analogously to people with command responsibility when crimes against humanity are committed, need to be held to account. This is important to ensure misdeeds are punished, victims are helped to achieve emotional closure, and future acts of comparable malfeasance are deterred.

Where is the accountability for Covid policy harms?[92]

Prof. Jayanta (Jay) Bhattacharya is a medical doctor (MD, Stanford), economist (PhD, Stanford) and epidemiologist (Stanford Medical School) all rolled into one, giving him a rare set of credentials to assess the multiple dimensions of Covid disease and policies. An academic with virtually no public profile before 2020, he emerged as an articulate and compelling voice against the errors and excesses of Covid policies from early 2020, culminating in co-drafting the Great Barrington Declaration (GBD) in October. He and co-authors Martin

[92] *Spectator Australia*, 8 October 2022, https://www.spectator.com.au/2022/10/where-is-the-accountability-for-covid-policy-harms/

Kulldorff (Harvard) and Sunetra Gupta (Oxford) were subjected by Anthony Fauci & Co. to a campaign to smear, discredit and "savagely take down" these "fringe epidemiologists" (Jay now proudly displays a business card describing himself as a fringe epidemiologist) that backfired spectacularly. The GBD is creeping up to a million signatures, including 63,000 public health scientists and medical practitioners. Jay's twitter followers have ballooned to 226,000 [443,900 in June 2023]: not bad for a fringe medico.

Jay was in Australia for a week recently with a punishing schedule of meetings and talks in Melbourne (Lockdown Ground Zero) and Sydney. I had the honour and pleasure of spending three days with him and taking part in a memorable evening panel on the 22nd in front of a sold out audience of 500 enthusiastic good folks. They rose in united adulation when informed he had charged no lecture fee beyond travel costs for his talks in Australia.

Jay was often asked: "Tell us about your critical take, as an epidemiologist, on lockdown." The implied question to me is: "You're no epidemiologist. Why should we listen to you." As a consequence of the experience of playing tag team with him, I concluded that my contributions to Covid policy debates since early 2020 have come not despite a lack of medical credentials but because of my particular background in conflict analysis and experience in the world of UN diplomacy. Let me explain.

In 2001, following heated controversy among UN member states over NATO's "humanitarian intervention" in Kosovo in 1999, an international commission formulated a new principle called the responsibility to protect. Former foreign minister Gareth Evans and I were the two principal writers and promoters of this concept which was unanimously adopted as the organising principle for the UN to respond to mass atrocities to help victims trapped inside sovereign state borders, with a careful balance between the permissive "licence" and the restrictive "leash" function of all laws and norms. The accompanying requirements for preventing mass atrocities and rebuilding afterwards highlighted the need for respecting universal human rights, embedding them in structures and institutions of national governance, recognising the importance of not demonising and "othering" different groups, and refraining from using controlled media to propagate enmity between "clean" and "unclean" groups.

I have argued previously about the abundance of early warnings on the range of grave harms that were likely to result from population-wide severe lockdown measures. The warnings came from established, credible and reputable bodies in the UN system (Unicef, World Food Programme), civil society (Oxfam), and intergovernmental organisations like the IMF and World Bank. India alone is feared to have created a 375 million-strong "pandemic generation" of children up to age 14 who are likely to suffer long-lasting impacts like increased child mortality, being underweight and stunted, and educational and work-productivity reversals. It's hard to see how these predicted harms do not constitute mass atrocity crimes.

If so, a third set of considerations arise. The responsibility to protect addresses the need to protect victims of atrocities. The twin principle of international criminal justice speaks to the need to punish the perpetrators: identify them, prosecute them and, if convicted, jail them. Hence Bishop Desmond Tutu's comment that, as a principal architect of the Iraq War, Tony Blair should be in the dock at The Hague, not on a podium in Africa.

The authors and enforcers of pandemic management policies and interventions, that have inflicted enduring health, mental health, civil liberties, social and economic damage, must be held to account. This is the one issue where Jay and I parted company in our discussions. He doesn't think vengeance serves any constructive purpose. I believe accountability is important firstly to punish, as distinct from seeking revenge, acts of harmful malfeasance when existing accumulated knowledge, science and pandemic preparedness plans were dumped in favour of authoritarian models imported from China.

Second, and listening to the reactions from the 500 people in Melbourne that unforgettable evening, it's going to be impossible to attain emotional closure, that alone can enable us as a community to move on, without an open and credible accounting. Perhaps most importantly, the best and most effective guarantee of "Never Again," a goal that Jay spoke passionately about, is to hold to account the authors of lockdown—a euphemism for the wholesale locking up of entire populations under house arrest even if healthy and not accused, let alone convicted, of any crime—and vaccine apartheid. Absent accountability, we could experience cycles of rinse and repeat.

Are lockdown zealots incapable of introspection?[93]

Writing in *The Atlantic* on 31 October, Brown University economist Emily Oster penned a pre-emptive plea for amnesty for Covid-policy hardliners. Why? Because they were all well-intentioned and their pronouncements rested on benign ignorance.

Judging by the numerous responses in print and social media and online commentary, the viral article lit the fuse on widespread, simmering but still raw anger. To many it suggests the lockdown zealots are incapable of introspection, of accepting culpability. Instead, they just want to move on to the next excuse to unleash blanket authoritarian control all over again.

Jessica Hockett has coined the word "Osterism" to describe the attitude of forgive, forget and move on from earlier finger-wagging, abusive and vile taunts because we didn't know but meant well. Abracadabra. Puff! it's all gone. "Twas but a bad dream, time to wake up and get going for the day's activities.

Sorry, but the whole Covid debacle needs to be turned instead into a parable with a moral for the ages, to show how easy it is for a

[93] Brownstone Institute, 13 November 2022, https://brownstone.org/articles/are-lockdown-zealots-incapable-of-introspection/

civilised society to be terrorised into believing blatant falsehoods and turn on one another with shocking savagery.

Covid malpractices were a moral failing

"Getting something wrong wasn't a moral failing." Oh, but it was, professor, and your lot owns it. In fact, considering sheer numbers, the society-wide breadth of enforcement measures, the depth of state intrusion into personal choices and economic activities, the magnitude of unethical edicts and practices, and the worldwide scope of the policies: this could well be the single biggest moral failing in the history of modern Western civilisation.

Oster, who endorsed vaccine mandates for universities and workers, says that in 2020–21, people couldn't have known that transmission is rare outdoors, masks are not very good at blocking viruses, and kids are a low-risk group for viral spread. Except these were mostly the conventional wisdom and departures from them was evidence-free radical experimentation. All those who pointed out these inconvenient facts were hounded from the public square by the baying mob that now wants to erase recent history.

Uh-uh, not so fast. Those responsible for our health and welfare chose to terrorise and harm us instead. There can be no closure until they've paid a price. Urging amnesty without admitting to wrongdoing is yet more gaslighting. When she noticed the harm that school closures were causing to her kids, Oster repositioned herself as a school moderate and tugged at our sympathy chords because she was called a "teacher killer" and a "*génocidaire.*" But is this really equivalent to "getting your head kicked in by riot police because you had the temerity to protest against indefinite population-wide house arrest?" asks Eugyppius.

Emily Burns speculates that Oster's primary motivation might have been to stop the bleeding of votes from Democrats in the midterms among educated suburban women who were infuriated by school closures and being called terrorists for wanting to influence school curricula.

A *Wall Street Journal* poll on 2 November indicated a 27-point shift since August to put support for Republicans ahead by 15% among suburban white women who make up one-fifth of the electorate. No deal, says Burns.

The midterm results did not quite work out quite as predicted for the Republicans. Nevertheless, Governor Ron DeSantis's resounding victory is surely a vindication of his hardline scepticism on lockdowns and pro-choice policy on vaccines. Florida has emerged as the state where not just woke, but also lockdown and vaccine dogma go to die.

Age-stratified Covid risks were exaggerated and lockdown harms downplayed

Check out this list of resources from Brownstone Institute of just how much we knew already in early 2020. *Spectator Australia* has gained a worldwide reputation for the scepticism expressed right from the start by several authors. As early as 7 May 2020, a mainstream outlet like the BBC published a chart showing the risk of dying with Covid closely tracking the "normal" distribution of death rates stratified by age.

In a recent review of several studies, John Ioannidis and colleagues conclude that the age-stratified survival rate of healthy under 70s infected by Covid-19 *before vaccines became available* is a staggering 99.905%, and furthermore, under 70s make up 94% of the world's population or about 7.3bn people. For children and adolescents under 20, the survival rate is 99.9997%.

Experts from Oxford University's Centre for Evidence Based Medicine used subsequent actual data to back-calculate a survival rate of 99.9992% for under-20s in Britain. Official data from the Office for National Statistics for 1990–2020 show that the age-standardised mortality rate (deaths per 100,000 people) in England and Wales in 2020 was lower in 19 of the previous 30 years. Remember, this is before vaccines.

The doomsday model from Imperial College London's Neil Ferguson in March 2020 that precipitated lockdowns estimated the survival rate to be twenty times lower.

Given his past record, why did anyone in authority give Colonel Chicken Little a platform to propagate "The sky is falling" yet again? Because of the criminal advice of health officials and decisions by relevant authorities, kids were masked for hours, vaccinated and deschooled. Forgive and forget the harms done to our precious children? Not in my name, thank you very much.

Early in the pandemic, reputable organisations warned about the extensive range and scale of harms. Members of the "we meant well and did the best we could under uniquely difficult circumstances" brigade have memory-holed what was known, thrown a cloak over the reliable data from the *Diamond Princess* cruise ship, ignored the taunts of mass murderers and granny killers that were hurled at nonconforming governments like Sweden and Florida, are studiously silent about their embarrassing embrace of the extremely dubious claims from China, and are in complete denial on their shrill denunciation of sceptical voices and the vicious, largely successful efforts to censor, humiliate and fire them. This included highly accomplished doctors and research scientists, as detailed in a recent article in *Minerva* by one Australian and four Israeli authors.

Would amnesty seekers like to go back in time, do some research on the scepticism expressed right from the early days, and then tell us again: which major ineffectual and harmful lockdown consequence was *not* predicted?

Are we there yet? Not quite

The policies are not all behind us. Many are ongoing. Several universities still require booster shots as a condition of campus or in-person classroom entry. People continue to suffer serious vaccine reactions that are studiously ignored by drug regulators.

There's no guarantee the whole sorry saga will not be repeated. To the contrary, there are indications that next time round, governments will move straight into the tried and tested measures knowing just how easy it is to manipulate public support for the most draconian edicts and enforcement actions.

For example, on 2 September, the European Commission published a plan to prepare for the return of Covid over the coming autumn and winter. The suite of measures—sorry, "set of tools"—include mask mandates, vaccination for school children, a EU Digital Covid Certificate, lockdowns, and the creation of a legally binding global pandemic treaty with a "reinforced WHO at its centre" in a strengthened "global health architecture."

The tactics developed during Covid to psychologically manipulate people's beliefs and coerce compliance with policy diktats are already being used by some governments, says Stephen McMurray, for the climate alarmism narrative.

Vaccine zealots like a columnist with the *Australian* persevere with their campaign of abuse and vilification toward *Covid* vaccine hesitants as "anti-vaxxers." Writing in the *Los Angeles Times* in January this year, Michael Hiltzik argued that it may be "a little ghoulish to celebrate or exult in the deaths of vaccine opponents," who received "their just desserts," but it is necessary to teach them the much-needed lesson that vaccines severely reduce hospitalisation, mortality and infection spread.

Tell us again why he deserves an amnesty? Instead, how about, as the lockdown bill comes due with major cost of living pressures and inevitable tax rises, we impose a specific levy on all those who clamoured for restrictions, closures and mandates?

In country after country, including Australia, cumulative excess deaths in the 2020–22 Covid era are running above pre-Covid averages. As the MSM slowly begins to report on this phenomenon, it's starting to raise the possibility that the measures to control Covid may indeed be causing more deaths than were saved, especially in the less vulnerable younger age groups.

But they still shy away from questioning the possible role of vaccines themselves in contributing to the elevated death toll. Lockdowns caused cascading economic disasters around the world and substantial economic damage has lasting and severe adverse consequences for public health.

Policy advisers and governments were wilfully blind to the reality that national wealth is an essential enabler of a first-world health infrastructure and services. They covered up their cussedness by vilifying lockdown critics as wanting to prioritise the economy over lives.

No rational public health harm-benefit analysis could justify the lockdown restrictions and mandatory mask and vaccine requirements. Not before 2020, not in 2020–22, not now. Rooted neither in science nor data but in smug self-righteous groupthink and assumptions-driven abstract modelling, the set of coercive restrictions and mandates made a metaphorical bonfire of hard-won and cherished liberties and freedoms.

All the institutions designed to check arbitrary abuses of power failed us miserably, from parliament and the judiciary to human rights machinery, media and professional associations.

The precautionary principle was flipped to enact policies that we knew would inflict harms, with inadequate knowledge of any positive good they would deliver. The self-aggrandising public health clerisy gravely damaged the common good. David Bell lists several conventional understandings that were upended with Covid and amount to a dozen little lies that together made up the Big Lie, ranging from masks to natural immunity via infection, misinforming the public, and abandoning quality adjusted life years as a key metric and informed consent.

The instantly-forged mass consensus on Covid policy has delivered a sicker, poorer and unhappier population in several countries. There is no better examplar than the "duplicitous" and furiously "backpedalling" Anthony Fauci of the pathology of denialism in hindsight, from lockdowns to masks, school closures and vaccines, plus the vicious efforts to crush dissent and destroy the professional reputation of critics. His early statements indicate he did know the existing state of knowledge that natural immunity through infection is useful in building herd immunity, masks in community settings are pointless, and lockdowns are incompatible with liberal democratic practices.

Not just individuals but public health institutions too resorted to ethically questionable gaslighting, half-truths and dissembling.[94] Explaining why Americans no longer trust the CDC, Dr Marty Makary from the Johns Hopkins School of Medicine points to the example of the CDC strongly recommending booster shots for all 24mn 5-11 year old Americans, despite a lack of outcomes data.

Philip Klein, commentary editor of the *Washington Examiner*, wrote confidently on 30 April 2020 that school shutdowns are intensely damaging to society and younger students in particular should be back at school. And Sweden did keep its primary schools open throughout.

Lockdown scepticism was foresight, not hindsight

Thus the prevailing uncertainty and lack of knowledge doesn't wash with the benefit of hindsight.

Professing ignorance now cannot excuse the brutality and severity of pandemic measures:

- Wholesale house arrest of healthy populations, massive transfer of wealth from the poor and the working class to the mega-rich while shielding the laptop class from any economic pain;

[94] On 20 June 2023, Bhattacharya tweeted newly released email under freedom of information access from Rochelle Walensky, the now departing head of CDC, from 30 January 2021 early in her tenure, showing that she, the head of the National Institutes of Health Francis Collins, and Fauci were all aware then, a month after the vaccination campaign began, of the reality of breakthrough infections. Yet they continued to push vaccine mandates anyway. For example Walensky said on MSNBC TV on 29 March 2021:"Vaccinated people do not carry the virus, don't get sick," and "it's not just in the clinical trials but it`s also in real world data."

- Violations of bodily integrity, "my body my choice," and informed consent principles, the suspension of the right to peaceful protest, the spread of the surveillance, administrative and biosecurity state;
- The transformation of citizens into snitches who boasted of reporting colleagues and neighbours for minor infractions of draconian and often confusing rules;
- The treatment of people as germ-ridden disease carriers and biohazards, the sheer dehumanization of people who just asked to be left alone;
- The cruelty of denying final goodbyes to dying parents and grandparents and the emotional closure of full service funerals;
- The state diktats of whom we could meet, how many, where and for how long; what we could buy, during which hours and from where;
- The theft of children's education and economic security by loading them with debt decades into the future;
- None of this really happened and if it did, it was all so long ago and we did it all for your own good, cross my heart.

Forgive and forget the harms done to our precious children? Hell no.

We were treated as disease-carrying vermin, as selfish ignoramuses, as right-wing nutjobs (but helping Big Pharma, Big Tech and Big Government is progressive?—go figure), while they corrupted science into a belief system with an infallible purity test. Having given us no quarter, they shouldn't expect any in return.

Seeing as how they copied Chinese style totalitarian edicts and enforcement, how about a Chinese-style public spectacle of self-criticisms as penance? Would that punishment fit the crime?

Covid crimes and amnesty, accountability and justice[95]

In the last section, I explained why Emily Oster's amnesty call for lockdown, mask and vaccine zealots has stirred up white-hot rage.

Figure 15.1: US opinion poll on Covid amnesty, November 2022

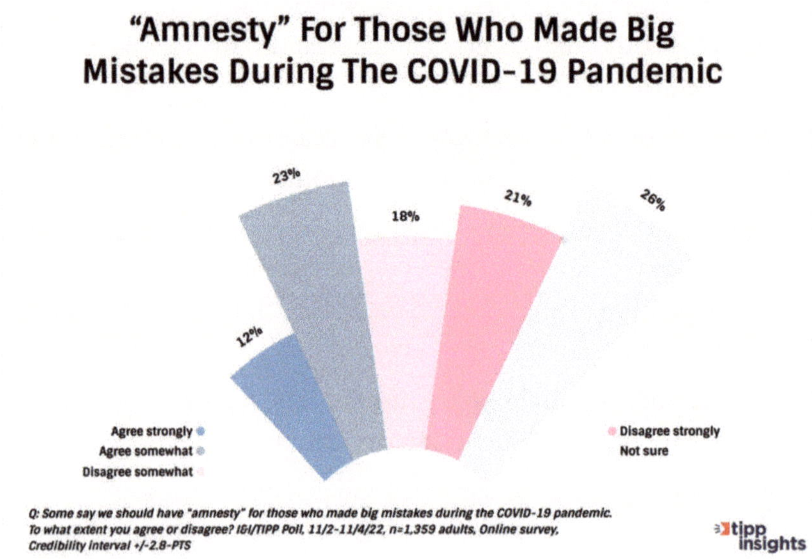

Source: TIPP insights, 14 November 2022

An I&I/TIPP Poll conducted on November 2–4 found 39-35 majority opposition to amnesty (Figure 15.1), and the stronger sentiment was negative by a lopsided 21-12 margin. While Democrats supported amnesty 48-30%, Republicans and Independents opposed it 49-27%. Support for amnesty dropped dramatically by age, from

[95] Brownstone Institute, 9 December 2022, https://brownstone.org/articles/covid-crimes-amnesty-accountability-justice/

52% among 25-44 year olds to just 17% among 65 and older. The age split is interesting,.

The victims of casual cruelty, capricious public health diktats and enforcement brutality are owed justice. But what type of justice? It might be helpful to look at examples from the theory and practice of international criminal justice. The sense of justice, fairness and equity is deeply ingrained in human beings.

Correct that. It's also deeply ingrained in some animal species. In the famous fairness experiments by primatologist Frans de Waal, capuchin monkeys were trained to trade pebbles for cucumber slices. When the monkey in the adjacent cage was given the more valued prize of a grape, the first threw its cucumber "reward" out of the cage in anger. Subsequently, even the second monkey refused to accept a grape until its companion was also given the same reward. This segment of the full TED talk by de Waal in 2011 has been viewed 22 million times, has been liked by 243,000 and commented on by more than 15,000. The full talk has nearly 5.5 million views.

The justice sentiment is expressed in collective norms and, in a general sense, in laws. If the dominant perception is that law mostly conforms to notions of fairness and justice, the odd anomaly will not pose a threat to the system of law. But if the opposite perception takes hold, and law is seen to have marched off on a tangent from justice, then the system of law—and the principle of a community based on the rule of law—will be brought into disrepute and collapse under the weight of illegitimacy.

That's the risk we run. The "deplorables" were arrested, cuffed, fined, tackled roughly to the ground, and had rubber bullets fired at them and assets frozen. If those responsible for these acts of criminality face no legal consequences, will faith in the rule of law and justice system survive undamaged?

Transitional justice

The purely juridical approach to justice can trap and suspend communities in the prism of past hatreds. Truth commissions, a halfway house between victors' justice and collective amnesia, take a victim-centred approach. They helped to establish a historical record and contributed to memorializing defining epochs in the national histories of Chile and South Africa.

The latter case is especially instructive because the apartheid state was an international *cause célèbre* for a long time. South Africa opted for a statutory body set up by parliament, not merely a presidential commission. The Truth and Reconciliation Commission (TRC) had subpoena powers that carried the carrot of full amnesty but also the stick of criminal prosecution. It held public hearings under shady trees in villages as well as in churches (with the attendant symbolism of repentance and forgiveness) that were televised to a global audience. For many victims it was the first opportunity to tell their stories. For 30 months the TRC was *the* national story: compelling, gripping, poignant—and cathartic.

Rwanda's version of transitional justice operated through the local *gacaca* system of people's courts, whose overriding goal was not to determine guilt but to restore harmony and social order. Mozambique also offers successful examples of communal healing techniques.

All three cases represented deliberate efforts through social and political channels to escape cycles of retributive violence coming out of decades of tumultuous political conflicts congealed around communal identity. Their record of bringing closure to legacies of systematic savagery in deeply conflicted societies is superior to that of institutions of international criminal justice.

Justice has many more roles to play beyond simply bringing wrongdoers to account: acknowledging the suffering of victims, educating the public, and deterring future criminal atrocities. Allied and

Axis powers from the Second World War are at peace not despite the Nuremberg and Tokyo tribunals, but also because justice cleared the path to reconciliation.

It's not possible to secure lasting peace without bringing criminal wrongdoers to account. However, these are not solely legal decisions but profoundly political choices with complex trade-offs.

Criminal trials for the architects, truth commission for the rest

How does all this apply to the Covid era?

There are indeed parallels to bitter civil wars and sectarian conflicts. We witnessed policy extremism, enforcement of tough lockdown measures and mask-cum-vaccine mandates with excessive use of force and instant hefty fines, and deeply fractured groups of populations where once had existed broadly cohesive societies. Families were torn apart and denied the opportunity to grieve together over the lonely death of loved ones, many friendships ruptured, and mom and pop businesses shuttered.

We need, firstly, criminal accountability for the top leaders and officials responsible for perpetrating the most egregious Covid policy outrages. Neither a Senate nor a Royal Commission in Australia and the UK, nor a presidential commission or Congressional investigation in the US, is likely to prove "fit for purpose." The duration of the emergency measures, the scale of damage, and the depth of trauma is much too great for that.

In addition, we also need the equivalent of a TRC for the bigger cohort of high profile "health influencers" of epidemiologists and medical experts, public intellectuals, CEOs of public sector organizations and private sector companies who imposed vaccine mandates, and media commentators who gave full rein to their inner bullies to shame, vilify, ostracise and otherwise traumatise all who dared to think for themselves and refused to go along in order to get along.

AHPRA: Public health watchdog, Big Pharma lapdog, or drug enabler[96]

A doctor dies by suicide

Mei-Khing Loo is a former practice manager whose 43-year old obstetrician-gynaecologist husband of 21 years, Dr Yen-Yung Yap, died of suicide in 2020 while under investigation by the Australian Health Practitioner Regulation Agency (AHPRA). He left behind three young children. Another speaker intimately familiar with the case explained how Dr Yap had his livelihood destroyed for having delivered two babies by suction rather than forceps in Adelaide in 2015 and 2019. There was no complaint to AHPRA, no litigation, no damage to the babies. In both cases "subgaleal haemorrhage" was suspected but never diagnosed and the babies were discharged and went home within five days. An internal audit resulted in an AHPRA notification.

Four doctors who knew Dr Yap told his legal team he had done nothing wrong in either birth. But the AHPRA-nominated expert (in gestational diabetes) claimed forceps should have been used and AHPRA imposed restrictions that effectively made it impossible for Dr Yap to continue his practice. "The ongoing harassment from AHPRA and the Medical Board will make me mentally and emotionally traumatised and professionally unable to care for my patients, and financially unable to care for our kids," he wrote in a letter to his wife shortly before his suicide.

Mei-Khing addressed a full audience in Sydney on 3 May about her grief, pain, and unsated anger, through bouts of sobbing and tears. Her speech was passionate, resonant, and yet also in the end inspiring, with a call to maintain the rage against the callous regulator.

---

[96] *Brownstone Journal*, 17 May 2025, https://brownstone.org/articles/ahpra-public-health-watchdog-big-pharma-lapdog-or-drug-enabler/

Only a change in the culture and institutional set-up of the regulator to make it more compassionate can best ensure that Dr Yap did not die in vain, she said. She was the only one of the roughly two dozen speakers at the conference to receive a standing ovation from the audience that had listened rapt in pin-drop silence to her presentation.

It also put in perspective another speaker who referenced an insensitive and "flippant" comment from a former Medical Board of Australia chair: "These doctors who are getting all stressed about a clearly frivolous complaint [to AHPRA] should really go and learn how to manage their stress a bit better" (In the series of podcasts from the Australian Society of Anaesthetists, Episode 84, 4 December 2023, at around the 29:40 mark).

Mei-Khing is the human face of some alarming statistics on health professionals' lack of confidence in AHPRA. According to Kara Thomas, Secretary of the Australian Medical Professionals Society, in a survey for AMPS 82.6% of healthcare professionals said that AHPRA lacks fairness and transparency in handling complaints and 78.5% reported unfair treatment at its hands because of a "guilty until proven innocent" approach to investigating complaints.

This is hardly surprising. In March 2023, AHPRA released the results of its own study on the distressing impacts of Australia's regulatory complaints process on doctors. The study resulted in a peer-reviewed article on 26 September 2023 in the *International Journal for Quality in Health Care*, an Oxford University Press journal. It's worth noting that the study team included Tonkin and AHPRA CEO Martin Fletcher, along with six other AHPRA staff. The study covered the four-year period 2018–2021 inclusive. Its major findings included the shocking fact that 20 healthcare practitioners involved in a regulatory process over the four-year period had committed or attempted suicide or self-harm resulting in 16 deaths, of which 12 were confirmed suicides and the other four were deemed likely suicides based on the information available. Few if any of the 20 practitioners were being investigated for a complaint regarding their clinical performance.

'The Misdeeds of AHPRA" conference

Adapting a popular saying against teachers, Dr Robert Malone wrote recently in the *Brownstone Journal*: "Those who can, do. Those who can't, regulate." An impressive number of health practitioners gathered for the day-long conference in Sydney on "The Misdeeds of AHPRA" on 3 May. The conference was oversubscribed, with many late registrants having to be turned away. Surprisingly, or perhaps not, no one from AHPRA seemed to be present although they had been invited.

In Australia, registered health practitioners across 16 professions are regulated by AHPRA and 15 National Boards as part of a national, multi-professional regulatory scheme. The goal is to streamline and standardise the regulatory system to ensure consistency, high quality, and national standards while protecting the public against medical malpractice and misconduct.

Driven by the profit-maximising motive of the pharmaceutical industry and the capture of lawmakers, health bureaucrats and regulators by lobbyists, the public health sector today is guilty of medicalising ordinary human suffering and pathologising the natural life cycles of human beings, including ageing. The entire system is built to put and keep people on medication, from the cradle to the grave. No one dies of old age any more. My GP would not accept, because the official form could not code, old age as the cause of death of my parents. I had to mention a specific cause that could be inputted for the computer to accept the answer.

One speaker listed the big criminal fines on Big Pharma that total $123 billion (unspecified but probably US currency) in just this century. Internal pharma documents confirm that they retain ownership and control of studies that they sponsor and that the purpose of the data collected is to support marketing of their product. They suppress adverse events data, cherry pick data on benefits, remunerate researchers generously but don't permit them to control use of data, draw up plans to influence regulatory agencies and health bureaucrats, liaise with media, and expand the market for their product through "disease-mongering" strategies. In this context, too many medical and scientific journals, especially those sponsored by the industry, are tainted and in effect an extension of the marketing arm of the pharmaceutical industry.

Over the course of the day, it became clear that we were in the midst of a roomful of people who had paid a price—some a small price, others a heavier price, and a few the ultimate price: financial, professional, and personal (strain on family, suspicions on the part of friends and colleagues, deteriorating health, toll on mental health). Yet all they had tried to do, in their opinion, was to stand up for patient safety and welfare as their primary, indeed overriding duty of care.

The conference was convened by AMPS and the Australian Doctors Federation. The discussions ranged widely over just what had happened, how it had all been possible, and what institutional safeguards can be recreated to avoid a repetition of the horrors of unscientific, unethical, and deeply corrosive health policy and practices.

An outsider to the healthcare profession is struck by the extraordinary complexity of the public healthcare provider and regulatory system. Little wonder that it's become a broken system in need of urgent repair or replacement. There has been a slow but steady shift from patient-centric care based on physicians' judgment and informed patient consent to protocol-governed compliance with rules and regulations set by bureaucrats. This has had the consequence and may indeed have been motivated by the desire to protect politicians and health bureaucrats, not the patients and certainly not the doctors.

The Covid legacy hangs heavy

The organisers in their introduction emphasised the importance of engaging in the conversation in a spirit of open dialogue in the hope of effecting positive change. But they did note that this would be in contrast to the behaviour of the regulator during the pandemic. The broad consensus among speakers and participants was that patient care suffered during the Covid years. Principles of good medical practice (non-maleficence or first do no harm, beneficence or do good, justice meaning equitable access to healthcare, individual autonomy, and personal agency as the basis for informed patient consent) were violated.

During the Covid years the cadre of public health technocrats deployed a lethal combination of fear and moralism to foment mass hysteria that overrode existing checks on their authority and rode roughshod over safeguards and liberties to gather in even more power to themselves. Yet, many official claims were either known from the start or subsequently shown to be at odds with the scientific evidence:

- Covid-19 could only have started in the Wuhan wet markets v. plausibility of Wuhan lab origin;
- Covid-19 kills healthy children, adolescents, and young v. negligible mortality of these cohorts;
- mRNA is broken down in minutes and doesn't pose long-term safety issues v. mRNA and spike protein detected in blood months and possibly years after injection;
- mRNA and adenoviral vectors are not gene therapies and required only the usual levels of regulatory scrutiny v. they were developed as gene therapies and should have received more rigorous scrutiny;
- mRNA vaccines contain minimal DNA contamination v. they were heavily contaminated and had potentially lethal side effects;
- Covid-19 vaccines prevent infection and community transmission v. they prevent neither infection nor transmission.

How many of us experienced being otherised while walking outdoors sans mask, with passers-by crossing to the lighted side of the street to escape from the vector of disease spread that any uncovered face symbolised? The arrival and mandating of Covid vaccines crystallised the moral landscape with even sharper clarity and bled over into a class bias that persists to this day.

For children especially the risk of severe illness or death from Covid is very slight. The risks of serious reactions to vaccines are higher. Protection against risk of reinfection is at least as robust and may last significantly longer for children who are infected but not vaccinated compared to the Covid-naïve who are vaccinated. The long-term effects of Covid vaccines are unknown. In the absence of other known treatments, existing antiviral inflammatory drugs with established safety profiles could and should have been repurposed to treat Covid-19.

Every one of these statements is contestable and subject to revision as the databank grows and more studies are published, but not one is so implausible as to be summarily dismissed.

In these circumstances, for health bureaucrats and regulators to claim a monopoly on scientific truth is just not good enough. The effort to shut down legitimate debates on pain of excommunication from the medical profession represents a clear and present danger to public health. I certainly have more confidence in my consultant's professional advice based on training, qualifications, experience, and knowledge of my medical history, free of pressures to conform to the zeitgeist from bureaucrats and regulators, the latter often with questionable links to industry. Those of us without medical credentials arouse understandable scepticism towards our critiques. This makes it all the more imperative not to silence medical professionals but to welcome and encourage contestable policy recommendations from them.

In recent times American and British authorities have admitted to the lack of any scientific basis for such mandatory lockdown-era measures as the two metre/six foot distance rule and school closures. Why did the Australian authorities adopt the rule? Did they have independent scientific advice to justify it or were they guilty of herd behaviour in mimicking what Europe, Britain, and America were doing?

We looked in vain for the emergence of an Australian equivalent of Anders Tegnell. Sweden's state epidemiologist showed remarkable courage of scientific convictions in standing against the herd and provided the world with the most instructive control group of all against the anti-scientific idiocy of lockdowns. In an interview with *Nature* early in the pandemic on 21 April 2020, Tegnell explained that the sole basis for the tough love of lockdowns was epidemiological modelling:

> *Closedown, lockdown, closing borders — nothing has a historical scientific basis .... We have looked at a number of European Union countries to see whether they have published any analysis of the effects of these measures before they were started and we saw almost none.*

AHPRA also has structural and operational links with the World Health Organisation (WHO). As a designated Collaborating Centre, AHPRA partners with WHO to promote best practice in health workforce regulation and promote access to quality health care, including by capacity building in other countries. More concerningly, AHPRA supports global regulatory capacity, implements WHO programs, and aligns with international (that is, not just national) priorities. Yet, whenever challenged, both WHO and AHPRA reject the claim that this dilutes national autonomy.

Practitioner concerns about AHPRA

The protracted crisis in Australia's medical regulatory system has developed over more than a decade. Every Australian is directly affected, either as a consumer of healthcare and/or as one of the 900,000 healthcare professionals. Practitioners have concerns regarding the judgment, consistency, proportionality, accountability, and independence of AHPRA as Australia's medical regulator. They believe its flaws and failures put at risk the integrity of Australia's healthcare system and the medical autonomy of doctors.

Two-tier justice meted out by AHPRA is indicated in several examples where serious misconduct or bad practice that harmed patients resulted in a mild slap of the wrist, whereas conduct that departs from the approved narrative, even when no patient has suffered harm, entangles the doctor in a costly and high-stress investigation that can involve suspension of the right to practice medicine for extended periods while the investigation proceeds at a leisurely pace.

In the complaints-driven system, AHPRA's KPI effectively seems to be not patient safety and welfare, but the number of doctors taken down. They demand moral purity of doctors, but exempt themselves from the same requirement. Ditto transparency and independent external scrutiny. They are meant to protect patient safety and promote patient welfare, but destroy the doctors on whom patients rely for safe medical care. "Independence" of the regulator in practice has been corrupted into meaning that they are not answerable to anyone else. They review and clear themselves whenever accused of overreach and responsibility for harming doctors. The system is durable and resilient because it allows governments to disclaim responsibility for the regulator's decisions, washing their hands Pontius Pilate-like for the fate of doctors harmed by their aloofness and callousness.

Notifications to alert AHPRA and the Boards to concerns about a registered health practitioner's performance, conduct, or health are central to the public protection objective. However, practitioners have many concerns about the prevalence and management of "vexatious" notifications that are disproportionately stressful and distressing. In particular, said one speaker, "AHPRA has weaponised anonymous complaints, to allow the process to be the punishment, without the need for proof." Several pointed to the potential for targeting doctors without supporting evidence by an AHPRA that takes an adversarial stance against practitioners under investigation, the virtually unlimited scope for investigations, the silencing of practitioners, and the fear-based compliance by practitioners.

Sometimes AHPRA tries to have it both ways. One speaker put up a slide that quoted a position paper from AHPRA and National Boards on 9 March 2021. It warned doctors, on pain of prosecution by AHPRA, not to promote anti-vaccination statements and health advice, and not to advise patients against Covid vaccination. Yet, the same guidance also required all health practitioners "to use their professional judgment and the best available evidence" in their practice of medicine. Another speaker cited examples of the medical literature often publishing contradictory conclusions drawn on vaccine safety and efficacy from study of the same data, for example in the *New England Journal of Medicine* and *Vaccine*.

Health practitioners particularly resent the two-tier justice which doesn't deploy the same process and standards of evidence for complaints levelled at AHPRA and the Boards. Given the undeniable reality that AHPRA investigations can cause harms that range from minor to serious, a key question is: How to hold regulatory bodies like AHPRA accountable for *their* actions? Who will watch the watchdogs?

A two-year review of the notifications framework by the National Health Practitioner Ombudsman Richelle McCausland on 9 December 2024 noted the tension between the function of AHPRA and Boards to ensure patient safety while also ensuring that practitioners "are treated fairly and not placed under undue stress." Her report acknowledged concerns that the complaints notifications process can be vexatious and "is being "weaponised" to harm practitioners." She made 17 recommendations to better resolve the tension between patient safety concerns and practitioners' rights to due process and their welfare.

A Queensland Supreme Court judgment on 13 December 2024 held that an extraordinary pandemic such as Covid-19 does not abrogate doctors" rights to "procedural fairness' before "an unbiassed tribunal," nor extend the Medical Board's "regulatory role to include protection of government and regulatory agencies from political criticism.'

Quo Vadis? The government, our enemy

There seemed to be broad agreement among the speakers and participants that the "subjugation" of the medical profession under AHPRA is failing both society at large as well as the healthcare professionals who come under its jurisdiction. It seems structurally and operationally unable to lift safety standards and health outcomes. To this end doctors owe a duty to patients to overcome fear, become strong, and unite against the budding tyranny of AHPRA.

To reverse the loss of proportionality and independence, AHPRA should be returned to being a registration and accreditation body. It should terminate its status as a WHO collaborating centre. Doctors must unite to defend informed consent, clinical discretion, and the sanctity of doctor-patient relationship. This can only come about if and when doctors, patients, and the public join forces to push back government intrusions into the clinic.

Many speakers and members of the audience raised important questions on where we go from where we are. Should Australia revert to state-based regulators or stay with a national regulator? In the US the system is chiefly state-based. In Canada, it operates mainly at the national level. This may be a false binary choice. The principle of subsidiarity would embrace both levels of regulation.

A question that arises with respect to any institution or bureaucracy that gradually descends into dysfunctionality is should it be reformed or abolished and replaced? Whatever the answer, advocates must understand the importance of framing the issue. In particular, their remarks and recommendations have to be patient-centric, and not focus on doctors' privileges and perks. Equally, they must articulate the key foundational principles like integrity, independence, professionalism, competence, transparency, informed consent, and scientific accountability. In addition, they need to explain why these matter for the health and integrity of the registration and accreditation system so that it can ensure the highest level of patient care.

The pathology of regulatory excess is more widespread and generalised than just the medical sector. Because the conference was focussed narrowly on the misdeeds of AHPRA, there was no linkage made to the broader societal and political trends that have resulted in the growth of the administrative, surveillance, and regulatory state. Quasi-autonomous NGOs (Quangos) are supposedly independent bodies that are nevertheless set up, wholly or partly funded, and appointed by governments. They have been delegated some legislative and some judicial functions that circumvent the formal machinery of government and end up exercising de facto governmental powers without any responsibility for the consequences of their actions, no clear lines of accountability, and seemingly unanswerable to anyone.

Elected politicians and unelected judges alike have seen their powers shift to unelected and unaccountable technocrats. AHPRA is part of that institutional landscape. Australian doctors as a class are among the victims of that power grab. Many—but not nearly enough—brave souls who stood up to AHPRA and other organisations in the brotherhood of medical regulators paid a heavy price in the form of censure, deregistration, and loss of professional jobs and status.

The uncontrolled proliferation of Quangos has unmoored the state from its democratic anchor and made it distant from the people. Increasingly, the state neither reflects our needs and aspirations nor responds to our concerns. More and more people are waking up to the reality of the administrative state that has slowly but surely captured almost all key institutions and is stealthily strangulating democracy. This is a major explanation for the success of Nigel Farage's Reform UK party in England's local elections on 1 May.

Key to the reforms will be rebalancing the doctor-regulator relationship in the boardroom, on the one hand, and re-sacralising the doctor-patient relationship in the clinic, on the other. And establishing a better balance between patient safety, doctors' rights and welfare, and regulatory reach. If the leviathan is to be defeated, the resistance will have to be much more broad-based than each sector taking on bits of the state apparatus piecemeal.

The question addressed in this article to Australia's medical regulator, as to whether the public health watchdog has been corrupted into a Big Pharma lapdog and drug enabler, is relevant for most countries. As in most areas in the current era, the United States has the heaviest normative weight and strongest gravitational pull of any country in the world. For better or worse, the presence of the likes of Robert F Kennedy Jr, Jay Bhattacharya, Marty Makary, and Vinay Prasad in the top echelons of public health decision-making in Washington DC is bound to have ripple effects in other countries in recalibrating the normative settling point of public health policy.

16: COVID INQUIRIES

The last chapter explained why accountability for the years of overreach by governments in the name of health security against the Covid pandemic is essential. One pathway to such accountability is to establish powerful commissions of inquiry with appropriate terms of reference and headed by a tough, experienced and widely credible chair. Under Australia's Royal Commissions Act of 1912, this is best pursued through a royal commission that has its special powers to compel witness testimony and require the submission of evidence. Refusing to establish one was among the earliest broken election promises of the Albanese Labor government.

Foreshadowing a coronavirus Royal Commission[97]

If ever there was justification for a Royal Commission, this is it. Its primary term of reference should not be to apportion blame, but to identify how we can prepare better for the next big one.

SARS-CoV-2 has not been even remotely as lethal as the Spanish flu of 1918–19 that killed the fit and young as virulently as it did the elderly and infirm. It infected 500 million people (one-third the world's population at the time) and killed around 50 million. Scaled up to the current global population, that would translate to around

[97] *Australian Outlook*, 11 June 2020, http://www.internationalaffairs.org.au/australianoutlook/foreshadowing-a-coronavirus-royal-commission/

200-250 million dead today. Yet authorities did not close down whole societies and economies in 1918.

SARS-CoV-2 will not be the last pandemic to hit us. There will be others, and next time Australia may not be fortunate in the timing (off flu season) or the geographical epicentre (North Atlantic). The choice of Commissioners should reflect modern Australian demographics and the reality that the best lessons to be learnt for successful responses are from East Asian countries.

The inquiry should focus on two broad areas: the relationship between science, modelling, and evidence that informed policy; and the lives saved by the strategies adopted against the lives lost and livelihoods destroyed by the lockdown measures.

Science, modelling and evidence behind coronavirus policy

Epidemiological modellers have not fared well in this crisis. Prior to this, the official position of the World Health Organisation (WHO) on the value of social distancing measures was published in an 85-page report last September. Its purported goal was to provide recommendations:

> *... for the use of NPIs [non-pharmaceutical interventions] in future influenza epidemics and pandemics based on existing guidance documents and the latest scientific literature. The specific recommendations are based on a systematic review of the evidence on the effectiveness of NPIs, including personal protective measures, environmental measures, social distancing measures and travel-related measures.*

There were two reasons for the WHO's sceptical conclusion on these measures. For one, "sufficient evidence" exists to show ineffectiveness of entry and exit screening; "weak evidence" that travel restrictions may delay the introduction of infections only temporarily and can adversely affect mitigation programs and disrupt supply chains, and border closures may work for small island nations in severe cases, "but must be weighed against potentially serious economic consequences." For another, "social distancing measures… can be highly disruptive, and the cost of these measures must be weighed against their potential impact."

Yet one after another, based on epidemiological modelling, governments introduced all these measures in a cascading rush. The pandemic was caused by a novel coronavirus. The public health community had little reliable existing knowledge and no time to have come to clear conclusions on the science behind its emergence, growth, curve, and retreat, let alone the best mitigation and suppression measures to fight it.

Accordingly, either the WHO guidance was not based in science and the epidemiologists have access to better scientific knowledge, in which case the public needs to know the basis of their confidence over that of the existing WHO advice. Or else the existing science behind the 2019 advice was sound, in which case the closures privileged abstract mathematical modelling over actual science based on observational data and medical scholarship. If so, the peoples of the world have been subjected to an unethical experiment in contravention of the science.

Consider what in itself is a trivial but nonetheless telling example. Official advice from different authorities on the recommended social distancing measure ranges from 1 metre, to 1.5 (Australia) and 2 metres (UK, USA). Which one of the three is based on science? They can't all be the scientific recommendation. As with many other elements of official advice, the choice has real-world consequences. In the case of the UK's absurd two-metre rule, Toby Young points out: "For most shops, the only way to keep customers six feet apart will be to introduce cumbersome one-way systems and force them to queue up outside…. how will people observe that rule on the pavement when there are queues outside every shop?"

The WHO messaging on face masks has also been confused and contradictory. In a video on 24 March, WHO recommended wearing them; in updated advice on 6 April, WHO said the "use of masks by healthy people in the community setting is not supported by current evidence and carries uncertainties and critical risks"; on 5 June, WHO reverted to advising mask wearing for everyone in public.

We have had similarly absurd, inconsistent, and even contradictory advice in Australia from federal and state authorities, all supposedly based on the best science. The tussle over state border closures is the most visible current example. But previous incidences included prohibiting a mother and daughter, who live in the same house, from going for a driving lesson together in a sealed car; playing solo golf, sitting alone on a park bench, or enjoying a solitary walk on the beach or swim in the ocean; and driving to in-state holiday homes. Staying cooped up at home with others is the healthier choice. Really? Meanwhile, it was permissible to wander around supermarkets and handle food and produce with no idea of how many others have handled it.

The randomness of the downward infection curves

Figure 16.1: Covid-19 reproduction rate (R)

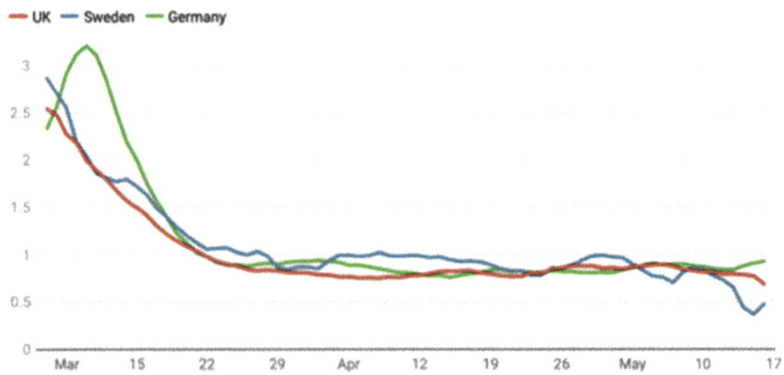

Source: Alistair Haimes, 'Lockdown and the R-number: Is Neil Ferguson right?', *The Spectator UK*, 11 June 2020.

The epidemiological experts have been sharply, and sometimes bitterly divided over the nature of the coronavirus curve, the comparative utility and futility of different mitigation and control measures, and how much weight to give to the collateral damage being inflicted on other public health, economic, and liberal goals that together represent the social purpose of the state. Jonathon Fuller discusses the contrasting philosophies of scientific knowledge between epidemiologists who prefer models and those for "evidence-based medicine" in clinical practice. The former advocate NPIs to flatten the curve; some of the latter subscribe to the notion of a "self-flattening curve," as Stanford's Nobel Laureate Michael Levitt put it. Oxford professor of theoretical epidemiology Sunetra Gupta holds that the strikingly similar patterns of the epidemic across countries (it grows, turns around, and dies away "almost like clockwork") is better explained by pre-existing immunities to related coronaviruses such as the common cold, than by lockdowns or government interventions. Figure 16.2 appears more consistent with the Levitt-Gupta thesis than the modelling thesis.

Contrasting Scandinavian examples

The best-known example of a country bucking the model is Sweden. Without compulsory lockdowns and with much activity as normal, the country has not been decimated by the disease. Applied to Sweden, it was projected that, without a lockdown *instituted by 10 April*, between 70,000-90,000 people would die by mid-May. The actual total on 30 May was 4,395—significantly higher than its Nordic neighbours but behind lockdown countries Belgium, Spain, UK, and Italy and about the same as France in deaths per million people (Figure 16.2).

Figure 16.2: Models vs reality in Sweden—No. of daily patients in ICU

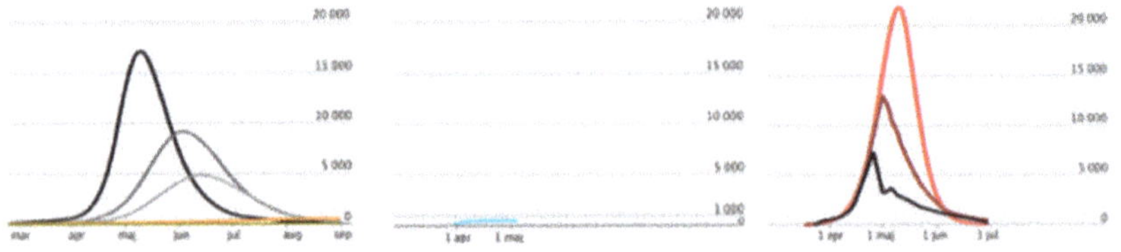

Source: Johan Norberg, 'Can we trust Covid Modelling?', *Spectator USA*, 13 May 2020

As with numerous other studies, that is, there is no clear evidence of the effectiveness of lockdowns. The two points of comparison—Nordic neighbours and other European countries—will be keenly watched over the coming months. Figure 16.2 is visually stunning in dramatising the discrepancy between two epidemiological models on either side of the chart and the empirical reality in the centre.

On 3 June, Swedish Radio published an interview with chief epidemiologist Anders Tegnell in which he acknowledged the perfectly obvious fact that in retrospect, they could have handled the crisis better and in particular taken better precautions to protect the care homes where more than half of Sweden's Covid-19 deaths have occurred. This "was spun pretty hard" in the international media as a mea culpa on lockdowns. It was not. Tegnell explained to Dagens Nyheter that knowledge about Covid-19 is much better now and would be useful for improved mitigation, but he still doesn't believe that lockdown would have been a better choice for Sweden: "the fundamental strategy has worked well."

Critics of Sweden's distinctive no-lockdown approach, some of whom seem almost to be willing Sweden to fail, resort to classic "whataboutery": But what about its 4,717 deaths compared to its closest comparable neighbour Norway's 239 deaths? One could counterpose: what about lockdown Belgium with 9,619 deaths and, at 842 deaths per million people, the highest death rate in the world?

Dr Camilla Stoltenberg, Director-General of the Norwegian Institute of Public Health, said on 22 May that the country could have controlled the virus without lockdown. Speaking to the state broadcaster about the release of a new report from her institute, she said: "Our assessment now.... is that we could possibly have achieved the same effects and avoided some of the unfortunate impacts by not locking down, but by instead keeping open but with infection control measures." Norway's reproduction number had fallen to 1.1 before the lockdowns were announced on 12 March. "The scientific backing was not good enough," she added, to warrant the hard policies, in shades of the WHO's 2019 advice.

We need real Covid inquiries[98]

Nearly four years on since the onset of the pandemic and the rash of public policy interventions to manage and contain it, many more people have become sceptical of the range of policy responses by health officials, governments and drug regulators. Yet, substantial numbers remain convinced that while mistakes might have been made, the interventions were mostly successful and generally well intentioned in unprecedently challenging circumstances of a fast spreading lethal new virus.

The sceptics feel vindicated on three counts: the gravity and universality of the threat from the disease were exaggerated, often deliberately; the efficacy of the policy interventions were overstated; and their collateral harms and risks were downplayed. The vilification, silencing and defenestration of genuinely concerned and well credentialled dissenters contributed to growing loss of trust in the good faith and competence of the authorities. In summary, over three years we witnessed the arrogance of know-all experts, the authoritarian

---

[98] Brownstone Institute, 19 January 2024, https://brownstone.org/articles/we-need-real-covid-inquiries/

instincts of governments and a surprising degree of timidity and compliance of publics.

The mantra of "Follow the science" has been unravelling. Testifying before Congress on 8–9 January, Anthony "I am science" Fauci confessed that the health authorities' six-foot distancing rule (1.5-2.0 metres for countries following the metric system) was "likely not based on scientific data." It "sort of just appeared." He also conceded that Covid vaccine mandates "could increase vaccine hesitancy in the future." The larger point of course is that the mandates contributed to a general loss of public trust in health and other institutions.

In an excoriating retrospective analysis of the Covid policies enacted by Drs. Fauci and Deborah Birx, Scott Atlas, who served as Covid adviser to President Donald Trump, wrote in *Newsweek* last March that the policies "failed to stop the dying, failed to stop the infection from spreading, and inflicted massive damage and destruction particularly on lower-income families and on America's children." He lists ten falsehoods that were promoted by health leaders, officials and academics.

Francis Collins, the former head of the National Institutes of Health, admitted last July that public health officials had shown an unfortunate narrow-mindedness in their single-minded focus on Covid to the neglect of other health, social and economic considerations. In his own words:

> *So you attach infinite value to stopping the disease and saving a life.*
>
> *You attach zero value to whether this actually totally disrupts people's lives, ruins the economy and has many kids kept out of school in a way that they never quite recover from.*

The UK Covid inquiry chaired by Baroness Hallett looks set to become the most expensive in British history, with one estimate from the Taxpayers' Alliance putting the total cost at £156 million. It has also proven farcical, devoting endless time on the equivalent of tittle tattle gossip on WhatsApp groups, and showing remarkable hat-doffing deference to the health officials and their top scientific advisers and rude indifference to equally eminent critics of the official narrative. Even by its own low standards, the nadir came with the testimony from the prime minister (PM), of all people. Presenting to the inquiry on 11 December, Rishi Sunak drew attention to a study which indicated that more quality-adjusted life years (QALY) would be lost by the first lockdown than by the Covid disease.

In a jaw-dropping response, Hugo Keith KC, counsel assisting the inquiry, quickly shut him down. He was not interested in "quality life assurance models" (*sic*), he said. Remember, this is the PM speaking, one moreover who was Chancellor under Prime Minister Boris Johnson at the time, suggesting that the cure might indeed have been worse than the disease. Professor Karol Sikora, an eminent oncologist and a former head of the cancer program at the WHO, called this "The single most revealing exchange in the Covid Inquiry."

Sir Patrick Vallance was the UK's chief scientist when coronavirus struck. Like Collins in the US, Vallance too conceded in testimony at the UK Covid inquiry on 20 November that science was given undue weight over economics: "The science was there for everyone to see. The economic advice wasn't."

In an astonishing open letter to PM Scott Morrison on 19 April 2020, many prominent Australian economists rejected commentators' calls for a rapid return to work and labelled the notion of a "trade-off" between public health and the economy a "false distinction." They said that while the measures adopted to contain the spread of Covid-19 had caused economic damage, those negative effects were far outweighed by the lives saved.

The letter was eventually signed by 265 economists. But it has not aged well and this might explain why the group's website with the full list of signatories is no longer accessible. This was astonishing because this non-economist was under the impression that cost-benefit analysis was integral to the discipline of economics.

For what it's worth, I wrote as early as 30 March 2020 in *Pearls and Irritations*:

> *"In responding to an epidemic, there is a trade-off between public health and economic stability. It is the duty of health professionals to focus solely on the former. It is the responsibility of governments to balance the two…*
>
> *"Public policy must be based on a balance of risks and benefits… The health of citizens and the health of the national economy are closely connected and interdependent."*

In a follow-up article on 17 April 2020, for the *Lowly Interpreter*, I wrote:

> *Health professionals are duty-bound to map the best- and worst-case scenarios. Governments bear the responsibility to balance health, economic, and social policies. Once these are included in the decision calculus, the political and ethical justification for the hard suppression strategy is less obvious.*

Albanese's Covid inquiry

In opposition Anthony Albanese and Labor had promised a Royal Commission, which has strong powers to compel witnesses to testify and demand relevant documents. In September Prime Minister Albanese announced the powers, composition and terms of reference of Australia's Covid inquiry. It failed every best-practice test of an open and independent public inquiry. It lacks statutory powers to gather documentary and oral evidence. With narrow and limited terms of reference, it will not examine decisions and actions of state governments, which formed the vast majority of pandemic management policies. Any self-respecting person approached to be on the panel would have politely but firmly turned down the invitation.

The three panellists are all women with public records of advocating lockdowns, masks and vaccines. Angela Jackson has past ties to the Labor Party. In June 2021 she tweeted that Melbourne's lockdowns had helped "to keep the rest of Australia Covid free," adding: "Time to bloody step up Sydney." The next month she said Victoria needed "a hard lockdown" to get through the pandemic. Catherine Bennett was also supportive of Melbourne's lockdowns in 2020–21. The third panellist is Robyn Kruk, director-general of the New South Wales Department of Health.

Defenders of the Albanese model were few and far between. The opposition party attacked it as a "half-baked" inquiry that would function as "a protection racket" for the mostly Labor state governments that had instituted some of the harshest unscientific measures in the world. Its scope should either be widened or else it should be disbanded, they said.

Peak aged-care bodies, unions and the pro-Labor government Greens added their voices to the chorus of criticisms of the decision to exclude actions by state governments. Even some Labor Party parliamentarians described the inquiry's narrow scope as "bizarre."

Human Rights Commissioner Lorraine Finlay said the inquiry will fail to do justice to the high human cost of the Covid policies, including family separations, school closures and Australians not permitted to come home from overseas. *The Australian* columnist Peter Van Onselen said Albanese's limited and toothless Covid inquiry was "base politics at its worst" and the PM had borrowed the playbook from the satirical British TV series *Yes, Prime Minister*. Paul Collits criticised the scope and all-women composition of the inquiry committee as a ."

Because of my work on Covid issues since March 2020, I was asked by several people to put in a submission (the closing date was 15 December), at least "for the record." I declined. Taking part in that sham exercise would imbue it with some degree of undeserved legitimacy.

On 21 September, a media release from Senator Malcolm Roberts derided the "betrayal of everyday Australians and small businesses" with the government "running away from a Royal Commission." He promised to request a Senate inquiry by the Legal and Constitutional Affairs Committee to recommend proper terms of reference for a Covid Royal Commission to be established in 2024. The Senate agreed to this on 19 October. The committee will report back by 31 March. Several groups, including some that I am associated with, have been busy preparing submissions to the Senate committee that had a closing date of 12 January.

A collaborative effort to draft a comprehensive people's terms of reference can be found here, with 45,000 signatories as at 17 January. It includes two organisations with which I am closely associated, Children's Health Defense Australia and Australians for Science and Freedom. (Full disclosure: I am one of the co-authors of the document.) It calls for answers to the scientific basis for some of the most intrusive and coercive pandemic management measures, the cost-benefit analyses behind the policies including an examination of the harms likely to result from both pharmaceutical and non-pharmaceutical interventions; and explanations for enacting and enforcing vaccine mandates despite knowing that they stop neither infection nor transmission.

Australian Senate to investigate excess mortality[99]

Some people claim that 60% of all statistics, like this one, is just made up out of thin air. All statistics in relation to Covid—numbers infected, infection and case fatality rates, deaths from and with Covid,

[99] Brownstone Institute, 15 April 2024, https://brownstone.org/articles/australian-senate-to-investigate-excess-mortality/

the number of lives saved by lockdowns, masks, and vaccines, the number of lives lost in the long term due to lockdown and mask harms and vaccine injuries, the widely-practised disinformation of misclassifying deaths in the first 2-3 weeks following vaccination as "unvaccinated" if the status is unknown or this was the second dose—are open to cherry-picked data being manipulated, with assumptions fed into models to produce pre-determined outputs.

This also makes cross-country comparisons exceptionally challenging, as countries use different definitions of key concepts and different methodologies to estimate the various counts. Still, we must work within these limitations as this is the only data we have.

Data don't back claims of vaccine success

'Success" of Covid vaccines in American public perception may arise from the chronological coincidence of the decline in Covid mortality rate that coincided with the vaccine rollout. But by this time sizable numbers of Americans had also been infected by the virus and built up natural immunity that is both more robust and longer-lasting than that conferred by vaccines. In time this eventuates into the public good of herd immunity.

Consider three examples—Australia, New Zealand, and India—that contradict the claim of the beneficial impact of vaccines in driving down the US Covid death rate. The data are drawn from Our World in Data and Worldometers. I will address the safety issues shortly. For now, the key takeaway is, following Karl Popper's falsifiability test, the three cases demonstrate the ineffectiveness of vaccines.

The US total Covid-related death toll as of 8 April 2024 is 3.6 times as many as died in pre-vaccine 2020. The explanation for this is that only one-third of all US Covid-related deaths were since 1 January 2022, by which date 63.4% of Americans had been fully vaccinated. By contrast, over 90% of Australia's Covid-related deaths occurred since 1 January 2022, when it had reached 75.5% full vaccination. In sharp contrast to the US, therefore, 27.1 times as many Australians died with Covid since 1 January 2022 as in 2020.

New Zealand deaths are even more disproportionately concentrated in the period since 1 January 2022, when 74.4% of the population was fully vaccinated. Only 25 people died with Covid in 2020, and by the end of 2021 the total was 50. Yet in April 2024 the total was between 4,000 (Our World in Data) and 5,700 (Worldometers—I have no insight on the discrepancy in numbers between these two data sources). That is, an astonishing 98-99% of all Covid-related deaths in the country occurred after hitting 74.4% full vaccination.

India's Covid mortality rate was higher than 1 death per million people for about 7-8 weeks from early May to the end of June 2021, peaking at 2.92 on 29 May 2021. This is the period in which the horrific tales of dumped corpses washing ashore and insufficient capacity of the cremation grounds dominated international news coverage of the dire Indian situation. In this time, India's full vaccination coverage was just 2-4% and the death rate peaked with only three percent of the population having completed the initial Covid-19 vaccination protocol. Thus Covid deaths rose and fell in symmetrical steepness according to some internal logic of the virus that had little relationship to the rollout of vaccines.

Measured by deaths per million people, Worldometers data as of 6 April show Australia with the 108th highest Covid mortality of 228 countries. However, countries that did better than Australia include South Korea, Japan, Vietnam, and India on the Asian mainland, in that order; and Taiwan, Iceland, and Singapore as island countries. Taiwan, of course, should have been a lot more exposed and vulnerable owing to winter conditions, proximity to China, and the volume of cross-strait travel before the alarm was raised in early 2020.

We know by now that the notion of an average Covid infection fatality rate (IFR) is highly misleading as a public health policy tool because of the great variability both by age structure and across the world's regions. Australia, possibly as an indication of the continuing hold of culture cringe that makes its leaders behave like poor relations of the Anglo-US "aristocracy," likes to compare itself to Europe and the US. Hence the interminable pats on the back by its officials for their brilliant Covid performance, ignoring the immeasurable advantages of the time bought by the good fortune of being in the Southern Hemisphere in the midst of summer when the disease broke in the Northern Hemisphere, the island geography as a natural barrier to the spread of the virus, the plentiful sunshine and outdoors leisure and recreational activities (though policies rather stupidly did their best to neutralise this natural asset: never underestimate the ability and moths-to-the-flame attraction of politicians for cock-ups), and housing and residential patterns.

Even so, if Australia can compare itself to Europe, then it is equally permissible to locate its performance in Oceania. Here Australia was the fifth worst of 18 countries in Oceania and New Zealand was the second worst (only French Polynesia fared worse).

On 26 March, the Australian Bureau of Statistics (ABS) published its monthly statistics for last year. The baseline average used is for number of deaths in the four years 2017–2019 and 2021. Because 2020 and 2022 were atypically lower and higher, respectively, than average years, they are not included in the ABS methodology for calculating the baseline average.

The first notable thing is the increase in the number of Covid-related deaths from 855 in 2020 to 1,231, 9,840, and 4,387 in the next three years. With assistance from heavy doses of coercion and compulsion for some sectors, the vaccine rollout from early 2021 had achieved extraordinarily high take-up and 95.5% of over-16s were double-vaccinated by the end of April 2022. Thus for practical purposes Australia had achieved universal adult vaccination.

And yet, there were 43% more deaths in 2021 and a staggering 11.5 times as many deaths in 2022 as in pre-vaccine 2020. In addition, there were more than five times as many deaths in 2023, by which time the pandemic was supposedly over, as in 2020. If this indicates vaccine success, I hate to think what failure would look like.

This contradicts all the bombastic claims of the public health clerisy about the great success of their pandemic management interventions centred on lockdowns, masks, and vaccines. How many times did Prime Minister Scott Morrison claim that his Covid management policies saved 40,000 lives, a made-up statistic that he continues to peddle?

Rather, it vindicates the two core claims of vaccine critics like Stanford University's Jay Bhattacharya, Oxford's Sunetra Gupta, and Harvard's Martin Kulldorff, the three eminent epidemiologists who wrote the Great Barrington Declaration in October 2020. They argued that once a virus is already seeded in the community, it cannot be eradicated but only managed until it becomes endemic and universal. And secondly, the various restrictions on social interactions could delay but would not be able to avoid the final toll. Consequently, the trajectory of the rise and fall of the coronavirus was likely to be policy invariant; that is, not much affected by the different policy interventions. And so it came to pass.

Sweden, take a bow

Among countries, the standout proof of this is Sweden, which took the sensible decision of staying with the existing science and policy recommendations based on a hundred years of research, data, and real-world experience, rather than risk the radical evidence-free lockdown and mask measures instituted by panicked governments. Ditto Florida among US states.

Their Covid health outcomes today are no worse than the average for European countries and US states. As per the Worldometers data, the case fatality rate of SARS-CoV-2 is 0.99% and the overall survival rate is 98.97%. The first may be overstated and the second understated, owing to the less than comprehensive reporting, recording, and data collection of infections among hundreds of millions in developing countries.

Measured by deaths per million people, Sweden was 23rd worst of 47 European countries and 35th worst globally and the US was the 14th worst in the world. Sweden's economic, educational, and social outcomes are substantially better.

On 11 February, Frederik NG Andersson and Lars Jonung from Lund University in Sweden published a study in *Economic Affairs* examining the benefits and costs of lockdowns across 25 countries in Europe, with a particular focus on Sweden as the outstanding contrarian on that policy. Their conclusions emphasise the importance of avoiding panic amidst a crisis and not letting short-term decisions undermine long-term outcomes.

Instead, measures introduced without a firm evidence basis as a temporary necessity lasted for two years and authoritarian China served as the model for curtailing civil liberties and citizens' rights. Europe's democracies instituted needlessly stringent lockdowns that produced negligible positive health effects but the decline in economic activity did correlate with the severity of lockdowns. This pathology was compounded by efforts to counter the downturn in economic activity with excessively expansionary fiscal and monetary policies that led to ballooning public debt.

By contrast, Sweden's lockdown restrictions were modest and mostly voluntary and its fiscal response was also restrained. This gave Sweden remarkably low cumulative excess mortality, small losses in economic growth, and continued strong public finances. Sweden's GDP today is around six percent bigger than in 2019. A 34-country study published in November in the US *Proceedings of the National Academy of Sciences* concluded that the US "would have had 1.60 million fewer deaths if it had the performance of Sweden.'

Let that sink in.

Figure 16.3: Australia's concerning excess deaths

Figure 1: Excess deaths by week (% change from average), Australia, Sweden and USA, 2020–23

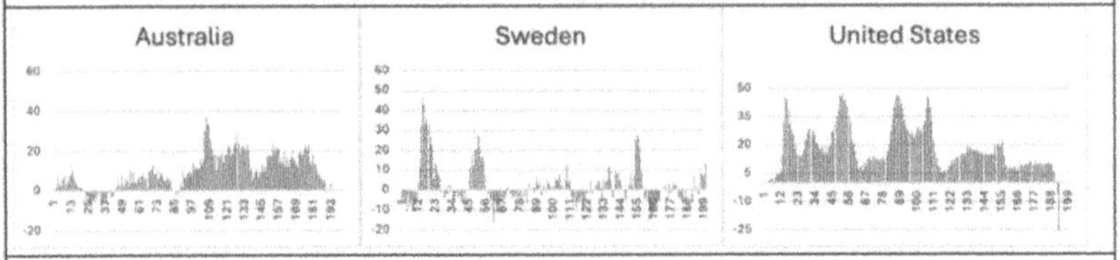

Drawn by the author using data from OECD.Stat (https://stats.oecd.org/index.aspx?QueryId=104676) as at 29 March 2024.

The second striking feature of the ABS data is the phenomenon of excess deaths, defined as "the difference between the observed number of deaths in a specified time period and the expected numbers of deaths in that same time period." Figure 16.3 is a snapshot of excess deaths in Australia, Sweden, and the US.

During the Covid years, the ABS explains, excess death estimates were "used to provide information about the burden of mortality potentially related to the Covid-19 pandemic, including deaths that are directly or indirectly attributed to Covid-19." Notice the sleight of hand (sleight of mind?) here. There is no mention of deaths resulting, either directly or indirectly, from the policies to deal with the pandemic, only from the viral disease itself.

Why does this matter? There is a medical term called "iatrogenic," defined by the *Cambridge Dictionary* as a disease or problem "caused by medical treatment or by a doctor." An example of its use in a sentence is: "Over 100,000 deaths occur in North America from iatrogenic disease, which means doctor- or drug-induced disease.'

There has been an extensive debate, out in the real world beyond the one inhabited by the top executives of the major vaccine manufacturers, public health bureaucrats, and the medical establishment, of the full magnitude and severity of Covid-19 vaccine injury, including deaths. Many studies, but not all, have found strong correlations between excess deaths and vaccination rollouts, rates, and number of doses.

Igor Chudov, for example, found that vaccination rates explain 24% of the excess mortality across 31 European countries, which is statistically highly significant. Charts produced by Fabian Spiker include three examples showing the temporal association of spikes in Covid-19 deaths across Africa, the strong correlation between boosters and Covid cases in Germany, and between the first doses of the vaccines and Covid deaths in 50–64-year-old women in US states (Figure 16.4).

Figure 16.4: Correlations between Covid-19 vaccines, cases and deaths in Africa, Germany and US states

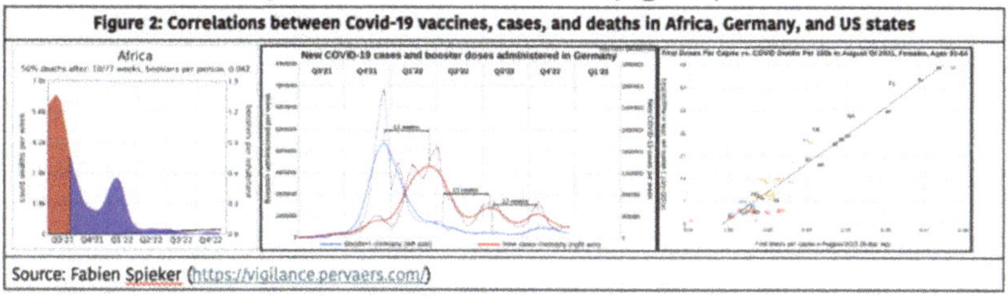

Because billions of Covid vaccines were administered by the revolutionary mRNA platform under emergency use authorisation before the traditional multiyear safety and efficacy tests normally required of new vaccines could be completed, public health authorities and drug regulators should have been extra vigilant about potential iatrogenic harms caused by vaccines. Instead too many seem to have operated as drug enablers rather than regulators.

A major risk-benefit assessment of vaccine boosters for 18-29-year-olds published in the *Journal of Medical Ethics* in January found that to prevent one Covid hospitalisation of a previously uninfected person, 22,000-30,000 people must be boosted with an mRNA vaccine. But for one hospitalisation prevented, 18-98 serious adverse events can be expected.

The net risk-benefit ratio is in fact even less favourable owing to the high prevalence of post-infection immunity in that population group and the lack of compelling public health benefits, since vaccines have only transient effectiveness against transmission. Mandates cause wider social harms like curtailing access to educational and job opportunities, reputational damage, threats of disenrollment and deportation, generating mistrust in society and public institutions, and fuelling vaccine hesitancy for life-saving paediatric and adult vaccines.

Another study published in February looked at death rates by vaccination status among hospitalised patients with Covid and found that in the over-50s, the vaccinated group had almost double the mortality rate of the unvaccinated group (70%-37%). Moreover, those with more doses had higher mortality rates.

Professor Carl Heneghan, director of the Centre for Evidence-Based Medicine at Oxford University, and Tom Jefferson ask why the UK Health Security Agency refuses to disclose to Parliament and the public data that it holds on mortality by number of vaccine doses. Could it be because data from the complementary Office of National Statistics show that excess deaths have been primarily in the vaccinated, suggesting but not proving that vaccines may be playing some role?

On 2 March, a cross-party group of 21 British MPs and peers criticised the "wall of silence" on the topic and wrote to Health Secretary Victoria Atkins about the "growing public and professional concerns" at the UK's rates of excess deaths since 2020. On 21 March, it was announced that the House of Commons will have a debate on excess deaths on 18 April.

Even with respect to any association between vaccination and excess deaths, however, Sweden is an outlier. It is among the most highly vaccinated countries, achieving 70% full vaccination in January 2022 (the US was at 65 and Australia at 77% at that time). Sweden's cumulative excess mortality from 1 March 2020 to 31 December 2023 was 21,260, compared to 51,007 for Australia and 1,313,492 for the US.

But here's the thing. According to Our World in Data, Sweden's total Covid-related deaths by 3 March 2024 was 27,219 and that for the US was 1,180,025 (Figure 3).

In other words, Sweden's non-Covid excess deaths were negative, lower than the baseline average. Because the dates between the two sets of figures are discrepant, I did some creative guesstimating using data from Our World in Data, OECD excess deaths statistics, and the provisional monthly statistics published by the ABS for 2020, 2021, 2022, and 2023. As per these non-authoritative calculations of date-adjusted data, by March this year the net non-Covid excess deaths were 29,367 for Australia, *minus* 4,574 for Sweden, and 222,016 for the US.

Figure 16.5: Sweden and US all-cause excess mortality and Covid-19 deaths

Excess mortality: Cumulative number of deaths from all causes compared to projection based on previous years

Our World in Data

The cumulative difference between the reported number of deaths since 1 January 2020 and the projected number of deaths for the same period based on previous years. The reported number might not count all deaths that occurred due to incomplete coverage and delays in reporting.

Table Map Chart Show selection only

Deaths from all causes compared to projection based on previous years

Country or region	Mar 1, 2020	Dec 31, 2023	Absolute Change	Relative Change
Sweden	-987	20,273	+21,260	+2,154%
United States	-14,790	1,298,702	+1,313,492	+8,881%

Screenshot 2024-03-30 at 0...

Cumulative confirmed COVID-19 deaths

Our World in Data

Due to varying protocols and challenges in the attribution of the cause of death, the number of confirmed deaths may not accurately represent the true number of deaths caused by COVID-19.

Table Map Chart Show selection only

Total deaths

Country or region	Mar 1, 2020	Mar 3, 2024	Absolute Change	Relative Change
Sweden	3	27,219	+27,216	+907,200%
United States	1	1,180,025	+1,180,024	+118,002,400%

What's interesting about Sweden, of course, is that this is exactly the result we would expect with Covid having killed substantial numbers of the vulnerable population of the elderly and the comorbid, thereby reducing the cohort at serious risk of death in the subsequent few years. Be that as it may, Sweden's example once again suggests that the enduring harms of lockdown restrictions might possibly have significant explanatory potency for the stubbornly persistent excess deaths. Or did Sweden just strike it lucky with its particular batches of the vaccines, as there seems to be some evidence that not all batches were equal in the quality control during the manufacturing process?

Returning to Australia, the non-Covid number of excess deaths was 16,046 in 2022 (9.7%) and 12,345 last year (7.5%). There's no conclusive evidence that vaccination is *a* or *the* primary cause of excess mortality. But there are enough concerning safety signals that the matter needs proper investigation in conjunction with the persistent patterns of harms from the lockdown social experiment. Refusing to investigate this is especially odd after the insistence since 2020 that even one avoidable Covid death is one death too many. Hence the insistence on shutting down an entire city or state with the detection of just one Covid case.

After repeated failed attempts, on 26 March the Senate voted 31-30 to hold an inquiry by the Community Affairs References Committee into factors contributing to excess deaths. Senator Ralph Babet, the prime instigator behind the motion, thinks this might be a world-first inquiry.

Remarkably, all the Green and Labor senators voted against this. Seriously? What do they fear will be revealed that they would rather keep hidden?

In striking contrast to the enthusiastic vaccine take-up in 2021–22, in the six months to March this year, only 3.3% of 18-64-year-olds had received a booster and in the much more vulnerable 65-74-year-olds, 21.4%, according to the Department of Health.

Clearly, most people are done with Covid and have stopped paying heed to the advice from public health authorities. This of course contains its own long-term dangers. Are Labor and the Greens not interested in knowing the vaccine truth and restoring public trust in the integrity of our public institutions, including Health and Parliament?

An Australian sceptical note on Covid-19 vaccine effectiveness

According to Our World in Data, New Zealand achieved 75% coverage of the initial COVID-19 vaccination protocol (two doses) on December 29th 2021, when its Covid-related death toll was just 44, and 80% (tantamount in effect to universal adult coverage) on June 8th 2022, by which time deaths had risen to 2,095. As at May 13th 2025, its death toll stood at 4,538. In other words, more than half of all New Zealand's Covid deaths occurred after effectively universal adult vaccination had been achieved and a scarcely believable 99% after 75% of the country's population had been double vaccinated.

Trust the government health experts as your single source of truth on anything and everything to do with Covid, including vaccines. They always prioritise your health over Pharma profits. And they are always right, even when they do a 180 degree about turn. Australia's Department of Health advice on June 3rd 2025:

> *COVID-19 vaccine is not recommended for healthy infants, children or adolescents who do not have medical conditions that increase their risk of severe illness. This is because the risk of severe illness was extremely low in this cohort over the course of the pandemic, and benefits of vaccination are not considered to outweigh the potential harms.*

Australian Government
Department of Health and Aged Care

Australian **Immunisation** Handbook

Healthy infants, children and adolescents aged <18 years are not recommended to receive COVID-19 vaccine

COVID-19 vaccine is not recommended for healthy infants, children or adolescents who do not have medical conditions that increase their risk of severe illness. This is because the risk of severe illness was extremely low in this cohort over the course of the pandemic, and benefits of vaccination are not considered to outweigh the potential harms.[1,2]

Related diseases:

COVID-19 (https://immunisationhandbook.health.gov.au/contents/vaccine-preventable-diseases/covid-19)

Page history

Last updated: 3 June 2025

Last reviewed: 3 June 2025

Never trust us non-experts, who said this all along.

Meanwhile Dr Sara Brenner, the US FDA's Principal Deputy Commissioner (and acting commissioner for a short period), revealed last month that she refused the COVID-19 mRNA vaccine while pregnant despite the FDA promoting it as "safe and effective" for pregnant women. Maryanne Demasi also reports on another FDA expert, Dr Janet Woodcock, who privately supported testing ivermectin's initial promise for treating Covid ("Wow—we should definitely test it") before doing an about turn and joining the FDA's mockingly public denunciations of ivermectin as a horse and cow medicine.

Setting aside questions about their safety, how anyone can claim that these statistics are compatible with the "COVID-19 vaccines are effective" narrative is mind boggling. Moreover, if we accept Karl Popper's criterion of falsifiability for disproving a scientific claim (if the claim is that all swans are white, and we find just one black swan, then the claim is empirically falsified and scientifically invalid), then the narrative is false not just for New Zealand but for the world.

The crucial period for looking at Australia and New Zealand in comparison to the UK is the nine months from November 12th 2021 to August 10th 2022. All three countries had achieved two-thirds double vaccination in their populations in November 2021. Despite increased levels of vaccination coverage after that date, over the next nine months Covid-related deaths jumped 6.9 times for Australia and a whopping 63 times for New Zealand, but only 1.2 times for the UK (Figure 1). The same variance can be seen in the second chart in Figure 1 that depicts the temporal correlation between vaccine doses administered and the Covid-related deaths per million people in the three countries. Meanwhile in Japan, after examining an 18-million strong database, Dr Yasufumi Murakami, Professor at the prestigious Tokyo University and Vice Director at its Research Centre for RNA Science, came to the sobering conclusion that "the more doses you get, the sooner you're likely to die, within a shorter period."

Clearly, leaving aside the question of their safety, COVID-19 vaccines were hardly effective at all in preventing Covid-related deaths. If someone believes as an article of faith that Covid vaccines are effective and Australia and New Zealand Covid deaths were low compared to high-income country averages because they refused to open their borders until after vaccination, then no amount of evidence will change their mind. For those who are prepared to look at the data with an open and critical mind, it is nonsensical to argue that a dramatic *fall* in Covid deaths after vaccination drive takes hold in Europe, UK and US is evidence of vaccine effectiveness, while an even more dramatic *spike* in Australia and New Zealand in the same period is also proof of vaccine effectiveness: heads you win, tails I lose.

Table 16.1: Selected Covid vaccination rates and deaths/mn people

	23 January 2021		25 July 2022		31 December 2022	
	Vaccination (%)	*DPM*	*Vaccination (%)*	*DPM*	*Vaccination (%)*	*DPM*
Australia	0.0	0.00	82.6	3.36	82.7	7.79
New Zealand	0.0	0.00	80.4	6.85	80.6	1.20
UK	0.69	20.35	74.0	2.25	74.5	1.95
Europe	1.17	7.59	65.9	1.28	66.1	1.16
USA	1.21	9.29	65.6	1.34	67.2	1.04

Table 16.1 and Figure 16.7 show that the deaths per million in July 2022 for New Zealand and in January-February 2023 for Australia were among the highest in the world. Yet, for both, the deaths were flat in the pre-vaccination period. By contrast, peaks for the other three I have used for reference in this chart (UK, US, Europe) were at their highest before vaccination took hold. This is why I remain surprised that Australia and New Zealand data have not figured far more prominently in the commentary by those sceptical of the narrative.

If not vaccines, what other factor might explain the difference in Covid mortality between the three countries? Well, thanks to their geographical remoteness in the southern and eastern hemispheres and their decision to close both inward and outward international travel before coronavirus was widely seeded in the community, as well as the good luck of summer season south of the equator during the initial virulence on the northern hemisphere, Australia and New Zealand avoided mass infections when Covid was first rampant. Many epidemiologists warned at the time, as indeed had the WHO in a report in September 2019, that this would delay but not avoid mass infections. In November 2021, compared to around 14% of the British population having been Covid-infected, the rates were only 0.7% and 0.2% in Australia and New Zealand, respectively. That is, the UK had a head-start over Australia and New Zealand in infection-induced natural immunity.

Thus a significantly higher proportion of the British population had immunity acquired through infection than their Australasian counterparts by the end of 2021. When, believing in the protective benefits of the vaccine, Australia and New Zealand opened up again, their Covid-naïve populations were vulnerable to the virus. By August 2022 the cumulative case totals were comparable in all three countries: slightly over one-third (35-37%) of the population. And by now there is a wealth of literature indicating that natural immunity is both more robust and longer-lasting than the weaker and shorter protective efficacy of Covid vaccines (which also rather changes the harms-benefit equation for healthy people under 70). Australia and New Zealand stand as stark demonstrations of this.

Is it any wonder that a dramatic erosion of trust in public health institutions has lowered Australia's childhood vaccinations to alarming levels, as the ABC reported on May 16th. This mirrors the situation in the UK, where the share of children being vaccinated against diseases, including measles and whooping cough, has likewise slumped to the lowest levels in more than a decade and below the 95% threshold said to be necessary for herd immunity.

Australia's Covid inquiry was not fit for purpose[100]

The 868-page report of the official inquiry into Australia's Covid-19 response, like the inquiry itself, is not fit for purpose. Bottom line: This is a report of, by, and for the public health clerisy. For example, the report recommends that the solution to state overreach and abuse of power during the pandemic is to increase the powers and resources of the same two groups (politicians and the public health bureaucrats) to control our behaviour in future health emergencies. As Manuel so gloriously said in Fawlty Towers: *Qué*?

---

[100] *Spectator Australia*, Flat White, 6 November 2024, https://www.spectator.com.au/2024/11/covid-inquiry-was-not-fit-for-purpose/

Instead of virtue-signalling obeisance to acknowledgment of country and lived experience, and a trigger warning that some may find the content distressing, how about this:

> *We acknowledge the great loss of life, liberty, and happiness caused by Covid-19 and the response to it. We strongly recommend a Royal Commission of Inquiry to establish the division of causal responsibility between the disease and government policies, so that the perpetrators of mass public harms may be held accountable.*

Granted, the inquiry was hobbled by tightly circumscribed terms of reference in yet another broken election promise that further eroded public trust in politicians and political institutions. Still, the panellists could have said no to the call to serve.

This article explores three important examples of where the inquiry fell short. In the first two on social distancing and face-masks, the non-pharmaceutical interventions departed radically from existing understandings with no scientific basis or evidence in justification.

In the third on vaccination, the response departed alarmingly from long-established protocols governing the approval and authorisation of vaccines after duly completed trials to determine their efficacy and safety, not just in an immediate timeframe, but over the long haul. To circumvent the full trials requirement, emergency use authorisation was necessary. This could not be granted if existing treatment was available. When physicians who claimed high success rates in clinical treatment of Covid patients with repurposed ivermectin and hydroxychloroquine, were ordered by regulators to cease and desist, suspicions were fuelled about industry capture of the regulators. There is also a plausible argument that the legal framework governing the approval process should have been that for genetically modified organisms. This wasn't done.

Social distancing

On May 31, the US Congress published the transcript of two days of testimony in January from Dr Anthony Fauci, the face of America's Covid response. On the second day of the closed-door testimony on January 10, Committee Staff Director Mitch Benzine asked about the origins of the six-foot social distancing rule applied at businesses, schools and all public settings. Fauci frankly admitted: "You know, I don't recall. It sort of just appeared." Pressed on relevant "studies that supported six feet," he said, "I was not aware of studies that—in fact, that would be a very difficult study to do." (pp. 183-84)

As early as April 25, 2020, Professor Robert Dingwall, a scientific adviser to the UK government as a member of the New and Emerging Respiratory Virus Threats Advisory Group (NERVTAG), said there has "never been a scientific basis for two metres," it was "conjured up out of nowhere" and it should more accurately be called a "rule of thumb." He also warned that the social distancing measures would cause "serious damage to society, to the economy and to the physical and mental health of the population." Was he right, or was he right?

A group of Oxford University scientists explained in June 2020 that the science behind the social distancing rule was complex while the rule was starkly binary. It assumed that the sole or primary transmission route was through physical contact or large droplets. This also explained the early phobia about constant use of hand sanitisers and disinfection of all potential contact surfaces like chairs and tables in restaurants and benches in parks. Yet, the really small viruses can also be aerosolised and spread through the air.

Our chief health officers and "experts" thus need to be interrogated on whether the adoption of the two-metre rule for Australia was an example of copycat idiocy or the persistence of culture cringe: where the Brits and Americans lead, we dutifully follow.

Masks

At the Congressional hearing on January 10, Benzine also asked if a cost-benefit analysis had ever been done "on the unintended consequences of masking kids versus the protection that it would give them." "Not to my knowledge," Fauci conceded. (p. 135).

Until 2020, "settled science" was clear. Masks are ineffective. They stop neither infection nor transmission. The UK Influenza Preparedness Strategy 2011, reaffirmed on February 27, 2020, encapsulated the prevailing consensus (paragraph 4.15):

> *Although there is a perception that the wearing of facemasks by the public in the community and household setting may be beneficial, there is in fact very little evidence of widespread benefit from their use in this setting. Facemasks must be worn correctly, changed frequently, removed properly, disposed of safely and used in combination with good respiratory, hand, and home hygiene behaviour in order for them to achieve the intended benefit. Research also shows that compliance with these recommended behaviours when wearing facemasks for prolonged periods reduces over time.*

This conclusion was reiterated in the WHO report published in September 2019 that summarised the best available studies to date, noting that "there is very little evidence of widespread benefit from their use" in community and household settings. It was repeated by senior WHO doctors Mike Ryan and Maria Van Kerkhove on March 31, 2020: "There is no specific evidence to suggest that the wearing of masks by the mass population has any potential benefit. In fact, there's some evidence to suggest the opposite in the misuse of wearing a mask properly or fitting it properly.'

Consider this poignant testimony to Scotland's Covid inquiry hearings from Alison Walker, a former BBC sports presenter, on

November 17, 2023. Having witnessed the trauma of her 89- and 90-year-old parents residing in care homes in 2020, she asked (around the 36-minute mark): "If you are surrounded by a group of people 24/7 wearing masks, and you don't see people smile for up to two years, what kind of effect is that going to have on your mental health and wellbeing?"

Care homes abandoned their duty of "care and compassion," she believed, and instead "operated under a veil of fear." (at 1:24:46) This was reinforced by the closing statement from the Care Home Relatives Scotland: "The evidence demonstrated that the use of masks caused distress, confusion and considerable difficulties with communication. Residents couldn't see smiles, had difficulty recognising relatives and those with hearing difficulties couldn't lip-read or read facial expressions or visual clues."

Masks also do cause some harmful side-effects in some people. Compulsory masking for everyone in all settings is a gross violation of fundamental human rights. It can be justified only if the evidence for their efficacy in community protection is compelling and the risk of harms is negligible. Instead, mask mandates were heavy on fear-mongering and virtue-signalling but light on data and science, overturning, in a couple of months, cumulative scientific consensus built over decades. The report mentions masks several times, but only in the context of the inconsistent application of mandates. It doesn't address the absence of high quality studies and data to contradict the pre-2020 consensus on their lack of efficacy in community settings, as confirmed in the Cochrane Review.

Vaccines

Part of the explanation for the tone-deafness towards the still smouldering white-hot rage in the community is the failure to address the fiasco of the efficacy and safety of Covid vaccines.

Table 16.2: Australia's vaccination coverage and Covid-related mortality, 2020–24

Date	*Per cent fully vaccinated*	*Cumulative total deaths*	*Deaths per million (7-day rolling average)*
21.ii.21	00	923	<0.01
11.x.21	50	1 541	0.65
25.x.21	60	1 754	0.59
21.xi.21	70	2 110	0.44
20.iii.22	80	6 482	0.76
10.x.24	83	25 236	0.00

Source for Table 16.2 and Figures 16.6–16.8: Our World in Data

From the start of vaccine rollout in February 2021 to 70% full vaccination on November 21, 2021, Australia's total number of deaths was 1,187 (2,110-923) (Table 16.2). From initial rollout until 80% full vaccination on March 20, 2022, it was 5,599 (6,482-923). Since achieving those landmarks, which for practical purposes amount to full adult vaccination, the numbers of Covid-related deaths are 23,126 and 18,754, respectively.

There are two ways to put these figures in perspective. More than 25 times as many people have died with Covid-19 since 70% full vaccination compared to the total number before vaccination; and more than 20 times since 80% full vaccination than before vaccination.

That is, 91.6% and 74.3% of Australia's Covid-related deaths occurred after 70% and 80% full vaccination, respectively. This contrasts with just 3.7% before the vaccines began to be rolled out. I really do hate to think what the statistics would be if vaccines were ineffective. And this is even without taking into consideration vaccine injuries or age-disaggregated Covid risks of hospitalisation and death for unvaccinated vs vaccinated and boosted healthy children, adolescents, and adults until age 60.

On October 23, the BBC said that AstraZeneca vaccines had saved 6.3 million lives and Pfizer another 5.9 million, just in the first year from December 2020 to December 2021, including 120,000 British lives saved until September 2021. Looking at Figures 1–2, one can see why they would make such a claim. Yet as per Popperian falsifiability, just the one contrary example of Australia is sufficient to falsify the hypothesis of the Covid vaccines having saved millions of lives.

Figure 16.6: Full vaccination rates, Australia, Canada, EU, UK, USA

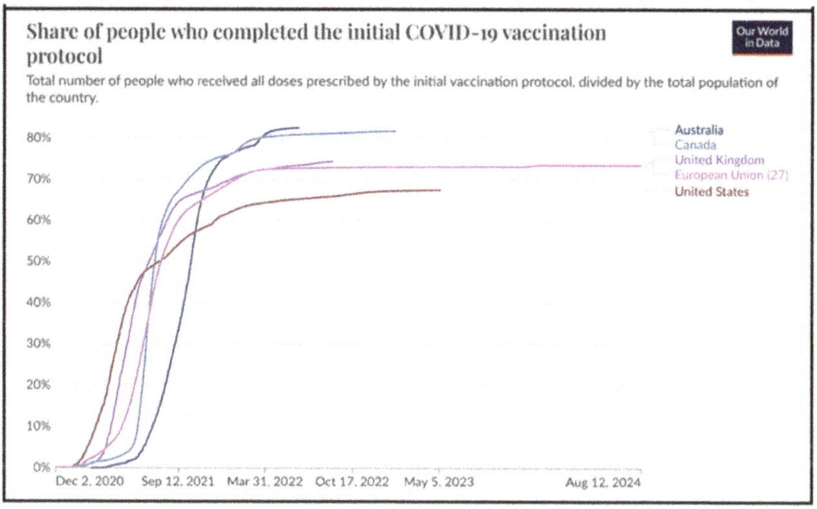

As can be seen in Figure 16.6, among the four countries plus the EU, Australia's vaccine rollout was the last to begin yet the most rapid and successful of all five in covering the population. Figure 16.7 shows that Australia's Covid mortality rate was above one death per million people almost continually for 17 months from January 9, 2022 to June 23, 2023, except for a brief period of three weeks in March–April 2023.

Figure 16.7: Daily new Covid-related deaths per million people, Australia, Canada, EU, UK, USA (7-day rolling average)

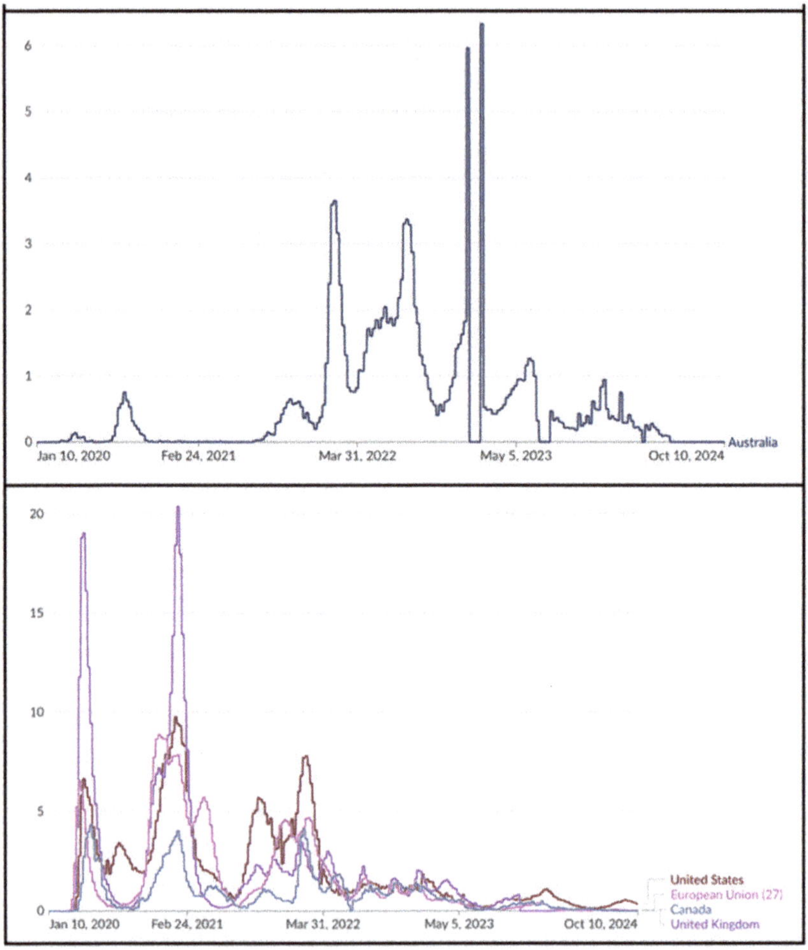

Figure 16.8: Cumulative Covid-related deaths per million people, Australia, Canada, EU, UK, USA (7-day rolling average)

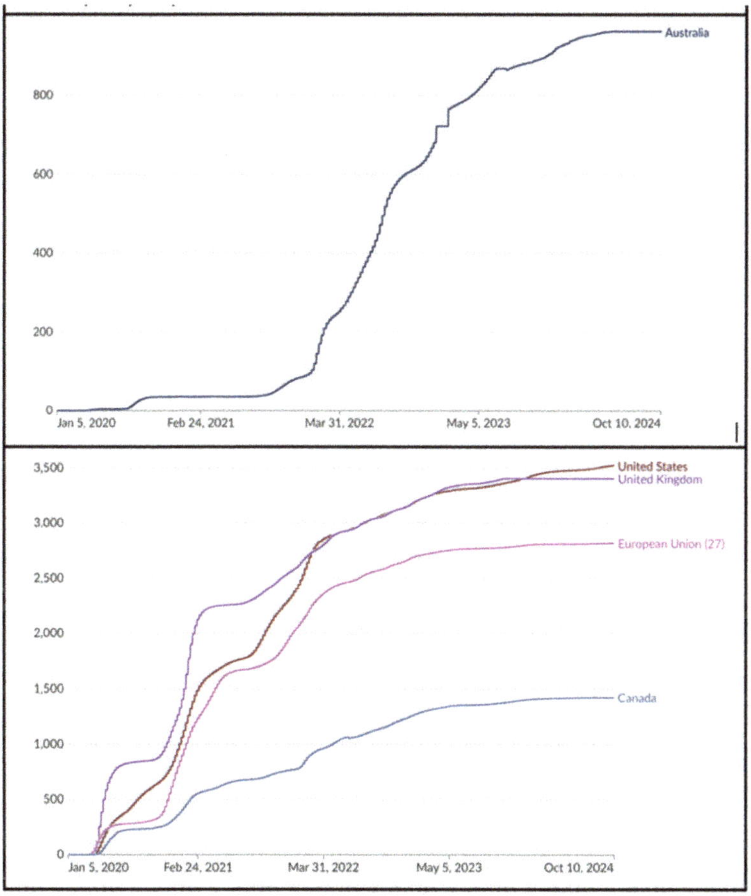

If we look at Figures 16.7 and 16.8 against the vaccination coverage in the five jurisdictions in Figure 16.6, two things become clear. For the four entities in the northern hemisphere, the heaviest Covid mortality toll both in terms of the daily and cumulative counts was in the first twelve months of the pandemic and the toll fell dramatically coinciding with the vaccine rollouts. For example, contrasting sharply with Australian data where the pre-vaccine deaths with Covid were under 4% of the total until October 2024, for the UK this was almost 40%. Confusing correlation with causation, authorities and vaccine-faithful advocates continue to attribute the fall to vaccines.

Yet, in the case of Australia, the relationship is reversed. Its Covid-related mortality rates and cumulative toll were exceptionally light in the first twelve months *before* the vaccine campaign was launched. For vaccine-sceptics, it's tempting to attribute this to vaccines causing the explosion in deaths. Yet such a conclusion is contradicted by the UK experience. Equally, however, the Australian experience refutes the hypothesis that vaccines saved millions of lives.

Instead, to my mind, taken together the divergent experiences powerfully indicate two other possible conclusions. Firstly, as was the case with lockdown restrictions and mask mandates, the rise and fall of the various coronavirus waves were policy-invariant, following a trajectory to some inner virus logic that was stubbornly indifferent to pharmaceutical and non-pharmaceutical interventions. Second, population-level immunity acquired naturally through infection likely played a more critical role in getting to herd immunity than vaccines. Hard border closures in Australia (and New Zealand) kept the virus at bay until such time as borders were reopened in the wake of rapid and high vaccine uptakes. This finally seeded the virus in the population and infection, hospitalisation and death rates rose sharply, herd immunity was achieved and the virus receded.

If this is so, then of course the benefit-harms equation for vaccines changes quite dramatically also. The failure—nay, the cussed refusal—to engage in cost-benefit analysis and publish the results, for an experimental product that may very well be contaminating our DNA (see Rebekah Barnett's comprehensive refutation of the charge that this is misinformation here), offers yet another bit of evidence that regulators have become vaccine enablers first, more committed to defend vaccines from criticism than protect people from harmful vaccines.

This article has weighed the report of the inquiry into Australia's Covid response and found it wanting on critically scrutinising the three measures of two-metre social distancing, masks and vaccines. One of the three inquiry panellists is Catherine Bennett, professor of epidemiology at Deakin University. In an interview with SBS on July 7, 2022, she said: "We have to ensure people have all their recommended boosters because the booster … reduces the risk of serious illness quite dramatically." She also recommended "people wear face masks and maintain social distancing." Make of this what you will.

Covid's abuse of power[101]

On 24 October, Jay Bhattacharya, once derided by Anthony "Mr Science" Fauci as a fringe epidemiologist, was awarded the Zimmer Medal for Intellectual Freedom by the American Academy of Sciences and Letters. The medal "is presented annually to a public thinker who displays extraordinary courage in the exercise of intellectual freedom." The 2023 winner was Salman Rushdie. Jay's citation recognises his "courage and firm commitment to intellectual freedom" and that he "resolutely refused… to compromise his scientific findings" and took "a stand for the public's right to unrestricted scientific discussion and debate." His writings and speeches are powerful examples of passion, courage and clarity of expression that reflects clear thinking. He toured Australia in 2022 and James Allan and I had the honour to share a packed townhall meeting with him (viewable online) in Melbourne in September 2022, and Rowan Dean likewise in Sydney. Sadly but not surprisingly, his tour was mostly ignored by Australia's mainstream media.

On 29 October 2024, the official panel inquiring into Australia's Covid-19 response submitted its 353,000-word report. It opens with

---

[101] *Spectator Australia*, 9 November 2024, https://www.spectator.com.au/2024/11/covids-abuse-of-power/

genuflections to political correctness: an irrelevant acknowledgment of country and lived experience ('We acknowledge that Covid-19 touched every person, every organisation and each sector in different ways"—you don't say); and content warning (in a report on Covid!). This is followed by turgid writing and bureaucratic analysis and recommendations. The Great Barrington Declaration of October 2020, co-authored by Bhattacharya, is still better big-picture value in both language and content and it might even profit PM Anthony Albanese to read its one page of 513 words, perhaps while sipping the bubbly in an upgraded first class cabin en route to a family holiday in Europe. At the granular level, the report has some positive features but these are outweighed by flaws of commission and omission, much like the response to the pandemic itself. Astonishingly, the words "cost-benefit analysis" do not appear. "Trade-off" gets four mentions.

The report confirms that lockdowns, state border closures, school shutdowns and vaccine mandates broke public trust in governments and science. They drove lower Covid vaccine take-up in the last two years and promoted cross-vaccine hesitancy. So did inconsistent advice, recommendations and enforcement practices across the states, compounded by the refusal to release health advice and its science and evidence base. The strong emphasis on human rights and the wider economic, social and mental health consequences of the pandemic policies is also welcome. So too discussion of the long-term damage to children's learning, development and emotional health, effectively punishing kids to protect the adults. All this is good, but neither new nor insightful. Several of us warned about precisely these downstream consequences in the pages of this courageous magazine from the start.

It's also simply not good enough. The report ignores how Australia's Covid response marked a radical departure from the prevailing consensus on science and policy as synthesised in the WHO September 2019 report. There is no clarity on why our own existing pandemic preparedness plans were ditched. Nor does the report explore the culture cringe whereby Australian health authorities mimicked American and British counterparts on made-up measures like the two metre social distancing, or why the regulators accepted results from the vaccine manufacturers' own trial results conducted overseas instead of requiring them to be done locally to our standards and satisfaction.

Critical flaws of commissions begin with paeans to leaders' courageous decision-making in conditions of mass fear and extreme uncertainty. The fear and hysteria did not match the data yet the government and media fed it. Experts who called for calm and responses proportionate to risks were ignored, censored and vilified. Early data, including from the *Diamond Princess* cruise ship in February 2020, confirmed that the risk from Covid was highly age-correlated and concentrated in the elderly. There was no reason to strip peoples and businesses of their liberties and freedoms, to put healthy populations under wholesale house arrest, treating them as germ-ridden criminals even if proven innocent.

Far from courageous, the leaders were cowardly and hypocritical. They had no skin in the game, suffered no financial penalty while decimating small businesses, paid no political penalty, got sugar highs on power tripping, hid behind health officials and typically exempted themselves from inconvenient restrictions they foisted on all others. Australia became fixated on the single, dubious metric of case numbers, exaggerating the Covid risks, downplaying the harms of interventions, heightening the fear, stripping people of rights and liberties, censoring dissent and cancelling critics. Regulators became vaccine enablers, more committed to defend vaccines from criticism than to protect people from harms.

The assumption of world-leading performance by Australia is rooted in simplistic and inappropriate European and North American benchmarks against which to assess our outcomes. Our southern hemisphere location, island identity, plentiful sunshine and open spaces, love of outdoors activities, relative paucity of high-density housing, etc. conferred immense advantages in coming through the pandemic with much better outcomes than Europe and America.

The most visible embodiments of courage through the pandemic public policy insanity were Florida Governor Ron Desantis and Sweden's state epidemiologist Anders Tegnell. Florida and Sweden resisted the lockdown groupthink, are in the mid-range of Covid metrics, avoided most of the health, economic, educational and social damage in European countries and US states with authoritarian approaches, including loss of public trust, and came out better on the balance of benefits versus harms.

Finally, the report vastly underrates public anger and cynicism. People were locked up at home on dubious data and science, forced to isolate from parents and grandchildren, unable to visit grandparents in their final days or attend family reunions, weddings, funerals and birthdays, coerced into taking the shot in order to shop, travel and keep jobs on false assurances of safety and effectiveness. Some of the worst offenders, responsible for the most egregious policies and thuggish enforcement measures, have been awarded the highest gongs going, promoted into governors' mansions and even promised a statue in their honour. The report's solution to the overreach and abuse of power by authorities during Covid is to create even more bureaucratic structures with more powers and resources, including an Australian Centre for Disease Control even as the US CDC sinks into ever greater disrepute by the month. Governments grabbed too much power, coming uncomfortably close to becoming police states. Who but the same experts would staff the CDC? It would incense many if those guilty of the biggest assault on Australians' health, and political and economic freedoms in history were to be rewarded with increased powers and resources to serially indulge their inner bullies.

Dealing with the past is a prerequisite for imposing justified punishment for crimes against the people, enabling closure for the many physical injuries and emotional trauma of the totalitarian responses and deterring future wrongdoers. This report doesn't take us far on the path we must, but are yet to, travel.

Hallett Inquiry Report: Of, by, and for lawyers[102]

On 20 November 2025, the Hallett inquiry into the UK Covid experience published its 800-page Module 2 report. An inquiry of, by, and for lawyers, it is a carefully curated political whitewash with no forensic exploration of the truth and no hope of any accountability. It collapses the most consequential public policy decisions in British history into a problem of mere timing caused by process failures. Far from revealing what happened, it is a testament to the refusal of the state to admit error. Many leaders are happy to engage in serial apologies and consider reparations in the name of the state they represent for incidents of alleged wrongdoings deep in the past well before their time, especially if these demonstrate their progressive pieties. But they seem incapable of acknowledging, saying sorry for, and offering compensation for instances of states behaving badly during their own time in office.

Far from mollifying critics looking for acknowledgment and accountability, the report will bring back the anger and rage associated with governments' Covid excesses. It reveals the chair, former Court of Appeal Judge Baroness Heather Hallett, to be science- and numeracy-illiterate, with an inability to grasp complex facts and little capacity for logical reasoning. "Had a mandatory lockdown been imposed" one week earlier, the report concluded, "modelling has established that the number of deaths in England in the first wave up until 1 July 2020 would have been reduced by 48%—equating to approximately 23,000 fewer deaths" (Vol. I, p. 5). This is a truly astonishing assertion. It demonstrates a complete lack of understanding of modelling.

---

[102] *Brownstone Journal*, 29 November 2025, https://brownstone.org/articles/hallett-inquiry-report-of-by-and-for-lawyers/

They do not "establish" any conclusions. Rather, they are built on assumptions and their outputs are speculative and often contentious forecasts—guesstimates—dressed in pretend mathematical precision.

Professor Neil Ferguson, whose modelling is relied on for the assertion, is widely discredited for a history of predictions on other diseases that proved to be excessively alarmist by orders of magnitude. Every time his Covid modelling was able to be measured against reality, it came up short. Sweden falsified the modelling which predicted the loss of 35,000 lives in the first wave without immediate lockdown; the actual figure was 6,000. It saved more lives than the UK. Rather than an exception that proved the rule, Sweden was the control case that falsified the narrative by sticking to the pre-pandemic script and therefore must never be mentioned.

Besides, Ferguson's paper on which Hallett relies also conceded that an earlier lockdown could have resulted in a larger second wave by deferring and not averting further infections. There is another way of showing that inconvenient truth. On 5 May 2021, in an article on the *Pearls and Irritations* site in Australia, I wrote that Figure 16.9 is "graphic evidence of the policy-invariance of Covid-19 with regard to non-pharmaceutical interventions, where the infection, hospitalisation, and mortality curves have followed their own logic and remarkably similar trajectories." A second interesting feature about the graph is the broad convergence of the end of the first curve by the end of summer in 2020. Czechia had instituted lockdowns early and its performance until that date, enthusiastically lauded in the MSM, appears to justify Hallett's claim that more lives could have been saved had the UK gone into strict lockdown a week earlier. But the explosion of Czechia's mortality toll in autumn 2020 is the truer picture, decisively invalidating Hallett's assertion of the net difference in mortality. As David Livermore, a retired Professor of Medical Microbiology at the University of East Anglia, comments in the *Daily Sceptic* in his article on the Hallett report: "At best [Czechia's] early lockdown delayed deaths; at worst it displaced the pandemic into the winter when people, with less sunlight and lower vitamin D levels, are more vulnerable to respiratory viruses."

Figure 16.9: Daily new Covid-19 deaths/mn people, UK, Sweden, EU, Czechia

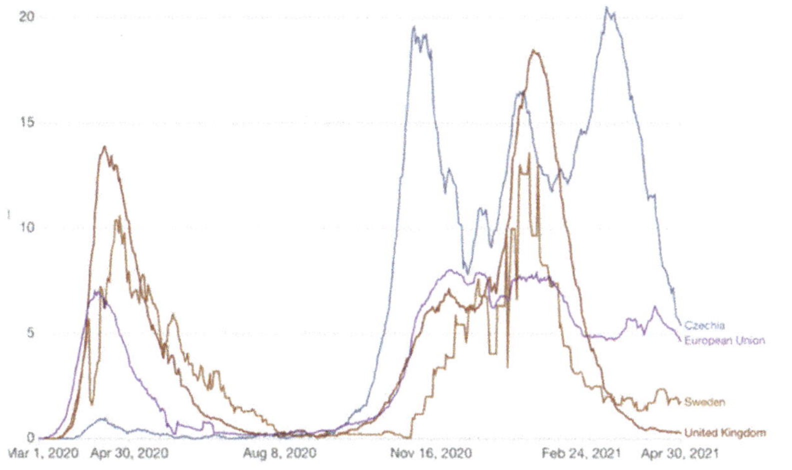

Source: Our World in Data.

Hallett's overall, seemingly predetermined conclusion, at a cost of £192 million (US $250 million), is that the lockdowns were too little and too late. Prime Minister Boris Johnson should have panicked sooner and deeper. She failed to engage with any cost-benefit analysis, refused to assess the full range of short and long-terms harms of lockdowns and wilfully ignored the contrary example of coercion-lite Sweden whose key pandemic control measures were recommended guidance, whose Covid and all-cause mortality metrics were not worse than average European results on any study and significantly better than almost all in most studies, but whose collateral harms were considerably less. Human beings are family- and community-oriented social animals. Sharing food and drink at home or in restaurants, enjoying the cinema, watching live sport, appreciating a concert or a play are not optional add-ons but fundamental to our daily life as human beings. The misnamed "social distancing" by contrast is profoundly anti-social and rubs against every fibre of human civilisation.

By way of analogy, consider deaths from road injuries. According to Our World in Data, in 2021 there were 1.2 million road fatalities worldwide: 52,800 in Europe, 41,300 in the US, 3,300-4,300 each in France, Germany, and Italy, 1,600 in the UK, and 218,400 in India. By definition, thousands, tens of thousands, and even hundreds of thousands of deaths could be averted in individual countries and over a million in the world by banning cars altogether. Such a ban is not even remotely on the agenda for consideration because of the absurdity of focussing on one single-cause mortality at the cost of all other social and economic variables that underpin modern social life. Yet, Baroness Hallett clearly believes that the Johnson government should have focussed solely on Covid deaths, collapsed the National Health Service into a Covid Health Service, and simply ignored the collateral costs and damage to the very fabric of British life just as she continues to do in her report.

Hallett is also critical of the 2021 Omicron variant lockdown that was rejected because had the variant been more severe or the vaccine less effective, "the consequences would have been disastrous" (Vol. I, pp. 8, 438). The scientists were wrong, the government was proven correct, but the Baroness is so much in awe of the former that she criticises the latter for its right judgment call. Remarkable. On this logic, we should never be permitted to cross the street even when the light turns green at a pedestrian crossing. *Quelle horreur*. Just because we made it across safely does not mean that we could not have been killed in the endeavour.

The long suffering British taxpayer may be owed a full refund of the £192 million expenditure racked by the inquiry thus far and the government should shut it down forthwith.

ABOUT THE AUTHOR

Ramesh Thakur, a Brownstone Institute Senior Scholar, is emeritus professor in the Crawford School of Public Policy, The Australian National University, Fellow of the Australian Institute of International Affairs, and a former United Nations Assistant Secretary-General. Born in India and educated in India and Canada, he has held full-time academic appointments in Fiji, New Zealand, Canada, and Australia and been a consultant to the Australian, New Zealand and Norwegian governments on international security issues.

Professor Thakur has served on the international advisory boards of policy-oriented research institutes in Africa, Asia, Europe, and North America. He is co-chair of the International Health Reform Project whose two-volume report, *The Right to Health Sovereignty,* is scheduled for publication in April 2026. His books include *Global Governance and the UN* (Indiana University Press), *The Oxford Handbook of Modern Diplomacy* (Oxford University Press), and *The United Nations, Peace and Security* (Cambridge University Press).

He has published opinion articles in *Asahi Shimbun, Asian Wall Street Journal, Australian, Australian Financial Review, die tageszeitung, Financial Times, Globe and Mail, Guardian, Hindu, Hindustan Times, Indian Express, International Herald Tribune, Japan Times, Newsweek, San Francisco Chronicle, Süddeutsche Zeitung, Times of India, and Washington Post.*

www.ingramcontent.com/pod-product-compliance
Lightning Source LLC
LaVergne TN
LVHW050906210926
848482LV00012B/358
9781763884571